Medicine, Health and the Arts

In recent decades, both medical humanities and medical history have emerged as rich and varied sub-disciplines. *Medicine, Health and the Arts* is a collection of specially commissioned essays designed to bring together different approaches to these complex fields. Written by a selection of established and emerging scholars, this volume embraces a breadth and range of methodological approaches to highlight not only developments in well-established areas of debate, but also newly emerging areas of investigation, new methodological approaches to the medical humanities and the value of the humanities in medical education.

Divided into five sections, this text begins by offering an overview and analysis of the British and North American context. It then addresses in-depth the historical and contemporary relationship between visual art, literature and writing, performance and music. There are three chapters on each art form, which consider how history can illuminate current challenges and potential future directions. Each section contains an introductory overview, addressing broad themes and methodological concerns; a case study of the impact of medicine, health and well-being on an art form; and a case study of the impact of that art form on medicine, health and well-being. The underlining theme of the book is that the relationship between medicine, health and the arts can only be understood by examining the reciprocal relationship and processes of exchange between them.

This volume promises to be a welcome and refreshing addition to the developing field of medical humanities. Both informative and thought-provoking, it will be important reading for students, academics and practitioners in the medical humanities and arts in health, as well as health professionals, and all scholars and practitioners interested in the questions and debates surrounding medicine, health and the arts.

Victoria Bates is a Lecturer in Modern History at the University of Bristol, UK.

Alan Bleakley is Professor of Medical Education and Medical Humanities at Plymouth University Peninsula School of Medicine, UK.

Sam Goodman is a Lecturer in Linguistics at Bournemouth University, UK.

Routledge Advances in the Medical Humanities

Medicine, Health and the Arts

Approaches to the medical humanities

**Edited by Victoria Bates, Alan Bleakley
and Sam Goodman**

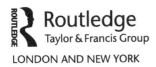
Routledge
Taylor & Francis Group

LONDON AND NEW YORK

First published 2014
by Routledge

Published 2014 by Routledge
2 Park Square, Milton Park, Abingdon, Oxfordshire, OX14 4RN

Simultaneously published in the USA and Canada
by Routledge
711 Third Avenue, New York, NY 10017

Routledge is an imprint of the Taylor and Francis Group, an informa business.

First issued in paperback 2015

British Library Cataloguing in Publication Data
A catalogue record for this book is available from the British Library

Library of Congress Cataloging in Publication Data
Medicine, Health and the Arts: Approaches to the Medical Humanities.
Edited by Victoria Bates, Alan Bleakley and Sam Goodman.
p. ; cm. — (Routledge advances in the medical humanities)
Includes bibliographical references.
I. Bates, Victoria, 1984- II. Bleakley, Alan (Alan Douglas) III. Goodman,
Sam, 1980- IV. Series: Routledge advances in the medical humanities.
[DNLM: 1. Humanities. 2. Philosophy, Medical. 3. Art Therapy.
4. History, 20th Century. 5. Humanities—history. 6. Medicine in
Literature. 7. Music Therapy. W 61]
RA425
362.1—dc23
2013013720

ISBN 978-0-415-64431-0 (hbk)
ISBN 978-1-138-96018-3 (pbk)
ISBN 978-0-203-07961-4 (ebk)

Typeset in Baskerville
by FiSH Books Ltd, Enfield

Contents

List of figures and tables

Figures

Tables

Notes on contributors

Victoria Bates is a lecturer in Modern History at the University of Bristol, UK. She recently had an article 'Sexual Trauma, Psychoanalysis and the Market for Misery' published in Springer's *Journal of Medical Humanities*, and is now beginning a new research project on the history of multidisciplinary medical education.

Jessica Beck is a freelance theatre director and Artistic Associate of The Bike Shed Theatre and Theatre 503. She completed a PhD at the University of Exeter entitled 'Directing Emotion: A Practice-led Investigation into the Challenge of Emotion in Western Performance' and is training as a Feldenkrais practitioner.

Alan Bleakley is Professor of Medical Education and Medical Humanities at Plymouth University Peninsula School of Medicine. He has a background in biological sciences, psychology and psychotherapy, and an international reputation in medical education and the medical humanities. He is widely published and is President of the Association for Medical Humanities.

Emma Brodzinski is a Senior Lecturer in Drama and Theatre at Royal Holloway, University of London. She is also a registered dramatherapist and works in private practice. She has researched extensively within the field of theatre and health and care and her publications include: *Theatre in Health and Care* (Palgrave 2010) and *Making a Performance: Devising Histories and Contemporary Practices*, in collaboration with Helen Nicholson and Katie Normington (Routledge 2007).

Sam Goodman is a Lecturer in Linguistics at Bournemouth University, UK. His research interests are in British fiction of the post Second World War period, national identity and fictional representations of colonial medicine. He is the editor, with Graham Matthews, of *Violence and the Limits of Representation* (Palgrave MacMillan 2013).

Fiona Hamilton is director of Orchard Foundation and tutor on Metanoia Institute's MSc in Creative Writing for Therapeutic Purposes. She specializes in creative, poetic and reflective techniques in healthcare and educational settings and is Chair of Lapidus.

Phil Jones is a Reader at the Institute of Education, University of London. He has held the roles of Director of Research and Reader at the University of Leeds, UK and visiting Professor to Leeds Metropolitan University, UK and Concordia University, Montreal, Canada. His publications include *Drama as Therapy* (Routledge 1996, 2007), *The Arts Therapies* (Routledge 2005), *Rethinking Childhood* (Continuum 2009) and *Rethinking Children's Rights* (with Sue Welch, Continuum 2010). His books on the arts therapies have been translated and published in China, South Korea and Greece. He has given keynote speeches in many countries including the prestigious Triennial World Congress for Psychotherapy in Sydney, Australia.

Therese (Tess) Jones is an associate professor in the Department of Medicine and Director of the Arts and Humanities in Healthcare Program for the Center for Bioethics and Humanities at the University of Colorado Anschutz Medical Campus. She is editor of the *Journal of Medical Humanities* and is widely published in the areas of literature, film and medical education. She is lead editor for the forthcoming *Health and Humanities Reader*, the first major text in the medical/health humanities published by Rutgers University Press.

Ludmilla Jordanova is Professor of History and Visual Culture at the University of Durham. She writes about historical practice, portraiture, public history and the cultural history of science and medicine since 1600. She is working on a book to be called *Traces of Life*, which approaches portraits, both historical and contemporary, from a medical humanities perspective. She is a Trustee of the Science Museum Group, which comprises five museums in London, Manchester, Bradford, York and Shildon, Co. Durham, and was a Trustee of the National Portrait Gallery, London, between 2001 and 2009.

Zack Moir is a teaching fellow in the Reid School of Music, University of Edinburgh. His research interests include the musical experiences of cochlear implant users, musical improvisation and music pedagogy in higher education.

Patricia Novillo-Corvalán is Lecturer in Comparative Literature at the University of Kent in Canterbury. She is the author of *Borges and Joyce: An Infinite Conversation* (2011). Her publications include articles on Modernism, Comparative and World Literature, and the Medical Humanities. She is currently editing a collection of essays entitled *The Art of Medicine in Iberian and Latin American Literature*.

Helen Odell-Miller is Professor of Music Therapy at Anglia Ruskin University, Cambridge, and an honorary therapist at Cambridge and

Peterborough Foundation Trust. She has published and lectured internationally and is co-author of *Supervision of Music Therapy* and *Forensic Music Therapy*. She is an elected member of the Professional Advisory Board on Allied Health Professions, to the Department of Health; a Board member for the International Centre for Research in the Arts Therapies; and The Music Therapy Charity.

Katie Overy is a senior lecturer and Director of the Institute for Music in Human and Social Development at the University of Edinburgh. Her research draws on music neuroscience, psychology and pedagogy to explore the role of music in human learning.

Paul Robertson was founder and leader of the Medici String Quartet. More recently he has been a Visiting Professor to the Copenhagen Business School, the University of Oxford and Peninsula Medical School. Following serious illness he has now largely retired from performance and is writing a book about meaning in music, in addition to running Music, Mind, Spirit (www.musicmindspirit.org) – a centre dedicated to music and the arts.

Anne Whitehead is Senior Lecturer in Modern and Contemporary Literature at Newcastle University, UK. She has published *Trauma Fiction* (Edinburgh University Press 2004) and *Memory: New Critical Idiom* (Routledge 2008). She is working on her next monograph, *Medicine and Empathy in Contemporary British Fiction*, which is contracted to Edinburgh University Press.

Ian Williams is a physician, comics artist and the initiator of the website GraphicMedicine.org. He is an Honorary Clinical Lecturer in the Faculty of Medicine and Human Sciences at the University of Manchester, UK and a member of the International Health Humanities Advisory Board. He is also joint Lead Editor for a forthcoming series of books on Graphic Medicine from Penn State University Press.

Louise Younie works as GP/Clinical Senior Lecturer at Barts and The London School of Medicine and Dentistry. She has been working in the field of arts-based inquiry within medical education for the last ten years both developing courses and researching learning through her masters (2006) and doctoral (2011) research.

Acknowledgements

The editors are very grateful to the Arts & Humanities Research Council for providing funding [AH/I50009X/1] for the 2011 conference and exhibition: 'From the Cradle to the Grave: Reciprocity and Exchange in the Making of Medicine and the Modern Arts'. The success of this Student-Led Initiative (Beyond Text) inspired us to pursue further multidisciplinary collaborations.

The dialogue that formed the basis of this collection also would not have been possible without the generous support of the Wellcome Trust. By providing funding [097508/Z/11/Z] for the 'Medicine, Health and the Arts in Post-War Britain' seminar series, they allowed us to share our ideas – with each other, and with a wonderfully varied public, professional and academic audience.

Our thanks must go to the Universities of Plymouth, Bristol and Exeter for helping to facilitate the collaborative seminar series. The Centre for Medical History at the University of Exeter has been particularly generous in supporting both of the above events, through its Wellcome Trust Strategic Award. The book also would not have been possible without a range of administrative and academic staff, who have provided invaluable professional advice throughout the process of organizing the events and editing this collection. Our thanks go to the National Portrait Gallery and various individuals for permission to reproduce images within the book. Finally, we are grateful for the enthusiasm and support of James Watson and the editorial team at Routledge.

Introduction

1 Critical conversations

Establishing dialogue in the medical humanities

Victoria Bates and Sam Goodman

In a 2003 issue of *Medical Humanities*, Stephen Pattison outlined his vision for the medical humanities as a field of study that:

> [W]ould prize diversity of forms...It should aspire to be a "broad church" of many languages and kinds of performance and analysis, in which bridges are built and conversations occur that reveal things to participants that they could not have learned within their own original limits and worldviews. By the same token...homogenisation and regularisation of thought, method, and practice would be actively resisted.
>
> (Pattison 2003: 34)

Pattison's comments were made in relation to his fear that the medical humanities would become marked by homogeneity rather than dialogue, particularly if they grew in popularity and were consolidated into an 'autonomous' discipline. To date, Pattinson's fears appear unwarranted. Since his article was published, international interest in the medical (and health) humanities has continued to grow and has manifested itself in new associations, research networks, university centres and funding opportunities. However, these new bodies continue to define themselves in terms of diversity. Even university research centres have been built as locations for exchange rather than standardization as, to cite just one example, the University of Glasgow notes on its website that the Medical Humanities Research Centre is advised by a committee 'drawn from various Schools and subject areas across the university' (University of Glasgow 2013). Many centres for medical humanities are also staffed by affiliates, who teach collaboratively across disciplines rather than being full-time staff who teach *only* medical humanities as an 'autonomous' subject.

Most forms of published literature also still await the building of 'bridges' and the 'conversations' to which Pattison referred over a decade ago. It seems difficult to imagine the medical humanities as homogenized, when so much multidisciplinary territory remains uncharted. A number of medical humanities journals were founded in the late-twentieth century including the US-based *Journal of Medical Humanities* (first published 1979) and *Literature and Medicine* (first published 1982) and later the UK-based *Medical Humanities* (first published in 2000, as an offshoot of the *Journal of Medical Ethics* first published in 1975). There is also a thriving e-journal *Hektoen International* published in Chicago by the Hektoen Institute of Medicine (first published in 2008). However, these journals remain relatively unusual in the extent of their multidisciplinarity. Rather than being characterized either by exchange between diverse perspectives or by homogeneity, much published work in the medical humanities has increasingly delineated its subfields.

Many monographs and edited collections have addressed specific aspects of the medical humanities such as medical history, representations of medicine in the arts, arts therapies and medical humanities in medical education.[1] These different approaches have been separated rather than merged or positioned in dialogue with each other. It is possible to find counter-examples to such claims, for example in a forthcoming *Health Humanities Reader* (Jones *et al.* 2014). Martyn Evans and Ilora Finlay's edited volume *Medical Humanities* (2001) also includes contributions from historians, philosophers, sociologists and practitioners. However, such publications remain the exception rather than the rule. The opportunities for truly multidisciplinary discussion thus remain largely unfulfilled, even in the form of edited volumes that inherently facilitate conversation and exchange. While no single publication can address the entire field of medical humanities, this volume seeks to make a step towards creating a climate in which such conversations are possible.

It is not our intention here to engage with the complexities surrounding definitions and redefinitions of the medical humanities, but it is worth noting that within this introduction we refer to the medical humanities in the plural and as multidisciplinary. Others within this collection refer to the medical humanities as interdisciplinary, and the editorial decision to leave these apparent discrepancies is a deliberate one. The question of whether the medical humanities is a 'multidiscipline', 'interdiscipline', 'discipline' or 'field' is by no means resolved (see Evans and Macnaughton 2004). Our decision to use the prefix 'multi' here refers to our conceptualization of the current edited collection as a dialogue between different approaches, rather than as a collaborative venture in which different disciplines work together to create a single 'interdisciplinary' approach. However, this is not to deny that in a different context the medical humanities can be truly interdisciplinary. Other authors have turned to terms such as transdisciplinary and circumdisciplinary, in an effort to best represent some complex forms of interdisciplinarity that are involved in medicine and the medical humanities (for example, Couturier *et al.* 2008; Austin *et al.* 2008; Wear 2009).

It is the malleability of the term 'medical humanities' that makes its definition so problematic and arguably even unnecessary; indeed, a clear-cut definition could remove the diversity of approach that makes the medical humanities so appealing in the first place. While the introductory chapters of Alan Bleakley and Therese Jones within this collection helpfully outline some important subfields of the medical humanities, it is noteworthy that there are contributions even within this collection that defy simple categorization. We use the term medical humanities but, like Jones, are in agreement with Rafael Campo (2005) that it is for 'lack of a better term'. We use 'medical humanities' here because it is the most recognizable and widely used term to describe the field, but in the recognition that neither 'medicine' nor 'health' humanities fully embraces all of the subjects covered within this book: medicine, health, well-being, science and technology. Although there are important debates to be had around terminology, to us it is not a matter of priority. The field of so-called 'medical humanities' incorporates a huge range of subjects and approaches, to the extent that no term will ever embrace them all. If such a term were to become possible, it would only be in consequence of an unfortunate narrowing of the field.

Instead of using this introduction to repeat the widespread debates surrounding use of the term 'medical humanities', we will use the space to explain three principles that underlie the volume as a whole: first, the medical humanities should be studied in a broad and inclusive way; second, history and context must not be eliminated from any study of arts/health relationships or the medical humanities in general; and third, the relationship between medicine, arts and humanities should be conceptualized in terms of reciprocity and exchange. These main principles were established through interdisciplinary dialogue over a number of years: first between medical history and literature scholars (Victoria Bates and Sam Goodman), then with arts for health practitioners and arts therapists,[2] and finally with a professor of medical education (Alan Bleakley). The contributors to this volume also presented at a seminar series to exchange ideas from their different disciplinary backgrounds.[3] Thus, the notion of conversation has shaped this collection from start to finish. The editors have encouraged authors to engage with the three common principles outlined above but otherwise have sought to avoid being overly prescriptive about the approaches that should be taken. Interdisciplinary and multidisciplinary conversations are only valuable if we seek common ground within difference, rather than using such conversations to eliminate difference.

The first principle outlined above relates to our overarching commitment to exchange and dialogue: a broad and inclusive approach to the medical humanities. Instead of trying to define the medical humanities or find a way to merge its different forms, this collection takes the diverse and discursive nature of the medical humanities as its starting point. We take medicine to include institutional medicine, health and well-being of the mind or body; the humanities to include history and the arts; and the methodologies for studying the medical humanities to include examining theory, practice, impact and representation. Indeed, the definition of humanities taken here could be expanded much further. It is primarily for coherence that the collection focuses on the recent history of the relationship between different art forms and medicine, broadly defined, rather than on other branches of the humanities such as philosophy. However, there is much scope for future work on these other aspects of the field.

The decision to focus on art and history relates to the second principle of this collection: the value of situating the medical humanities in history and context. In order to demonstrate this principle and to allow for comparison between chapters, the book focuses on a case study of the UK since 1945. In combination, the book's chapters identify a range of ways in which the medical humanities have been shaped by national and international developments such as; the creation of the National Health Service (NHS), the challenges posed by treating veterans after World War Two, new technology, funding bodies, a growing interest in narratives (the linguistic turn), and the rise of brain sciences (the cognitive turn). Many of the chapters situate these UK trends in Anglo–American and global contexts, while also demonstrating the importance of locality. This book can really only skim the surface of such a complex subject, but seeks to present a methodological case for the value of time and place in studying the medical humanities.

It is of course possible to trace a much longer history of the relationship between the arts and medicine, not least the long-held notion that medicine itself is an art. However, the aim of this book is not to provide a comprehensive history of the medical humanities. Such an approach would defeat the spirit of multidisciplinarity with which the collection has been developed. While the book includes one contribution by a historian, its other contributors draw upon history in a variety of ways and with differing emphasis. Some chapters focus on specific periods in history, while others use history as a background from which to understand current-day practice. Each of these approaches is appropriate to the author's respective discipline and is valuable for demonstrating the different ways in which history and context can be used in studying the medical humanities. Overall, the collection seeks to demonstrate the socially contingent nature of both the arts/medicine relationship and the medical humanities. While this collection focuses on the UK, these methodological concerns have international relevance.

The final guiding principle of this collection relates to the importance of recognizing reciprocity in the relationship between medicine and the arts. This theme of reciprocity ties in with the matter of dialogue and conversation, as already discussed above, in terms of bringing together authors who study uses of art in medicine and those who study the impact of medicine on art. It is a central theme of the volume and consequently has informed both its subject matter and structure. The volume focuses on four main art forms in order to allow space for three chapters on each. This structure is important for demonstrating the dynamic and bidirectional nature of relationships between medicine and the arts. The chapters are organized around the subjects of visual art, literature, performance and music. Each section contains an introductory overview, addressing broad themes and methodological concerns; a case study of the impact of medicine, health and well-being on an art form; and a case study of the impact of that art form on medicine, health and well-being. This structure is conceptual and does not operate so clearly in practice. This lack of clarity is important in itself for highlighting the interwoven nature of medicine, health, well-being and the arts. The question of impact overlaps heavily with that of representation, while separating the arts from health, medicine and well-being could be seen as a false dichotomy. The material is organized to bring out these issues.

Outline of chapters

In recognition of the transatlantic history, development and continual reciprocity of medical humanities, the volume contains an introductory section entitled 'Britain and Beyond'. The first chapter within this section by Alan Bleakley focuses on the twentieth-century emergence and development of the medical humanities. He draws upon his experience as a medical educator to show how the field has been shaped by key individuals and by the contexts from which it has emerged. He also sets out a future programme for the medical humanities, which would operate to democratize medical practice. It would also provide an aesthetic and critical basis for medicine by drawing upon the avant-garde in the arts and humanities to develop an 'aesthetics of resistance'. Bleakley concludes by arguing that a critical medical humanities offers skepticism towards utilitarian models of well-being, seeing meaning in illness.

Many of Bleakley's themes are picked up in the second introductory chapter, which focuses on international aspects of the medical humanities. In 'Oh, the Humanities!': Dissent, Democracy, and Danger', Therese Jones explores the development of humanities scholarship and teaching in the US and beyond. Building on her work as editor of the *Journal of Medical Humanities*, Jones considers the increasing diversity of scholarship in the field and the growth of medical humanities educational programmes in colleges and universities throughout the US. Like Bleakley, she uses this subject matter to consider the future development of medical humanities. Jones' chapter not only shows the internationalization of the medical humanities but also questions some of the major assumptions at its core – like Bleakley she calls for a more critical approach to terms such as 'humanism' and 'humanities'. Jones argues that engaging with the unsettling aspects of medical practice can aid the personal and professional development of healthcare workers. She also argues for the importance of recognizing the authority of patients, which anticipates other chapters within the volume such as Fiona Hamilton's chapter on Expressive and Reflective Writing (ERW).

The second section of the book relates to visual art, with an overview chapter by Ludmilla Jordanova. Jordanova considers medicine in its broadest forms – including sickness, health, healthcare professionals and disability. Her chapter examines the roles of medicine as art, art as medicine and both as forms of culture. Jordanova uses her expertise in modern history to present an analysis of the links between medicine and the visual arts since 1945. She shows that the visual arts have increased the social and cultural prominence of medicine in British society and thus addresses a major theme of this volume, by situating the relationship between art and medicine in its shifting historical contexts.

The first case study within the visual arts section of the book analyzes and evaluates the impact of medicine and health on visual art, particularly in terms of how healthcare and illness has been represented in popular visual narratives. Ian Williams, a doctor and graphic artist, explores the medium of comics and its development throughout the twentieth century. Building on Jordanova's overview, which discusses some of the most important and prominent links between visual art and medicine over the last 70 years, Williams presents an alternative representation of medicine in visual art through the example of the underground comics movement. Like Jordanova, he situates such developments in their social and political contexts. Williams shows how comics and graphic pathographies constitute a source of alternative knowledge about the body, health and disease. His work thus complements the discussion of literary pathographies elsewhere in the volume and shows the overlaps between different art forms and between medicine, the arts and culture.

Louise Younie provides an alternative case study for the visual art section, examining the role of visual art in medical education as part of the medical humanities movement. As both doctor and educator, Younie considers the potential practical outcomes for trainee healthcare workers through the creation of and engagement with artwork. In the same way as Williams, she shows the importance of symbols, metaphors and imagery in visual art as a means of producing and representing meaning. She also discusses the challenges presented by integrating visual art into the undergraduate medicine curriculum, particularly matters surrounding surveying and quantifying outcomes – a timely debate that connects with a number of chapters throughout the volume. This chapter can be situated productively against Williams' chapter, which shows the role of new types of visual art in energizing existing fields, including the medical humanities in medical education. In dialogue, the two chapters also show that both new and existing fields need to pay critical attention to aesthetic and practical links between the visual arts and medicine in order to ensure their development and survival.

The third section of the volume focuses on literature and writing. In the overview chapter for this section, Anne Whitehead traces the shifting relationships between literature and medicine in the period since 1945. Her chapter provides a useful counterpoint to the chapters by Ludmilla Jordanova and Ian Williams, as it considers the work of John Berger (also addressed by Jordanova in relation to its visual aspects) and the rise of the literary genre of pathography in the late 1980s and 1990s (considered by Williams in its graphic form). In addition to this history of the field, Whitehead offers an analysis of current-day and potential future practice for using writing as a healthcare education tool. Whitehead thus returns to concerns raised by Alan Bleakley's introduction, questioning what a shift towards the critical medical humanities might indicate for the future direction of the field.

The first case study within this section is provided by Patricia Novillo-Corvalán, whose chapter engages with the impact of medicine and health on literature. Novillo-Corvalán uses literary analysis to explore the myth of Philoctetes and its twentieth-century reception and reinterpretation in Britain and beyond. The chapter focuses on literary appropriations of Philoctetes by the poets Seamus Heaney and Derek Walcott. It highlights the importance of the myth to the medical humanities throughout the twentieth century, particularly in relation to the representation of wounds and pain. Novillo-Corvalán also shows how the reinterpretation of the myth has been influenced by different cultural and political contexts, as the wound of Philoctetes provides a useful literary metaphor. This argument thus highlights the importance of context and history for understanding the relationship between medicine and the arts, which is a key theme of the volume as a whole. It also supports comments made by contributors to the visual art section about the particular value of art for representing health, illness and suffering through symbolism and metaphor.

The second case study is provided by a facilitator of an arts-for-health programme, providing a practice-based perspective on the relationship between literature, writing and medicine. Fiona Hamilton examines ERW as a therapeutic process for patients, with a focus on the centrality of the patient's voice and perspective. The chapter engages with a range of writing techniques and examines the historical development of ERW, particularly in relation to its grassroots origins. It thus connects with other chapters within the volume that highlight how developments in the relationship between medicine and the arts are often driven from below rather than from above. Together, the chapters within this section show the importance of literature in giving voice to a range of social, cultural, political and individual concerns about health. They also indicate that the relationship between medicine, health and literature is conceptualized differently when writing is considered (and valued) as process rather than product, a matter that is relevant to all of the art forms considered in the volume.

The fourth section of the volume moves from literature to the place of drama and performance within the medical humanities. In the overview chapter in this section, Emma Brodzinski provides a conceptual framework for understanding the reciprocal relationship between medicine and performance. Brodzinski takes a broad view of the notion of performance and addresses matters such as body art, stage performance, television dramas and the blurring of performance with that of everyday life. The chapter considers the different manifestations of the relationship between what Brodzinski identifies as 'social' and 'aesthetic' drama in relation to medicine and health. She demonstrates the value of examining performance as medicine and medicine as performance, which builds upon themes raised throughout the volume about the interconnectedness of medicine and the arts.

The ways in which medicine and performance intersect are demonstrated further in Jessica Beck's case study chapter, which considers the influence of neuroscience on theatrical practice. Beck draws upon both her research in drama and her theatre practice, which uses a technique called Alba Emoting, to consider the role of emotions on the stage. She examines the history and context of this subject throughout the twentieth century and up to the present day, highlighting the shift from psychology to the neurosciences, as well as the move in theatre towards collaboration with scientists. Beck argues that, in response to theories of emotion and cognitive neuroscience, in the last 70 years a number of important theatre directors have educated their actors to use physiological cues for emotional responses. This case study demonstrates the direct impact of medical and scientific thought on theatrical practice, as well as fitting broadly with Brodzinski's emphasis on reciprocity. It provides an example of the role of physiology in performance and the role of performance as physiology.

Phil Jones provides the second case study chapter in the performance section, considering dramatherapy from a conceptual rather than a purely practical perspective. Jones is particularly concerned with the relationship between arts therapies and the medical humanities, arguing that the intersection between the two is valuable and productive. The chapter also addresses a concern raised by many other contributors to the book about measuring the impact of arts therapies, noting that approaches of the medical humanities could provide a means to resolve such anxieties. In combination, these three chapters show the broad forms that the relationship between performance and medicine can take and the importance of bringing these diverse forms together. There is value in understanding performance as incorporating everyday life, medicine as including the mind–body relationship and the medical humanities as including all of its subtopics in dialogue (a notion that also forms the basis of the volume as a whole).

The final section of the volume deals with the intersection between medicine and music. The overview chapter of this section represents a departure from the preceding format; Paul Robertson presents an opinion piece from the viewpoint of a musician and educator who has worked closely with music therapists for over 40 years, thus who has been a part of its contexts, developments and history. Returning to one of the defining themes of the volume, Robertson's chapter explores the tension between quantitative measures and qualitative experience in evaluating the impact of music on health. He also considers how new technologies such as brain scanning methods have influenced the perceived relationship between music and medicine over the last 70 years. His discussions of measurement and brain science connect with many of the issues raised in relation to other art forms, as noted above. Robertson also draws upon his own experience as a virtuoso musician and ensemble leader to discuss the beauty of music as an ancient form that can 'alleviate suffering and enhance the quality of life'.

Robertson's discussion of technological innovations leads directly to the case study on the impact of medicine and health on music by Zack Moir and Katie Overy. Moir and Overy consider the historical emergence of Cochlear Implant (CI) technology and the musical experience of CI users. They show that, while such technology improves hearing, it does not necessarily improve the hearing of music that is currently available. Moir and Overy argue that as musical experience is important socially as well as aesthetically, there is value in developing a new kind of music specifically for the different requirements of CI users. They also consider the design of software to manipulate the sound of recorded music in order to improve musical experience. Thus, they provide a case study that demonstrates some of the complex ways in which technology can shape musical experience, both negatively and positively.

In the final chapter of this section, Helen Odell-Miller considers changing trends in the professional practice of music therapy in Britain since 1945 and situates these trends in international contexts. Odell-Miller writes from the perspective of a clinician, researcher, trainer and developer of the profession. In this chapter she considers how changing trends in clinical practice and research have contributed to the current professional identity of music therapy. Odell-Miller also examines clinical material to show how the relationship between music and health is expected to work in psychological practice, demonstrating that there is no 'one size fits all' approach to therapy. Her chapter completes the section of the volume on medicine and music, which, as a whole, raises complex questions about how to define the success of medicine for musical experience and of musical experience as medicine.

Concluding comments

These brief chapter summaries allow for some comments on the main themes that emerge from this edited volume as a whole. One such theme is the value of thinking broadly and critically about relationships between arts, health and well-being. Rather than simply examining the aesthetic or practical value of this relationship, this volume also focuses on the complexities of its nature. Its chapters show that using the arts for self-reflection may be unsettling for patients, even as part of the path to the promise of improved 'well-being'. They also show that artistic representations of health and medicine can be political and challenging, as well as aesthetic and therapeutic. The nature of this relationship is variable and highly dependent on the context in which art and – or as – medicine is produced and consumed.

This volume also demonstrates that value judgements and debates about evidence-based healthcare are unavoidable in many subfields of the medical humanities. However, it indicates that the question 'does it work?' might helpfully be supplemented by a historical analysis of *why* the question 'does it work?' has become an increasingly central one. Many of the chapters outlined above make reference to recent debates about the need for quantitative evidence of the (often qualitative) links between art, health, well-being and medicine. While showing that such debates are legitimate and important, these chapters also demonstrate the potentially restrictive nature of questions around evidence-based healthcare. They indicate that there may be an alternative to the qualitative/quantitative binary, which would focus more on understanding processes than on measuring outcomes. Such understanding is only possible through genuinely open, rather than defensive, dialogue between medicine and non-scientific or non-practice-based disciplines.

Such multidisciplinary dialogue holds further value in breaking down artificial divisions between categories such as impact and representation, practice and aesthetics, process and product. Many of the overlaps between such categories have already been addressed above and are demonstrated throughout the volume, but remain worthy of note here as main themes. This volume also indicates the value of understanding how history and context has shaped the medical humanities as both objects and fields of study. Its chapters make some steps towards addressing the history of the emergence and development of the medical humanities, but this subject still awaits rigorous scholarly examination. Such contexts also include matters that are beyond the remit of this book but which would benefit from further study, such as how medical humanities can be understood through the lenses of gender, class, ethnicity and age.

Overall we would encourage this collection to be read in its intended spirit: as a multidisciplinary conversation between artists, doctors, historians, literary scholars, medical educators, arts therapists and more. This collection combines chapters that survey and consider the limitations of existing fields with case studies of new ways in which the medical humanities can be approached. It is therefore intended neither as a collection of pioneering essays nor as a simple survey of the field. Instead, the book presents a conversation between the past, present and future of the medical humanities. This book seeks to stimulate questions rather than provide answers but, if we accept Pattison's vision of the medical humanities cited at the start of this introduction, its value lies therein.

Notes

1   The range of literature related to these areas of study is extremely broad and varied. It would therefore not be possible to attempt a literature review, nor would it be reasonable to reference any single text as a representative example of any of the subfields noted here. The extent of this diversity is in itself an important point as it illustrates the lack of homogeneity in the medical humanities.
2   The authors of this chapter collaborated with a number of arts and health practitioners and arts therapists from Devon (UK) for an exhibition, in association with the Arts and Humanities Research Council (AHRC)-funded conference ' "From the Cradle to the Grave": Reciprocity and Exchange in the Making of Medicine and the Modern Arts', University of Exeter, 2011.
3   These seminars were funded by the Wellcome Trust, which has played a significant role in encouraging and shaping medical history and medical humanities in the UK.

References

Austin, W., Park, C. and Goble, E. (2008) 'From Interdisciplinary to Trans-disciplinary Research: A Case Study', *Qualitative Health Research*, 18: 557–64.

Campo, R. (2005) ' "The Medical Humanities," For Lack of a Better Term', *JAMA*, 294: 1009–11.

Couturier, Y., Gagnon, D., Carrier, S. and Etheridge, F. (2008) 'The Inter-disciplinary Condition of Work in Relational Professions of the Health and Social Care Field: A Theoretical Standpoint', *Journal of Interprofessional Care*, 22: 341–51.

Evans, M. and Finlay, I. G. (eds) (2001) *Medical Humanities*, London: BMJ Books.

Evans, H. M. and Macnaughton, J. (2004) 'Should Medical Humanities be a Multidisciplinary or an Interdisciplinary Study?', *Medical Humanities*, 30: 1–4.

Jones, T., Wear, D. and Friedman, L. D. (eds) (2014) *Health and Humanities Reader*, New Jersey, NJ: Rutgers University Press.

Pattison, S. (2003) 'Medical Humanities: A Vision and Some Cautionary Notes', *Journal of Medical Ethics: Medical Humanities*, 29: 33–6.

University of Glasgow (2013) 'Medical Humanities Research Centre'. Online. Available: www.gla.ac.uk/schools/critical/research/researchcentresandnet works/mhrc (accessed 12 February 2013).

Wear, D. (2009) 'The Medical Humanities: Toward a Renewed Praxis', *Journal of Medical Humanities*, 30: 209–20.

Section One

The medical humanities

Britain and beyond

2 Towards a 'critical medical humanities'

Alan Bleakley

In Mark Haddon's (2012) novel *The Red House* a junior doctor diagnoses a rare condition that causes a mother's baby to be stillborn. Disconcertingly, the doctor not only 'seemed pleased with himself for knowing the biology behind such a rare syndrome', but also 'gave the impression that she [the mother] was meant to feel pleased too, for having won some sort of perverse jackpot' (Haddon 2012: 103). Observations such as Haddon's seem to confirm the intuitive rationale for the inclusion of the medical humanities in medical education – to educate for sensitivity, so that we do not produce doctors who place cases and smart diagnoses before persons and feelings.

The term 'medical humanities' may appear to be exclusive of healthcare professionals other than doctors. For this reason, the 'health humanities' and the 'humanities in healthcare' are becoming preferred terms, especially in North America (Jones *et al.* 2014). However, in this chapter, I use 'medical humanities' because I refer specifically to medicine and medical education. The medical humanities offer four contested and fragmented fields – all of which are addressed to some extent within this edited volume:

- The humanities studying medicine: such as history of medicine or the critical evaluation of medicine in literature.
- Arts and humanities intersecting with medicine in medical education: 'medicine as art'.
- Arts for health: for example, art in hospitals and arts activities with patients – often called 'arts as medicine'.
- Arts therapies: sometimes linked with arts for health, but usually associated with mental health interventions using arts media within a psychotherapeutic framework.

This chapter considers the emergence of the medical humanities as a complex field of study with emphasis upon the different trajectories of 'arts for health' and medical education. It shows that different aspects of the medical humanities emerged together but have been since been shaped by contexts such as funding opportunities and intellectual collaboration. The chapter then provides an overview background against which the detailed case studies throughout the volume may be considered.

In the period since 1945 the medical humanities have been developed increasingly in medical schools in North America, Britain and beyond (for example, Crawshaw 1975; Banaszek 2011). The perceived benefits of such an approach are still hotly debated, not least the potential reduction of the ongoing problem of iatrogenic illness through improved clinical team communication (Bleakley and Marshall 2013) set within a wider project of the democratizing of medical culture through medical education.

The medical humanities in North America

It can be seen from the timeline (appendix, Bleakley and Jones) that the medical humanities first developed an identity in the US, where the term was coined in 1947. Barr (2011) argues that US doctors in the 1870s, who had visited Germany particularly to study laboratory sciences, started a long revolution in medical education that was brought to a head by the Flexner Report in 1910.

Commissioned by the Carnegie Foundation, Flexner's report exposed a lack of adequate scientific and clinical education across many US medical schools and recommended a root-and-branch overhaul, including the standardization of curricula. Unfortunately, this led to closures of underfunded schools catering for minority students (Hodges 2005).

Wujun Ke (2012) offers a standard critical reading of Flexner, suggesting that Flexner's emphasis on the importance of the biological sciences in early medical education led to a bias towards curative rather than caring medicine, where basic science teachers rather than clinicians have a formative influence on students. Life sciences teachers are the first to shape the identities of students, particularly anatomists who educate through the ritual of dissection, while clinicians primarily shape students' identities in the later clinical years. The voiced skepticism of many basic science teachers towards the humanities may contribute to students' 'empathy decline' – a process by which medical students develop cynicism (Neumann *et al.* 2011). New celebratory readings of Flexner, however, suggest that his interest towards ethical and humane practice has been overlooked. Flexner was an admirer of John Dewey, sharing the latter's democratic and humanitarian values. Garrett Riggs suggests that '[i]f history is a guide, medical education could be on the cusp of another set of great advances by renewing interest in medical humanities... The time is ripe to embrace the rest of the Flexner Report' (Riggs 2010: 1669).

Kenneth M. Ludmerer (1999) traces the history of twentieth-century US medical education as a cycle of erosion then regaining of public trust, in which doctors must engage with wider social concerns as well as empathy for individuals. Political consciousness-raising in the US in the 1960s and early 1970s, spanning the Vietnam War and the Civil Rights movement, led to medical schools becoming more responsive socially and engaging with educational reform. A knock-on effect was to introduce more humanities teaching in medical education (Ludmerer 1999: 237–59). This involved innovations such as the introduction of professional actors playing 'standard' patients for the purposes of student learning and assessment in simulated clinical contexts (Hardee and Kasper 2005).

However, as medicine became increasingly driven by a profit motive during the 1960s and 1970s, framed as a business with patients as consumers, so insurers became more adept at litigation for medical error in protecting consumer rights (Mohr 2000). Medicine had to regain its human touch. The early hegemony of science studies and anatomy helped to de-sensitize medical students through objectifying the body, with such anaesthetizing driving out any lingering interest in the aesthetic. By the 1990s the 'inhumanity' (Weatherall 1994: 1671) of scientific medicine was deemed to be endemic.

A series of papers throughout the 1970s developed this critical discussion around the need to restore sensitive, humane medicine in a time of unprecedented explosion of scientific understanding and social concern (Clouser 1971; Banks and Vastyan 1973; Leake 1973; Pellegrino 1974; Reynolds and Carson 1976). Skeptics responded vigorously towards these suggestions. For example, J. D. Wassersug argued that 'real medical progress has not been made by humanitarians but by doctors equipped with microscopes, scalpels, dyes, catheters, rays, test tubes, and culture plates' (quoted in McManus 1995: 1144). Skeptics also gained a tactical high ground by demanding that proponents of medical humanities offer scientific evidence of impact.

The need to reconnect with an alienated public expressed itself in the consulting room as a need to listen closely to patients' stories. Also, the rising wave of litigation demanded that medical ethics take a central place in medical education. Literature offered a rich medium for teaching ethics. Interest in the history of medicine was supplemented by an interest in restoring the art of 'taking a history' from the patient. 'Narrative medicine' became the most popular form of the early medical humanities, challenging the dominant values of evidence-based medicine by turning attention away from generalized population statistics to the meaning of illness for the individual in context. A bioethicist, Kathryn Montgomery Hunter (1991), wrote the first book on narrative medicine.[1] She argued that doctors learn to diagnose and treat from repeated exposure to patients' stories, thinking narratively and drawing on science where necessary. Montgomery Hunter suggested that science education in contemporary medicine was overemphasized, where medicine is a 'science-*using*' practice (Montgomery Hunter 1991: 25; author's emphasis). Montgomery Hunter placed narrative clinical reasoning in the genre of the detective story – a pragmatic focus that appealed to doctors as they use the senses to discriminate among clues (Bleakley *et al.* 2003). It is received wisdom in medicine that doctors make their diagnoses largely on the basis of what is in a patient's story outside of the physical examination and clinical tests, and recent research confirms this (Mylopoulos *et al.* 2012).

Development of the medical humanities in the United Kingdom

The nascent UK medical humanities culture embodied three strands. First, the arts for health movement had developed from arts therapies – conceived in the UK at the end of the Second World War – and became a vibrant culture by the early 1990s, attracting funding from the Nuffield Trust. Second, the Wellcome Trust established the academic study of the history of medicine. Such funding has fundamentally shaped the writing of medical history and the medical humanities. And third, the development of the medical humanities in medical education, which had taken a foothold in the US by the early 1970s, was seeded. I now consider this latter development, with particular attention to the period from the early 1990s in which the field was consolidated.

In 1993, entering new territory, the Wellcome Trust funded a seminar looking at the relationships between the arts and health. In the same year, the General Medical Council (GMC) published the first edition of *Tomorrow's Doctors* (1993) that set out a curriculum framework for UK medical schools. The GMC encouraged provision of optional special study components (SSCs) beyond the core undergraduate curriculum. These would be mainly in sciences, but modules in history of medicine and literature were also encouraged. However, Deborah Kirklin later pointed out that no extra funding was available to medical schools to support this initiative, while in 2002 'only three dedicated medical humanities academic posts exist in the UK' (Kirklin 2002: 101). As Victoria Bates and Sam Goodman note in the introduction to this edited volume, in the UK the medical humanities have often relied on multidisciplinary collaboration rather than providing truly interdisciplinary job roles.

Ludmerer (1999: xxi) suggested that '[i]t would be a great error to view the history of American medical education as devoid of people or personalities', and the same can be said for the development of the medical humanities in the UK. Two figures – Robin Philipp and Kenneth Calman – offered a formative influence, with particular interests, respectively, in arts in health and medical humanities in medical education. Calman was the Chief Medical Officer (CMO) for Scotland (1989–1991) and then England (1991–1998), a member of the Nuffield Council on Bioethics (2000–2008), and had strong links with the Wellcome Trust. Philipp, a public health consultant working within the NHS, was interested in health inequalities, the area in which 'arts for health' was having its greatest impact (Coats 2004). Philipp had come from New Zealand where he was involved in the first medical humanities and narrative medicine conferences organized outside the USA, in 1994 and 1996. Arts for, and in, health, however, refused to be 'medicalized', supporting a range of psychological and therapeutic approaches from its association with arts therapies, and had little to do with the training of doctors (Hamilton *et al.* 2003; Health Development Agency 2000). In the wake of the GMC's 1993 initial recommendations about study of humanities for medical students – certainly influenced by Calman as CMO for England – Calman met with the Minister of Health in 1996 to discuss the initiative of the 'humanities in medicine'.

The first major UK conference organized by Philipp and Calman, the first 1998 Windsor conference (Philipp *et al.* 1999), embodied a dual approach of arts in health and humanities in medical education, setting out explicitly to 'promote the arts from the margins into the very heart of healthcare planning, policy-making and practice' (Philipp *et al.* 1999: 8). It was supported by the Nuffield Trust, who later also supported the development of the first institute for the medical humanities in the UK at Durham University, where Calman was by then Vice Chancellor. The 1998 and subsequent 1999 Windsor conferences downplayed those aspects of the medical humanities that constituted an academic study of medicine, particularly through disciplines such as history, philosophy and literature. The lack of attention given to this form of medical humanities was ironic as it would later become the dominant medical humanities approach, with strong funding support from the Wellcome Trust.

A manifesto emerged from the first Windsor conference, with a rhetorical tone of urgency. The medical humanities would lead to medical students becoming 'more "rounded" people' who would develop the values and skills of compassion and empathy for both patients and colleagues (Philipp *et al.* 1999: 115). The pedagogical plan, however, was confused. While medical schools 'should' include humanities such as moral philosophy, theology and literature, and perhaps history, creative writing and painting (implying core and integrated provision), it was proposed that this approach *could* be introduced through an intercalated BA degree (implying elective choice).

The report from a second Windsor conference in 1999 contained a warning from the philosopher Robin Downie that '[a]rt can be counterproductive if it is done for the wrong reasons. The typical artist is for example, not a good health role model!' (quoted in Philipp *et al.* 2002). This stereotype is revealing, as it made the UK medical humanities initiative suddenly look reactionary. The two Windsor conferences, under the influence of utilitarianism rather than skepticism,[2] framed the medical humanities as a 'healing' force in the service of medicine, rather than problematizing the ideal of 'healing'.

Kenneth Calman famously suggested that the Department of Health should become a 'Department of Health and Happiness' (quoted in Health Service Journal, 22 April 1999). As a grand narrative, this utilitarian view would set the tone for the development of the medical humanities in the UK into the new millennium. It mirrored the dominant North

American approach to the medical humanities as self-evidently positive through alignment with the ideals of 'life, liberty and the pursuit of happiness' embodied in the Constitution and the Declaration of Independence as 'self-evident truths'. Paradoxically, this alignment was not pursued to its logical conclusion, where the medical humanities offer a means for democratizing medicine (Bleakley 2012), for example, in challenging the ingrained hierarchies that lead to poor teamwork and ineffective patient consultations compromising patient safety (Bleakley and Marshall 2013). Perhaps more importantly, the medical humanities were not seen as having potentially negative unintended consequences such as the paradoxical imperative 'you will be humane!' (Petersen *et al.* 2008).

The heart of the medical establishment sought support for the Windsor conferences, which were endorsed by the President of the GMC. Such lobbying would have an effect. In the 2003 edition of *Tomorrow's Doctors*, the GMC encouraged inclusion of the 'humanities related to medicine' through SSCs that would constitute 25–33 per cent of the curriculum (GMC 2003: A12). However, the revised 2009 edition made no specific reference to humanities, while recommended SSCs provision was cut to 10 per cent (GMC 2009: 50).

Fault-lines gradually emerged within the medical humanities movement in the UK, which originally tried to contain the interests of three disparate groups mentioned earlier: arts in health practitioners who aligned with psychological views of health and illness and refused to be 'medicalized'; humanities scholars who took medicine as their topic and were not necessarily interested in medical education; and medical educators, often clinicians, who were interested in how medical practice could be humanized, but not in psychological therapies or academic scholarship. At the 2002 inaugural conference of the Association for Medical Humanities (AMH), Martyn Evans and David Greaves asked 'how "medical humanities" would be – and *should* be – understood' (Evans and Greaves 2002: 1; author's emphasis). 'Medical humanities' were not framed as problematic – the conference consensus was that both the medical humanities in medical education and the arts in healthcare 'were not its central concern[s]' (Evans and Greaves 2002: 1). The medical humanities were defined rather as 'the literary, anthropological, historical, or philosophical engagements (among others) with medicine' (Evans and Greaves 2002: 1).

As noted earlier, this was to become a dominant view, despite being strongly contested within the association and its executive committee, and debated at subsequent AMH annual conferences. Such a position was instrumental in lobbying the Wellcome Trust, with its early interest in history rather than pedagogy, to commit to providing major grant awards in 2008 for the development of centres in the UK for medical humanities research. Both of the successful centres focused upon themes of health and well-being, aligning with utilitarianism. The University of Durham Centre for Medical Humanities addresses the themes of 'health', 'well-being' and 'human flourishing', while the University of London King's College development is a 'Centre for the Humanities and Health'. The recent widening scope of Wellcome Trust research funding, which has changed from 'history of medicine' to 'medical history and humanities', may, however, serve to broaden the field in coming years. Following a review in 2008–2009, the Wellcome Trust has presented a new vision that explicitly embraces critical conversations between artists, academics and practitioners. This active interest in promoting a more critical form of medical humanities is indicated by the provision of Wellcome Trust funding for a multidisciplinary seminar series (2012) that formed the basis of this edited volume.

What does the future hold for the medical humanities in medical education?

This chapter has focused on the USA and UK, where the medical humanities have been formally progressed. However, there are many recent global developments in the field (Batistatou 2010), especially in Canada (Kidd and Connor 2008; Banaszek 2011). These developments reveal the same themes identified in the brief histories above, such as utilitarian bias. However, a concern that is rarely addressed is just what *kinds* of arts and humanities are employed in medical humanities provision. In this section, looking to the future, I argue that the medical humanities culture can be seen as conservative, failing to draw on the powerful interventions that the avant-garde in the arts may provide.

I argue that the arts and humanities, particularly as employed in medical education, have merely nuanced medical practice, rather than offering fundamental critique and resistance. Explicit engagement with the avant-garde, or 'the incessant clash of the movement of art against established boundaries' (Guattari 1995: 106) has been avoided. Such art includes radical performance that draws on bodily and medical themes to give meaning to illness (Orrell 2010) within a tradition of skepticism, questioning ideals such as 'health' and 'well-being' that underpin the utilitarian outlook, as noted earlier.[2] Macneill argues that medical humanities present a 'tame' approach, offering medical students 'soft' relaxation, celebratory supplement or diversion from the 'hard' stuff of biomedical science and evidence-based clinical practice (Macneill 2011: 86). The medical humanities employed uncritically can merely serve to reinforce medical dominance (Rees 2010).

Catherine Belling (2010) refers to the more radical stream of thinking within the medical humanities, noting unintended and paradoxical consequences of humanities-based medical education. For example, Wear and Aultman (2005) show that exposing medical students to narrative approaches can produce discomfort, defensiveness and resistance to confronting political matters such as inequality and oppression. Students readily tolerate benign plots and characters in literature, where transgressive and challenging plots and characters at first produce resistance rather than empathy. Belling stridently suggests that 'we must attend to resistance, even provoke it, if humanities teaching is to promote critical inquiry as well as neutral reflection', as 'rigorous humanities teaching can develop an orientation toward uncertainty, knowledge, and action that characterizes the best physicians' (Belling 2010: 939).

Greater humility may be needed to balance the rapidly developing intellectual swagger of the field of the medical humanities. Johanna Shapiro (2011) rightly warns against narrative medicine becoming inflated through smart textual approaches that question the authenticity or reliability of patients' stories, calling for 'narrative humility' from researchers. Further, Claire Hooker and Estelle Noonan (2011) point out that the medical humanities show western imperialistic tendencies. An emergent 'critical medical humanities' must also be self-critical.

Summary

This overview of the development of the medical humanities traces the emergence of a dominant utilitarian and artistically conservative model. By contrast, the 'critical medical humanities' affords skepticism towards utilitarian models of health and well-being. Taking a more critical approach allows us to see meaning in illness and provides a point of resistance to reductive biomedical science. It also draws on the avant-garde in arts and humanities to provide deep critical impact. Such an approach is political and practical, as well as aesthetic and ethical, where it provides a potential democratizing force for medical culture (Bleakley 2012) as an 'aesthetics of resistance' (Weiss 2005).

Notes

1   'Narrative medicine' was introduced into the UK by Greenhalgh and Hurwitz (1999).
2   The debate between skepticism and utilitarianism is neatly formulated in Voltaire's *Candide*.

References

Banaszek, A. (2011) 'Medical Humanities Courses becoming Prerequisites in Many Medical Schools', *Canadian Medical Association Journal*, 183: E441–2.
Banks, S. A. and Vastyan, E. A. (1973) 'Humanistic Studies in Medical Education', *Journal of Medical Education*, 48: 248–57.
Barr, D. A. (2011) 'Putting the Flexner Report in Context', *Medical Education*, 45: 17–22.
Batistatou, A., Doulis, A., Tiniakos, D., Anogiannaki, A. and Charalabopoulos, K. (2010) 'The Introduction of Medical Humanities in the Undergraduate

Curriculum of Greek Medical Schools: Challenge and Necessity', *Hippokratia*, 14: 241–3.

Belling, C. (2010) 'Sharper Instruments: On Defending the Humanities in Undergraduate Medical Education', *Academic Medicine*, 85: 938–40.

Bleakley, A. (2012) 'The Humanities Offer a Democratizing Force for Medical Culture', *Ars Medica*, 9: 1–6.

Bleakley, A. and Marshall, R. J. (2013) 'Can the Science of Communication Inform the Art of the Medical Humanities?', *Medical Education*, 47: 126–33.

Bleakley, A., Farrow, R., Gould, D. and Marshall, R. J. (2003) 'Making Sense of Clinical Reasoning: Judgement and the Evidence of the Senses', *Medical Education*, 37: 544–52.

Coats, E. (ed.) (2004) *Swallows to Other Continents: Creative Arts and Humanities in Healthcare*, London: Nuffield Trust.

Clouser, K. D. (1971) 'Humanities and the Medical School: A Sketched Rationale and Description', *Medical Education*, 5: 226–31.

Crawshaw, R. (1975) 'Humanism in Medicine – The Rudimentary Process', *The New England Journal of Medicine*, 293: 1320–2.

Evans, H. M. and Greaves, D. A. (2002) ' "Medical Humanities" – What's In a Name?', *Medical Humanities*, 28: 1–2.

Flexner, A. (1910) *Medical Education in the United States and Canada*, New York, NY: Carnegie Foundation for the Advancement of Teaching.

GMC (2009) *Good Medical Practice*, London: GMC.

GMC (2003) *Tomorrow's Doctors*, London: GMC.

GMC (1993) *Tomorrow's Doctors*, London: GMC.

Greenhalgh, T. and Hurwitz, B. (1999) 'Narrative Based Medicine: Why Study Narrative?', *British Medical Journal*, 318: 48–50.

Guattari, F. (1995) *Chaosmosis: An Ethico-Aesthetic Paradigm*, Bloomington, IN: Indiana University Press.

Haddon, M. (2012) *The Red House*, London: Jonathan Cape.

Hamilton, C., Hinks, S. and Petticrew, M. (2003) 'Arts for Health: Still Searching for the Holy Grail', *Journal of Epidemiology and Community Health*, 57: 401–2.

Hardee, J. T. and Kasper, I. K. (2005) 'From Standardized Patient to Care Actor: Evolution of a Teaching Methodology', *Permanente Journal*, 9: 79–82.

Health Development Agency (2000) *Art for Health: A Review of Good Practice in Community-Based Arts Projects and Initiatives which Impact on Health and Wellbeing*, London: Health Development Agency.

Health Service Journal (22 April 1999) 'Send in the Clowns'. Online. Available: www.hsj.co.uk/news/send-in-the-clowns/29709.article (accessed 1 March 2013).

Hodges, B. (2005) 'The Many and Conflicting Histories of Medical Education in Canada and the USA: An Introduction to the Paradigm Wars', *Medical Education*, 39: 613–21.

Hooker, C. and Noonan, E. (2011) 'Medical Humanities as Expressive of Western Culture', *Medical Humanities*, 37: 79–84

Jones, T., Wear, D. and Friedman, L. D. (eds) (2014) *Health and Humanities Reader*, New Brunswick, NJ: Rutgers University Press.

Ke, W. (2012) 'Healthcare Reform: Using Medical Humanities as an Alternative Solution', Online. Available: http://triplehelixblog.com/2012/03/healthcare-reform-using-medical-humanities-as-an-alternative-solution (accessed 1 March 2013).

Kidd, M. J. and Connor, J. T. (2008) 'Striving to do Good Things: Teaching Humanities in Canadian Medical Schools', *Journal of Medical Humanities*, 29: 45–54.

Kirklin, D. B. (2002) 'Acquiring Experience in Medical Humanities Teaching: The Chicken and Egg Conundrum', *Medical Humanities*, 28: 101.

Leake, C. (1973) 'Humanistic Studies in US Medical Education', *Journal of Medical Education*, 48: 878–9.

Ludmerer, K. M. (1999) *Time to Heal: American Medical Education from the Turn of the Century to the Era of Managed Care*, Oxford: Oxford University Press.

Macneill, P. U. (2011) 'The Arts and Medicine: A Challenging Relationship', *Medical Humanities*, 37: 85–90.

McManus, I. C. (1995) 'Humanity and the Medical Humanities', *Lancet*, 346: 1143–5.

Mohr, J. C. (2000) 'American Medical Malpractice Litigation in Historical Perspective', *Journal of the American Medical Association*, 283: 1731–7.

Montgomery Hunter, K. (1991) *Doctors' Stories: The Narrative Structure of Knowledge in Medicine*, Princeton, NJ: Princeton University Press.

Mylopoulos, M., Lohfeld, L., Norman, G. R., Dhaliwal, G. and Eva, K. W. (2012) 'Renowned Physicians' Perceptions of Expert Diagnostic Practice', *Academic Medicine*, 87: 1413–7.

Neumann, M., Edelhäuser, F., Tauschel, D., Fischer, M., Wirtz, M., Woopen, C., Haramati, A. and Scheffer, C. (2011) 'Empathy Decline and Its Reasons: A Systematic Review of Studies With Medical Students and Residents', *Academic Medicine*, 86: 996–1009.

Orrell, P. (2010) *Marina Abramovic and the Future of Performance Art*, London: Prestel.

Pellegrino, E. D. (1974) 'Educating the Humanist Physician: An Ancient Ideal Reconsidered', *Journal of the American Medical Association*, 227: 1288–94.

Petersen, A., Bleakley, A., Brömer, R. and Marshall, R. (2008) 'The Medical Humanities Today: Humane Health Care or Tool of Governance?', *Journal of Medical Humanities*, 29: 1–4.

Philipp, R., Baum, M., Mawson, A. and Calman, K. (1999) *Beyond the Millennium: A Summary of the Proceedings of the First Windsor Conference*, London: The Nuffield Trust.

Philipp, R., Baum, M., Macnaughton, J. and Calman, K. (2002) *Arts, Health and Wellbeing: From the Windsor I Conference to a Nuffield Forum for the Medical Humanities*, London: The Nuffield Trust.

Rees, G. (2010) 'The Ethical Imperative of Medical Humanities', *Journal of Medical Humanities*, 31: 267–77.

Reynolds, R. and Carson, R. (1976) 'The Place of Humanities in Medical Education', *Journal of Medical Education*, 51: 142–3.

Riggs, G. (2010) 'Commentary: Are we Ready to Embrace the Rest of the Flexner Report?', *Academic Medicine*, 85: 1669–71.

Shapiro, J. (2011) 'Illness Narratives: Reliability, Authenticity and the Empathic Witness', *Medical Humanities*, 37: 68–72.

Wear, W. and Aultman, J. M. (2005) 'The Limits of Narrative: Medical Student Resistance to Confronting Inequality and Oppression in Literature and Beyond', *Medical Education*, 39: 1056–65.

Weatherall, D. J. (1994) 'The Inhumanity of Medicine', *British Medical Journal*, 309: 1671–2.

Weiss, P. (2005) *The Aesthetics of Resistance*, Durham, NC: Duke University Press.

3 'Oh, the humanit(ies)!'

Dissent, democracy, and danger[1]

Therese Jones

Several years ago, after Rafael Campo – writer, physician, teacher – returned from a conference on the medical humanities in London, he published a commentary in the *Journal of the American Medical Association*, which he titled: ' "The Medical Humanities," for Lack of a Better Term' (Culler 2005). In this commentary Campo organizes the discussion around a disarmingly simple, albeit incredibly thorny, question put to him by a medical student: 'So, what are the medical humanities, anyway?' (Campo 2005: 1009). Despite his success as an essayist and poet and his commitment to critical and pedagogical pursuits in the academy, Campo discovers that he can neither gracefully nor satisfactorily answer that question for the student, for his clinical colleagues and health administrators, or even for himself. He stumbles between two poles: 'knowing intuitively that the way medicine is now taught and practiced is simply *wrong*, that the human is being supplanted by unfeeling science and uncaring economics' and the 'need to articulate rationally…just what it is that I do – and that this work is not amorphous and merely sentimentally gratifying, but can be productively studied and harnessed' (Campo 2005: 1009).

In this chapter, I will briefly examine how the medical/health humanities – for lack of a better term – in education and clinical training for health professions continues to be divided along the fault lines of dualistic and mechanical thinking most frequently captured in the use and misuse of the words, 'humanism' and 'humanities'. As Jonathan Culler notes, it is not at all surprising that the human in the humanities leads us astray: 'The crisis of the humanities might even be linked to the fact that our language proposes a strong link not just between the humanities and the human being but between *humanistic* thinking and even *humane* behavior' (2005: 8). Thus, there has been and continues to be a tension between the instrumental justification for the humanities in medicine, which ostensibly enables and promotes more caring professionals and better caring practices – what Jeffrey Bishop deems the 'dose effect' of the humanities (Bishop 2008: 17) – and the intellectual practice of the humanities with all of its democratizing energies and dangerous possibilities, which enable and promote fearless questioning of representations, challenges to the abuses of authority and a steadfast refusal to accept as the limits of enquiry the boundaries that medicine sets between biology and culture.

Those of us in the medical/health humanities often feel beleaguered and diminished by the demands to calculate the value of what we do in terms of quality improvement (such as producing more empathic, compassionate and reflective professionals) or measurable outcomes (such as demonstrating more effective communication and reduced spiritual distress). However, there are notable indicators that, in spite of our internal battles over who we are and what we do and external battles over why we matter, ground-breaking scholarship and educational initiatives are actually increasing. Thus, the remainder of this chapter will include a discussion of the development of humanities scholarship and teaching inside and outside the US. Most noteworthy, for example, is a significant increase in the geographic diversity of authors who have and who are submitting their work to the *Journal of Medical Humanities*, of which I have been editor since 2003, as well as the dramatic proliferation of medical/health humanities educational programmes in colleges and universities throughout the US. Finally, the creation and implementation of the International Health Humanities Network at the University of Nottingham is bringing together scholars, professionals, artists and patients in order to develop new approaches to enhance health and well-being.

The 'ethical imperative' of the medical/health humanities to improve the caring in medical care (Rees 2010: 267) is still entrenched and still evident in pedagogical trends such as narrative medicine, reflective writing rubrics and reading lists dominated by physician-writers whose work is often read as clinical reality rather than textual representation. It is, nevertheless, being contested and rejected. As Culler writes, one thing the humanities are good at is 'seeing situations in another light' (Culler 2005: 37) – re-presenting, re-describing and re-contextualizing – whether it be Alan Bleakley's (2012) prediction that as a democratizing force, the medical humanities will play a bigger role than we might imagine or Geoffrey Rees' call for the 'dangerous possibilities organized through collective engagement in the work of the medical humanities' (Rees 2010: 277).

The humanities and the health professions: Why? What? How?

Why? Development and dissent

Why introduce and integrate the humanities into science- and clinically-based curricula such as medicine, nursing, pharmacy and allied health programmes? Why aren't the scientific basis of knowledge and the apprentice model of training adequate for healthcare practitioners to enter their chosen professions? K. Danner Clouser, the first philosopher to teach ethics at a medical school in the US, attempted to answer such questions in a 1980 keynote address at a conference on the role of humanities in health education:

> Where...do we train for understanding, suffering and joy? Where do we gain ideals and models – for motivations, for patterning our lives, for fashioning our goals, emotions, attitudes and character? Where do we think about and entertain purposes, goals, and styles of life? Where do we gain perspective on our own life, on others, and the relationships between them?
>
> (Clouser 1980: n.p.)

At the time, Clouser was espousing one of the most commonly advanced political and pedagogical justifications for the still nascent medical humanities 'movement' – the belief that something vital and fundamental was missing in health professions education and that the humanities could fill in those gaps and omissions.

As Bleakley notes in his introductory chapter to this volume, such ideas and opinions had been simmering since the educational reforms of the 1960s, when relatively modest medical schools in the US were dramatically expanding to become vast academic medical centres. With a broad mandate to reform the curriculum, medical educators hurried to incorporate new knowledge and accommodate larger changes affecting clinical practice, such as shifting disease patterns and emerging methods and technologies for diagnosis and treatment (Ludmerer 1999: 197). However, although biomedical content continued to evolve dramatically, the ongoing struggle to encourage student compassion and empathy, to include family and community health needs in addition to those of the individual patient, and to emphasize reasoning and analysis over rote memorization remained remarkably similar to what had already been undertaken in the previous century. With the 1970s came the emergence of seemingly miraculous but morally troubling medical and technological advances such as organ transplantation, standards of death, *in vitro* fertilization and complex pharmaceuticals. Educators inserted humanities materials and methodologies into medical curriculum and clinical practice with the intention of remedying the growing imbalance between the technological aspects of healthcare and the human aspects of caregiving (Hawkins and McEntyre 2000: 3–4).

During the inaugural session of the Institute on Human Values in Medicine, physician and ethicist Edmund Pellegrino would declare the hope of bringing:

> [S]ome of us in medicine who are concerned with issues involving human values into close discourse with those...in the disciplines outside of medicine who have interest in, and perhaps a desire to help

us with, the human problems that arise in medicine for the patient and the physicians.

(Pellegrino 1972: n.p.)

He noted that on almost every medical campus a 'subterranean current of interest in exploring potential contributions from the humanities' already existed, a current that has not only remained strong at health sciences centres but that has continued to grow as the number and quality of programmes across the country now demonstrate.

However, nothing in the early proceedings and publications of this burgeoning field prescribed which areas of academic study should be 'invited' into the curriculum although the usual ones – history, literature, philosophy – were consistently mentioned. In fact, presenters at this first Institute were mindful about casting a wide net to include all humanities disciplines as well as the social sciences, confident and excited about what such a collective and interdisciplinary presence might bring to medical education. Clouser suggested that 'each [humanities] discipline should be working to interrelate conceptually with some discipline of the medical world. It is an interdisciplinary enterprise aiming for new insights and understanding' (1972: n.p.). Yet, then and now, one fundamental question remains: what *particular* knowledge and skills do humanities disciplines bring to the enterprise of educating healthcare practitioners?

Literature offers a compelling illustration of how that question can evoke both inventiveness and defensiveness among its practitioners. Over 20 years ago, Anne Hudson Jones (1990) described two major approaches to teaching literature and medicine, each with the same goal of improving patient care. What she calls the 'aesthetic' approach focuses on the literary skills of reading, writing and interpretation for use in medical practice. Joanne Trautmann Banks, the first literature scholar to join the faculty of a medical school in 1972, writes from this orientation in 'The Wonders of Literature in Medical Education', in which she argues that 'to teach a student to read *in the fullest sense* is to train him or her medically' (Trautmann Banks 1982: 26; original emphasis). She refers to the interpretive skills necessary for the exploration of literary texts which require students to study subtle, ambiguous and rich detail; to fill in gaps; to understand relationships; to look at 'what is being said' and to approach 'words in their personal and social contexts and when several things are being said at once' (Trautmann Banks 1982: 26). The imparting and practising of literary analysis and critical reading has instrumental value by virtue of supplying specific intellectual tools to the multiple dimensions of medicine.

The other approach, also in the service of patient care, has more to do with moral reflection rather than with merely introducing medical students to basic literary elements such as point of view, plot, imagery and setting. This approach engages students with cultural perspectives on health and illness, social justice and the moral dimensions of patient encounters through literary works that 'illuminate a particular set of human experiences and...encourage moral reflection in treating patients confronting these experiences' (Hunter, Charon and Coulehan 1995: 789). Those favouring this approach often cite the work of philosopher Martha Nussbaum, known for her exploration of literature in developing the moral emotions. In the preface to *Poetic Justice* (1995), she argues that the ability to imagine the concrete ways in which people different from us grapple with their disadvantage can have practical and public value given the deep prejudice and rampant oppression in the world enacted through sexism, racism, classism, able-ism, homophobia and ethnic discrimination.

Arising from, and enmeshed with, Nussbaum's view that attending carefully to the nuances and complexities of literature can sharpen and deepen moral sensibilities is a third approach – the focus on empathy. This approach suggests that studying literature has the potential to enhance a student's ability to understand others' feelings, plights and values, requiring the reader 'to suspend his or her own point of view and enter the reality of another character or another world' (Hunter, Charon and Coulehan 1995: 789). However, this approach has become increasingly challenged, particularly when humanities inquiry is tied directly and specifically to the development of humanism and humanistic professionals. Just as medical/health humanities scholars and educators have become less willing to adapt their research interests and pedagogical practices to the exigencies of clinical practice and classroom education over the past 40 years, so too have they become less comfortable with (even overtly hostile to) the tacit assumption that teaching literature to health professions students is the means of enlightenment and empathy. To return again to one of the original articulations of and justifications for the medical humanities, *Literature and Medicine: A Claim For a Discipline,* Jones challenges and cautions against any notion that studying the humanities makes one more humane:

> This expectation makes me very uncomfortable. This expectation is a burden, not just for literature, for all of the humanities. We all hope that it will [make one more humane], but there have been too many examples to the contrary for me to believe in any guarantee.
>
> (Jones 1987: 32)

In fact, increasing numbers of theoretical justifications for humanities in health professions education suggest that the 'ethical imperative' of the humanities has been either simply outgrown or deliberately discarded.

What? Expansion and accessibility

The humanities disciplines traditionally represented and integrated in health professions education include history, literature, philosophy, bioethics and comparative religion as well as those aspects of the social sciences that have humanistic content and employ humanistic methods relevant to medical inquiry and practice, particularly sociology, anthropology and psychology. The field has been further developed and influenced by such philosophical and pedagogical projects as postmodernism, feminism, disability studies, cultural studies, media studies and biocultures. Moreover, the influence of narrative inquiry on the medical/health humanities cannot be overstated, in particular physician and literary scholar Rita Charon's pioneering work in the theoretical development of narrative in medicine. Arguing that physicians must have the ability to listen to patients' stories, to understand the meanings of such stories and to be stirred in order to act in support of patients, Charon proposes that narrative competence is what humans use 'to absorb, interpret, and respond to stories... [which] enables the physician to practice medicine with empathy, reflection, professionalism and trustworthiness. Such a medicine can be called *narrative medicine*' (Charon 2001: 1897; original emphasis). She writes that:

> [N]arrative knowledge is what one uses to understand the meaning and significance of stories through cognitive, symbolic, and affective means. This kind of knowledge provides a rich, resonant comprehension of a singular person's situation as it unfolds in time, whether in such texts as novels, newspaper stories, movies, and scripture or in such life settings as courtrooms, battlefields, marriages, and illnesses.
>
> (Charon 2001: 1898)

Narrative in the contemporary health professions curriculum is interdisciplinary in both nature and application: its tenets appear in patient interviewing, in making deeper sense of the medical record, in acts of diagnosing and in psychosocial aspects of patienthood. Moreover, narrative inquiry is also the source of an explosion of reflective writing across the curriculum.

As the field of medical/health humanities and its practitioners have become less a novelty in health professions education (over 60 per cent of medical schools in the US currently report both required and elective humanities courses), the benchmarks by which academics chart the successful growth of a field of study have been slowly and steadily met. These include several well-respected peer-reviewed journals; professional societies; annual meetings in the US as well as international conferences; active listservs (such as Mersenne Digest and NYU Literature, Arts and Medicine), blogs, resource databases and networks; and graduate programmes awarding both masters degrees and doctorates.

A simple inventory of submissions to the *Journal of Medical Humanities* demonstrates a trend that may very well indicate both the growing interest in and global spread of the medical/health humanities. From 2004 to 2009, roughly 20 per cent of all submissions to the journal came from authors outside the US with 60 per cent of those representing the UK, Canada and Australia and the remainder representing a handful of European countries including Finland, France, Germany, and the Netherlands. However, from January 2009 to December 2012, roughly 40 per cent of all submissions came from authors outside the US with about the same percentage (60 per cent) of those representing the UK, Canada and Australia. In addition to those countries listed above, European authors now hail from Italy, Poland, Spain, Sweden, and Switzerland. South American scholars and educators from Brazil, Chile and Colombia are represented as well as authors from Hong Kong, India, Israel, Japan, Malaysia, Nigeria, South Africa, Taiwan and Turkey.

The most common disciplinary perspectives among authors outside the US are literature and language (including rhetoric and narrative); philosophy and bioethics; history and cultural studies. The number of ethical analyses of medical practices and patient care (abortion, reproductive technologies, eugenics, pain research and immigrant health) are nearly equivalent to those submissions foregrounding literary theory and criticism of authors such as Virginia Woolf and William Faulkner as well as historical research and analysis on topics such as syphilis in Renaissance Europe or the regulation of Canadian midwifery. Medical education, both pedagogical theory and classroom practice, is also a very prominent content area among these submissions with topics such as the need for narrative and teaching the delivery of bad news as well as sample curricula. Moreover, as in the US, disability studies is becoming an important area of enquiry with submissions on cognitive disabilities (autism and mental illness), physical impairments and the significant connections between disability studies and medical humanities. In all, scholars and researchers from outside the US are tackling similar topics and posing familiar questions especially in regards to medical education and patient care as their American counterparts.

Moreover, the development and implementation of undergraduate programmes in the medical/health humanities has been nothing short of phenomenal in the US, as many colleges and universities now offer undergraduate majors, minors, concentrations and/or certificates as a valuable complement to science-based curricula and as independent programmes that address current and complex matters in the humanities and social sciences. At the time of this writing, Sarah Berry, a colleague from Hobart and William Smith Colleges, New York State, and I are analyzing preliminary information gathered from a survey of US institutions with medical/health humanities programmes already in place. Our unpublished data currently show that 10 liberal arts colleges and major universities currently offer a major in medical/health humanities; 31 offer a minor; and seven offer either a certificate or concentration. All programmes are interdisciplinary, requiring course work in the sciences as well as the humanities.

These academic endeavours are gaining in popularity and garnering special attention from both educators and students in light of revisions to the Medical College Admission Test (MCAT), a prerequisite for admission to US medical schools. Beginning in 2015, the MCAT will include sections on behavioural and social sciences as well as critical analysis of texts that raise ethical concerns and foreground cross-cultural studies. There will be questions about gender, about cultural influences on expression, about poverty and about how people process and express emotion and stress – all in a day's work for the humanities (Rosenthal 13 April 2012).

However, this marked expansion in scholarship and curriculum has prompted demands for inclusiveness. As an inter- and multidisciplinary field, the medical humanities have become increasingly complex with multiple identities and myriad challenges, not the least of which is the demand for measurable outcomes or identifiable competencies. But by its very disciplinary descriptor, *medical*, it retains a narrow frame, largely concerned with the value of history, literature, philosophy, art and media to medical education and medical practice. Scholars such as Paul Crawford, the driving force behind the International Health Humanities Network, are arguing for a 'more inclusive, outward-facing and applied discipline, embracing interdisciplinarity and engaging with the contributions of those marginalized from the medical humanities' such as allied health professionals, patients, and informal carers (Crawford 2010: 4).

As we near the half-centenary of the field, there has also been a movement in the US to adopt the more encompassing, contemporary and accurate label of the current academic enterprise – the health humanities. For some scholars and educators, the terminological shift from 'medical' to 'health' humanities might feel like just an academic exercise or a mere distraction; while we all know that nomenclature matters, this shift will likely have little effect on our daily work. However, mirroring the dynamic but deliberative process that fostered and shaped the original disciplinary project over 40 years ago, timely and robust discussions have emerged about the political, ethical, rhetorical and cultural implications of such as shift. For example, in a lively and recent conversation on a medical humanities listserv, reactions to such a suggestion ranged from simple expressions of appreciation for inclusiveness from a nurse-educator to practical considerations around community engagement and public policy – 'the notion encompasses more than the individual's experience of disease, illness and health, but the community perspective of these issues including equity, funding, policy, resources allocation' (Klugman 1 November 2012) – to nuanced and informed perspectives addressing a more contemporary focus on global health:

> Many sick people are not actively patients, may not engage biomedicine much if ever, and perhaps more importantly, overwhelming evidence suggests that health and its distribution in human populations is mostly

not the result of medical care...Thus, I would suggest that any definition of the health humanities cannot be limited to the field of medicine,
medical care, or medical professionals, and also ought not have as its
central goal the advance of the practice and science of medicine. I also
believe our primary goal should be directed to health and human flourishing rather than to the delivery of medical care; the two objectives are
actually not nearly so tightly interwoven as most tend to think, even if
both are independently of great worth.

(Goldberg 31 October 2012: n.p.)

Indeed, the variety of disciplinary identities and academic affiliations of the
scholars and educators in our field simply and persuasively model the kind
of inter- and multidisciplinary enquiry and innovative collaboration that is
the hallmark of current health humanities scholarship and education
worldwide.

How ? Practical applications and dangerous possibilities

In the US, the humanities are found throughout health professions curricula in various forms and with a full range of complexity regarding content
and pedagogy. In the most instrumental approaches, humanities content is
inserted into lectures for the purpose of illustrating a phenomenon: a film
or YouTube clip, an excerpt from a poem or short story, a paragraph lifted
from a *New Yorker* article. The content itself is likely not explored through
the methodologies of literary criticism or media studies but more often
used to exemplify something, even to liven up a class. Frequently, such an
approach finds its way into smaller formats such as group discussions where
the aesthetics of a short story or the elements of a film are bypassed for the
examination of the clinical or bioethical relevance of its content. There is
the tendency here to view the text as an instance of clinical reality rather
than a linguistic or imagistic construct.

Teaching humanities disciplines with increasing complexity involves a
fuller engagement with whatever text is under study – a documentary film,
an historical essay, a bioethics case, a legal document, or a classic work of
fiction. This kind of critical practice has the potential to alert students to
language in ways they would not have recognized otherwise: the words that
caregivers and patients use when attempting to understand each other; the
plots of the stories patients tell; the themes and tones of various narratives;
the pervasive but unspoken issues surrounding power in healthcare
settings; the layers of complexity in seemingly uncomplicated decisions; the
unspoken world views and values informed by religion and spirituality.

Over the past 20 years, cultural studies and disability studies have influenced many disciplines and pedagogies including the medical/health
humanities. With these orientations, students encounter texts that might
be literary, historical or media-produced and that include arts-based and

cultural artefacts. These materials raise matters related to power, authority and justice in healthcare and challenge the hegemony of a biomedicine that contributes to disparities and the discrimination of persons who do not quite fit the codified and naturalized norms of health. Such approaches offer teachers and students an opportunity to examine critically the origins and nature of their personal beliefs and values, the beliefs and values embedded in the curriculum and the learning environment as well as institutional policies – all of which intersect and which influence the quality of care they give to patients. They also require that teachers and students step out of their comfort zone in order to pose difficult and complex questions, scrutinize their own biases and prejudices and disturb their reliance on a biomedical approach to healthcare – in other words, by embracing and enacting the 'pedagogy of discomfort', noted as well by Bleakley in his own introduction (Wear and Aultman 2005: 1056). Finally, in addition to engaging them in such critical and political inquiry, the materials and methodologies of the medical/health humanities can reinforce students' sense of agency in developing their own professional identities; understanding their own special influence on healthcare practice and delivery; and accepting their own responsibility in how care giving is both taught and modelled. Such enquiry rarely leads to simplified clarity or snap decision-making; rather, it produces uncomfortable ambiguity.

For those professionals already in practice, exposure to the health humanities offers both the challenge and opportunity to deconstruct norms; to help and heal patients by recognizing them as individuals with complex identities embedded in networks of friends and family, community culture, and society; to tolerate their own discomfort; and to develop a respect for patients as authorities on their own experiences of illness and disability. Professionals can also recognize that the biomedical model is only one source of knowledge about illness and disability and only one source of authority – even while it remains the dominant source of power in the clinic. Bodies are not only biological but also socio-cultural, and caring for persons demands clinical knowledge and skills, narrative knowledge and skills and cultural knowledge and skills (see Garden 2013 [in press]).

As a disparate but devoted community of scholars and educators, I would argue that we have moved well beyond Campo's feeling that 'no conception of the medical humanities compels, caught somewhere between manifesto, mushiness, and marketing lingo' (Campo 2005: 1009). Publications such as this one both tackle and transcend the familiar justifications and passionate assertions borne out of the ethical imperative of the medical/health humanities. The rigorous analyses and creative work found here and elsewhere actively resist treating the humanities as a 'refuge from difficult questions' and instead, decisively offer them as a crucible for difficult questions, replete with all of the dangerous possibilities that Rees and others envision (Rees 2010: 269).

Note

1   Portions of this introduction will be published in the *Health and Humanities Reader*, edited by Therese Jones, Delese Wear and Lester D. Friedman (in press; Rutgers University Press, 2014).

References

Bishop, J. (2008) 'Rejecting Medical Humanism: Medical Humanities and the Metaphysics of Medicine', *Journal of Medical Humanities*, 29: 15–25.

Bleakley, A. (2012) 'The Humanities Offer a Democratizing Force for Medical Culture', *Ars Medica*, 9: 1–6.

Campo, R. (2005) ' "The Medical Humanities," For Lack of a Better Term', *JAMA*, 294: 1009–11.

Charon, R. (2001) 'Narrative Medicine: A Model for Empathy, Reflection, Profession, and Trust', *Journal of the American Medical Association*, 286: 1897–1902.

Clouser, K. D. (1972) 'Humanities and the Medical School', in L. L. Hunt (ed.), *Proceedings of the First Session, Institute on Human Values in Medicine*, Philadelphia PA: Society for Health and Human Values.

Clouser, K. D. (1980) Keynote Address for a Conference Entitled 'The Allied Health Training Institute on the Role of the Humanities in Allied Health Education', Thomas Jefferson University. Online. Available: http://weberstudies.weber.edu/archive/archive%20A%20%20%20.%201-10.3/Vol.%203/3.1Clauser.htm (accessed 23 February 2013).

Crawford, P., Brown, B., Tischler, V. and Baker, C. (2010) 'Health Humanities: The Future of Medical Humanities?', *Mental Health Review Journal*, 15: 4–10.

Culler, J. (2005) 'In Need of a Name? A Response to Geoffrey Harpham', *New Literary History*, 36: 37–42.

Garden, R. (2014 [in press]) 'Social Studies: The Humanities, Narrative, and the Social Context of the Patient-Professional Relationship', in T. Jones, D. Wear and L. D. Friedman (eds) *Health Humanities Reader*, New Jersey: Rutgers University Press.

Goldberg, D. (31 Oct. 2012) Posting to ASBH LitMed List. Online. Available: litmed@listserv.com

Hawkins, A. H. and McEntyre, M. C. (2000) 'Teaching Literature and Medicine: A Retrospective and a Rationale', in A. H. Hawkins and M. C. McEntyre (eds) *Teaching Literature and Medicine*, New York: Modern Language Association.

Hunter, K. M., Charon, R. and Coulehan, J. L. (1995) 'The Study of Literature in Medical Education', *Academic Medicine*, 70: 787–94.

Jones, A. H. (1987) 'Reflections, Projections, and the Future of Literature and Medicine', in D. Wear, M. Kohn and S. Stocker (eds) *Literature and Medicine: A Claim for a Discipline*, McLean VA: Society for Health and Human Values.

Jones, A. H. (1990) 'Literature and Medicine: Traditions and Innovations', in B. Clark and W. Ayock (eds) *The Body and the Text: Comparative Essays in Literature and Medicine*, Lubbock TX: Texas Tech University Press.

Jones, T., Wear, D. and Friedman, L. D. (2014 [in press]) 'Introduction', in T. Jones, D. Wear and L. D. Friedman (eds) *Health Humanities Reader*, New Jersey: Rutgers University Press.

Klugman, C. M. (1 November 2012) Posting to ASBH LitMed List. Online. Available: litmed@listserv.com (accessed 23 February 2013).

Ludmerer, K. M. (1999) *Time to Heal: American Medical Education from the Turn of the Century to the Era of Managed Care*, Oxford: Oxford University Press.

Nussbaum, M. C. (1995) *Poetic Justice: The Literary Imagination and Public Life*, Boston: Beacon Press.

Pellegrino, E. (1972) 'Welcoming Remarks', in L. L. Hunt (ed.) *Proceedings of the First Session, Institute on Human Values in Medicine*, Philadelphia PA: Society for Health and Human Values.

Rees, G. (2010) 'The Ethical Imperative of Medical Humanities', *Journal of Medical Humanities*, 31: 267–77.

Rosenthal, E. (13 April 2012) 'Pre-Med's New Priorities: Heart and Soul and Social Science. Online. Available: www.nytimes.com/2012/04/15/education/edlife/pre-meds-new-priorities-heart-and-soul-and-social-science.html (accessed 23 February 2013).

Trautmann Banks, J. (1982) 'The Wonders of Literature in Medical Education', *Mobius*, 2: 22–31.

Wear, D. and Aultman, J. M. (2005) 'The Limits of Narrative: Medical Student Resistance to Confronting Inequality and Oppression in Literature and Beyond', *Medical Education*, 39: 1056–65.

Section Two

Visual arts

4 Medicine and the visual arts

Overview

Ludmilla Jordanova

'Medicine' is a notoriously hard term to define. In this chapter I will be considering many different aspects of medicine – from ideas about sickness and health to the activities of professionals and representations of disability. There is little advantage to be gained from struggling towards a simple definition of a word that is best thought about in terms of the centrality of health for human beings, the concern to respond somehow to illness, pain and suffering, and the wide range of people, remedies and institutions at the forefront of those responses. In other words, however we define it, medicine is everywhere. It should come as no surprise, then, that it is *in* the visual arts too. Nor that medical practice, for which highly honed visual skills are central, generates forms of visual art.

I take the visual arts to be more straightforward to define than medicine, but no less ubiquitous. Visual art is made by those with distinctive constellations of skills, including manual dexterity and visual intelligence, producing work that is intended to evoke a response by virtue of its visual properties. Reactions of pleasure, awe, shock, interest, revulsion, admiration or puzzlement may all be elicited by drawings, paintings, sculptures, prints, photographs and so on, as well as by work in new media. The visual arts are not confined to galleries and museums, but are also on display in books and magazines, on posters and billboards, and in a range of public places, including hospitals. Some art items will command both high prices in international markets and the attention of well-known critics, while others lead more modest lives, but may provoke widespread comment, for example, when they are generated for the purposes of advocacy. Disability rights movements, to take one important case, are particularly interested in public imagery and the ways in which it can be used to change attitudes.

The focus of this volume is the medical humanities, a field that has been taking shape in recent decades. Here, I use examples from Britain after the Second World War, a period of dramatic change with respect to both medicine and the visual arts. The inauguration of the National Health Service in 1948, along with the development of comprehensive welfare policies, was of fundamental significance for British society; so too was the rise of leisure industries, rights-based political movements, and legal changes relating to sexuality and reproduction. For many commentators, the 1960s were a decisive turning point (for example Marwick 1998). Major shifts included more experimentation in, and public engagement with, the visual arts. Visiting museums and galleries is now a major activity to be construed not just in terms of post-war patterns of consumption, but of government 'access' agendas. 'Widening participation' has become a watchword in culture as in education. In a climate of increasing 'permissiveness', it has become possible to speak about, and to represent, intimate aspects of health, disease and disability. Artists working in a wide range of media have participated in these trends, which are international in character even as they are inflected by local and national contexts.

It is vital to keep the breadth of 'medicine' constantly in mind throughout this chapter. And in that spirit, to think of bodies, health and sexuality as bound up with it, that is, as integral to the health-and-medicine domain. I can put the same point another way by pointing out that the political movements that have dominated the post-war period have had 'identity' at their heart, generating wide interest in the concept (for example Appiah and Gates 1995). 'Identity' has been explored in many different ways, but the body, mind, sexualities and well-being of the group in question, such as women or the disabled, lay at the core of that exploration (for example Hevey 1992). Feminist artists were interested, among other things, in the representation of women's bodies, and hence developed a critical discourse on the conventional, even hegemonic, ways in which such representation occurred, in the present as in the past (Parker and Pollock 1987). How, then, could 'medicine', the shorthand I am using in this chapter, *not* be a major theme, and how could subjects such as childbirth, menstruation, breast cancer, and sexuality be ignored?

One important trend from the 1960s onwards was the exploration of health and sickness from a variety of perspectives outside what was perceived as mainstream medicine. Alternative approaches to well-being are increasingly tolerated and economically significant, as is evident in many forms of visual culture, including items designed to promote alternative approaches to health. Thus the oppositional dimension present in many of the post-war confluences between diverse forms of medicine and the visual arts needs to be acknowledged and sympathetically understood. But this is not the only way in which we can approach the highly intricate relationships between medicine and the visual arts. It is vital to recognise how strong forms of professionalization have been in this period, including among those who work with the visual arts in medical settings. Important work is undertaken *within* the medical establishment by practitioners who are also artists, and by professional artists participating in medical life – I consider some of them in this chapter. Other forms of practice, psychoanalytically-based therapy that encourages patients to make art, and the use of art in educating medical students, for instance, suggest further ways in which the zones of medicine and the visual arts have become entwined.

I have alluded to three kinds of links between medicine and the visual arts, two of which are addressed further within the case studies in this section. First, there are visual artists who use medical themes in their work – the graphic novels discussed in Ian Williams' chapter provide an example. Second, medicine may draw on the help of visual artists or technologies in the process of education or diagnosis – Louise Younie's chapter shows that this includes art forms ranging from traditional drawing to installations, sculpture and photography. In a third type of link, visual art may be used therapeutically – particularly in psychiatry and in hospitals. Thus, we can appreciate the ubiquity of medicine *in* art, medicine *as* art, art *in* medical practice, and art *as* medicine.

To understand British culture and society since 1945, including its international context, some attention needs to be paid both to 'medicine', seen in a generous way, and to the visual arts, which in recent decades are enjoying a glamour, prestige and commercial success that are particularly noteworthy. We may want to connect these phenomena to, on the one hand, an unprecedentedly open environment with regard to the human body, and on the other, with confessional and celebrity cultures that exploit the body. I want to note the surprising fragmentation between scholarly writings on the three key areas addressed here: medicine, the visual arts, and contemporary Britain. Distinct specialized literatures have grown up in each one, and they seem to be unconnected in terms of themes, sources, theories, approaches, guiding assumptions and target audiences. One possible mission, then, for the medical humanities is to act as a bridge between medicine and any other discipline that relates to and bears upon it. Writings in this spirit might succeed in bringing together historiographies now separated, thereby showing how fundamental visual phenomena are for understanding the recent history of medicine as well as the societies for which health and medicine are central concerns. Standard medical history works pay little or no attention to visual culture (for example Cooter and Pickstone 2003; Jackson 2011).

Medicine may productively be considered as a form of culture; since 1945 its cultural prominence has increased through its presence in the visual arts. These trends need to be seen in historical context, which includes broad shifts in politics, economics and society. Books about contemporary Britain hardly mention the areas I am considering in this chapter (for example Addison and Jones 2005; Clarke 2004; Hollowell 2003; Morgan 2000). Many writings on the visual arts feel little need to engage with social trends, although they certainly acknowledge the role that second-wave feminism, for instance, has played in the art world (Parker and Pollock 1987; Archer 2002). Furthermore, scholarship on museums, galleries, heritage and leisure forms yet another distinct field. Thus, we lack a basic map of the principal shifts, confluences and trends for the multiple relationships between medicine and the visual arts since the war. This chapter sketches in some of the main issues, and mentions a few of the most striking examples of medicine and visual arts coming together. It does not dwell on art in hospitals and the rise of art therapy, important phenomena though these are. Rather it takes a range of examples and draws more general points out of them, concluding with brief reflections about the opportunities for medical humanities in this area.

A brief sketch map

At this point I need to list, all too baldly, some of the ways in which medicine and the visual arts intersect. It is not possible to pursue all of them; rather in this chapter I lay special emphasis on the visual arts as arenas within which medical issues are mediated, which enables them to be shared with the public. *Within* medicine, the visual arts are present not only through the skills of some practitioners as artists, but through the rich visual culture that is an integral part of medical practice itself: scans, x-rays, clinical charts and diagrams, for example. To produce and interpret such items requires visual skills, and aesthetic criteria are adopted in making them, even if these criteria differ from those adopted by professional artists. Art more conventionally defined is commissioned and bought by hospitals and other medical institutions. These practices are many centuries old, but have achieved new prominence in recent decades, when 'hospital art', for instance, has become a recognizable phrase, even if it encompasses a wide range of practices (Cork 2012). Then *making* art is also a part of medical practice, a form of therapy offered to certain kinds of patients, and, as we see from Younie's chapter in this section, making art is also being used experimentally in medical education (Gilroy and McNeilly 2000; Hogan 2001). Medical practice in general requires honed visual skills to be applied to the human body and representations of it; this in part accounts for the affinities between art and medicine. There is also funding for those wishing to explore and express these affinities (for example Anderson 2010). When this comes from medical sources, such as the Wellcome Trust, we may infer that some form of the public understanding of medicine is involved. Thus, we might observe that artists are useful to those who want to present medicine to lay audiences. Given that being an artist is generally rather precarious financially speaking, such opportunities are valuable.

Artists for their part are omnivorous, often keen to comment on and criticise contemporary trends, even as they are dependent on collectors, galleries and museums, agents, dealers and auction houses. If part of a self-conscious avant-garde, they may well want to take on what are perceived as establishment values, and to challenge conventions and taboos; as a result, medicine and health are appealing areas. Both sides – the art world and the medical world – recognize the importance of identity. Self-portraiture, understood as a form of autobiography, offers opportunities for the scrutiny of issues that can be legitimately termed 'medical'. Academic and medical establishments also want images of their brightest and best, hence the production of portraits, which affirm and shape collective identity, remains a healthy activity (Jordanova 2000). Portrait artists need commissions from individuals and institutions. Thus, there can be few organizations, whether medical or artistic, that are not touched by the multiple intersections between medicine and the visual arts. This includes hospitals, medical schools, universities, colleges and academies, museums and galleries, as well as specialist organizations, such as the Wellcome Trust.

Given the massive growth of leisure industries in the period since 1945, there are many chances for non-specialists to encounter the medicine-art intersection. One example is in public art, such as the Carrara marble statue of a disabled woman, *Alison Lapper Pregnant*, by Marc Quinn (born 1964), shown first on the fourth plinth in Trafalgar Square between 2005 and 2007, and then used prominently in giant replica form at the London 2012 Paralympic Games. Marc Quinn is regarded as a leading contemporary artist, one of the so-called YBAs (Young British Artists) associated with the Saatchi collection. But this intersection was also brought to the public when a famous portrait of the physician William Harvey (1578–1657) was repatriated in the early 1970s – having been illegally exported some years earlier – to be hung on the walls of London's National Portrait Gallery, amidst much comment in the press. Yet there is a difference to be drawn out here. Sir Geoffrey Keynes (1887–1982), the distinguished surgeon who was chairman of the NPG Trustees at the time, wanted to affirm the public face of medicine through a historic artefact, a work of art, a portrait of someone he openly heroized (Keynes 1966; 1985 [1949]). Charles Saatchi (born 1943), by contrast, is a collector with the means to buy and display new art that elicits a range of reactions from the public. The relationships between audiences, the visual arts, and spaces for display have certainly shifted in complex ways since 1945. Medical subjects have played a central role here, partly because the shifting ways in which artists use their own bodies invite changing responses on the part of viewers.

The preceding paragraphs have given the briefest of sketches about where the medicine/art nexus arises, and hint at ways it has changed in the last 70 years or so. The huge success of the London venue, the Wellcome Collection, with its exhibitions, café, bookshops and activities, gives a sense of how this nexus has become glamorous and widely appealing, in a way that earlier generations would have found perplexing. At a more populist level, we might note the extraordinary interest elicited by Gunther von Hagens (born 1945) and his spectacles of human anatomy. What I have said so far indicates not only how large the subject matter of this chapter is, but also how full it is of rich research possibilities.

I pursue some of these themes through a series of examples, organized chronologically, starting with 'drawings' by the sculptor Barbara Hepworth, who was working around the time the National Health Service was being born in the late 1940s, through John Berger and Jean Mohr's *A Fortunate*

Man, first published in 1967, to John Bellany's remarkable work from the 1980s during his experience of liver disease and receiving a successful transplant. I then move on to the more self-consciously radical work of the Young British Artists and their contemporaries, most of whom were born in the 1960s, stressing the importance of figures from earlier generations, such as the photographer Jo Spence (1934–1992) and Helen Chadwick (1953–1996), who is sometimes described as a conceptual artist. I consider work in a range of media – painting, drawing, print-making, photography and sculpture. One advantage of focusing on prominent artists is that we can gauge more easily the level and nature of public reaction to and inter-est in them, although this chapter is not, it should be stressed, concerned with the critical reaction to contemporary art works.

My examples give particular prominence to the ways in which artists have engaged with medical themes since 1945. This is a phenomenon of excep-tional importance, and it deserves sustained scholarly attention. Such artistic engagement has taken many forms, including performance art, as Emma Brodzinski shows in her discussion of Orlan – one of the best-known exponents of the genre. Successful and high-profile artists have the capac-ity to reach large audiences, to shape ways of thinking and responding to major human phenomena. They do so through exhibitions that attract attention, even if, like *Sensation* at the Royal Academy, London in 1997, they also provoke anger and criticism (Rosenthal *et al.* 1997). It is possible to argue that the exhibition was deliberately provocative, designed to shock audiences, even while being staged at an institution at the heart of the British establishment, yet there is more to be said, in particular about the medical themes that were present in many works. Thus, we need to recog-nize the character and status of the visual arts in contemporary Britain, the prominence that they enjoy, and their capacity to make forceful public statements, as Marc Quinn's *Alison Lapper Pregnant* has done. Lapper (born 1965) is herself an artist who engages with these issues. She is portrayed naked, heavily pregnant, with her incomplete limbs, caused by the congen-ital disorder phocomelia, fully displayed. However disturbing some works of art dealing with medical themes are, they deserve careful analysis by virtue of their status as commentaries, produced by the distinctive visual intelligence that artists possess. It is vital then to move away from thinking about works we 'like' or 'dislike', too often the terms in which *Sensation* was discussed. The alternative is to reflect on the distinctive types of interven-tion that the visual arts are capable of offering. It is precisely because the issues surrounding health and medicine touch everyone that artists explore them. This broad phenomenon is not new. The human body has, so far as is known, been shared terrain for medicine and art since records began. What has changed is both the level of explicitness with which human bodies, whatever their state, can be represented, and the desire to engage in a critical manner with dominant, normative discourses concerning health and illness. These two trends, in both of which second wave feminism played a major role, made possible the moving and provocative photographic work of Jo Spence, who charted her experiences of breast cancer with both humour and a sharp eye for the depersonalization of patients and sufferers. I return to her work later in the chapter.

Hepworth's 'Hospital Drawings'

The sculptor Barbara Hepworth (1903–1975) produced an extraordinary body of two-dimensional work in close collaboration with medical personnel, several of whom were either active as artists or deeply interested in the visual arts (Hepburn 2012). These are what she called her 'Hospital Drawings', executed in a range of materials, including oil paint and pastel, depicting surgical operations in Exeter and London that she was invited to witness. Her initial entree came via one of her children, who had been treated for osteomyelitis. Hepworth developed a warm and long-lasting friendship with Norman Capener (1898–1975), a surgeon and artist, who pursued sculpture with her encouragement. She became a special kind of witness to medical procedures, able to articulate forcefully, in both images and words, the relationships between her own artistic practices and those of the operating theatre, between her drawings in two-dimensions and her sculptures in three, and between her understanding of hands and their deployment in the operating theatre. These beautiful works, which interpreted what she saw through her own visual and tactile experiences, contain apparently simple flowing lines and soft colours – yellows, blues, greens – that give them an otherworldly air. And while the gowns and masks, along with other details, locate them securely in an operating theatre, the figures also appear angelic, almost ghost-like. Certainly they give viewers access to a setting, which carries a certain mystique, and which is inaccessible to most lay people. If the doctors and nurses seem like ministering angels, Hepworth is not, I think, idealizing them as medical heroes, but connecting them with the forms she was exploring in her other work. Furthermore, her interest in surgery was rooted in the materiality of bodies in use, and in substances deployed in medical practice, such as plaster for making casts. Learning and practising medicine involve the constant translation between two and three dimensions, as it did in Hepworth's work, in which drawing played an important role.

Hepworth was particularly interested in hands, and specifically in the actions and gestures that make up an operation. This interest is clear in her sculpture, and she used her own hands in highly distinctive ways, feeling with the palm of her hand rather than with her fingertips, and developing her own understanding of the roles of the right and left hand respectively. The hand is a long-established point of intersection between art and medicine (for example Schupbach 1982; Jordanova 1992). It is striking that Henry Moore (1898–1986), with whom Hepworth is frequently compared, produced an exquisite drawing in 1978 of deformed hands, those of

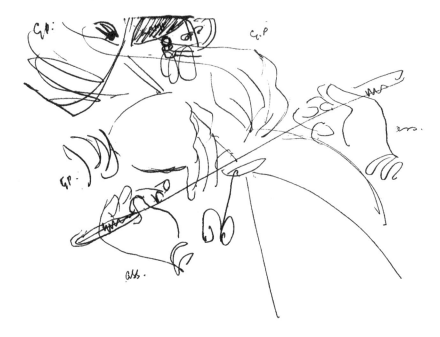

Figure 4.1 Barbara Hepworth, *Sketchbook for the Fenestration of the Ear Operation*, 1948, pencil on paper, 26 × 20.7cm

Source: Science Museum, © Bowness, Hepworth Estate

Dorothy Hodgkin (1910–1994), the only British woman so far to have won a Nobel prize for science (Jordanova 2000: 156). One way of pursuing these themes then is to examine the intense engagement with the body among artists attuned to abstraction, which had been evident much earlier in the century in the work of artists working in a range of media, including photography (for example Clarke 1997: 171). It takes only a very few lines to evoke not only the viewer's recognition of a human body, but their understanding of its key features, for example, that a skilled action is being performed with intense concentration, or indeed that something is amiss with it. By setting this body of work in context, we can appreciate the complex relationships between the people and the institutions involved. For example, in 1953, Hepworth gave a lecture about her 'Hospital Drawings' to a group of surgeons in Exeter, and such encounters, like her correspondence with Capener, help flesh out our understanding of one manifestation of the art-medicine nexus and its audiences (Hepburn 2012: 81–117).

If we consider this nexus from the point of view of the widest possible audiences, traditions of documentary photography have certainly had an extensive impact. Furthermore, since at least the interwar period, magazines and photographic books, often on sensitive social subjects, such as abject poverty, established traditions of engaged photographic practice (Clarke 1997: ch. 8; Jordanova 2012: 130–53). One of the most celebrated books concerning medicine to come out of the post war period is best seen in this light.

A fortunate man?

A Fortunate Man (1967), which was produced in a number of editions, is a meditation on the life and work of John Sassall, a country GP prone to depression, who later committed suicide. The text is by John Berger (born 1926), an influential thinker and acclaimed writer in many genres, including fiction. It is often referred to in literary contexts, as in Anne Whitehead's chapter within this volume, and internet searches reveal comments by practitioners who have been profoundly moved by the book. What Berger has to say about Sassall and his practice is indeed eloquent, emotional and evocative – it gives readers not only a strong sense of a particular practitioner, but of his patients, their rural setting and the complex relationships between these elements. But *A Fortunate Man* was actually a collaborative enterprise, involving the Swiss photographer Jean Mohr (born 1925), who has worked particularly on humanitarian issues. Berger and Mohr have produced five books together. Happily, it is no longer necessary to defend the inclusion of documentary photography in a discussion about 'art'. For decades leading art museums have collected such work, and shown major exhibitions dedicated to it (Jordanova 2012: 130–53). Any discussion of medicine and the visual arts in the post-war period needs to engage with this medium, which may be set in the context of the longstanding interest in photographs of medical subjects (Fox and Lawrence 1988). Indeed, we should remind ourselves that medical practitioners and scientists were at the forefront of the early uses of photography in the mid-nineteenth century. As a medium, photography continues to appeal to those working on the relationships between art and medicine. Nonetheless, even taking the long and complex relationships between medicine and documentary photography into account, *A Fortunate Man* stands out.

Perhaps it is useful to see it in relation to another remarkable collaboration, between the writer James Agee and the photographer Walker Evans, which produced *Let Us Now Praise Famous Men* (1941), a book documenting their time living with poor white families in the American South (Agee and Evans 1988 [1941]). The comparison brings three shared features into focus. First, in both cases we witness profound identification with the subjects of the book. This identification is expressed both visually and verbally. Second, the books have been published in a number of editions, where the paper, page size, layout and tones vary. Thus, visually speaking, there is no single, stable object in either case, even if the text remains the same in all editions. As a result, publishers and designers are also significant collaborators in these projects, and our settled ideas about agency and authorship are disrupted. I may refer to Mohr's photographs or to Berger's text, but this can be no more than pragmatic shorthand. The point is germane to our understanding of the relationships between medicine and the visual arts in *A Fortunate Man*. The book taken as a whole portrays a particular and somewhat heroic view – created by many hands – of general practice in the UK in the 1960s. Third, text and photographs are woven together without recourse to captions. For example, we do not know the names of the patients whose images are included, nor why these rather than any others were selected. Thus, the reader must work to link text and image, and to interpret the pictures, and they are likely to do so as much through their emotional responses to the photographs as by conscious reflection on the text.

The text of *A Fortunate Man* expresses Berger's understanding of Sassall's personal philosophy of medical practice, which was developed and deployed in a specific historical context – one which was striving to understand health and illness in relation to the whole person, hence there is much about the setting and the community in which patients, like their doctor, existed. More specifically, we can refer to Michael Balint's influential book, *The Doctor, His Patient and the Illness*, which adopts a psychoanalytically informed approach to medical practice and is explicitly invoked by Berger (Balint 1957; Berger and Mohr 1967: 68). Berger is keen to convey Sassall's depth of understanding of his patients as people, his role within the community, and above all his own personality, beliefs and suffering. I have just made all these points in words; Mohr offers a visual engagement with and commentary upon these complex themes. There are more than 70 photographs in the book, many of which seem to have no medical content, but they serve precisely to make the points about setting and community that lie at the heart not just of Sassall's practice but of Berger's account of it. It could be argued that Mohr merely *illustrated* the themes to which Berger and Sassall gave priority. Even if this were the case, which to me is implausibly reductive, we should find the photographs worthy of discussion. Berger and Mohr became long-term collaborators. Mohr possesses a honed *visual* intelligence by virtue of being a professional photographer. There was no preordained or obvious way in which Balint-style general practice would be conveyed visually. Mohr created an imagery that expressed the multiple collaborations between artist, doctor, writer, and community, using his visual and technical skills. It is only through a close analysis of the images in question that we can begin to understand how this complicated mediation works.

Since Berger focuses on Sassall's practice and on his entire way of life, it comes as no surprise that Sassall is shown actually at work (for example Berger and Mohr 1967: 79–81), capturing not only the quality of his engagement, but a medical ballet in which doctor, nurse and patient play the main roles. Another group of photographs show him working, but less obviously practising medicine – speaking on the telephone or into his dictaphone, entering or leaving rooms, for instance (Berger and Mohr 1967: 75, 77, 139), while others show him with 'patients', but talking with them, not examining or treating them (Berger and Mohr 1967: 67, 145, 148). I put patients in inverted commas to signal that these were people Sassall knew well, his friends and neighbours, even as his class background and education set him apart from them. These photographic strategies help us to experience Sassall and his setting holistically. But, at a more detailed level, we cannot help but be struck by the attempt to show suffering, pain and despair, for example, by sequences of photographs of the same subjects (Berger and Mohr 1967: 107–11, 119–22), which focus on their faces. We see here something that is characteristic of the book, taking pictures from a low angle, and sometimes from behind Sassall's back so that the viewer sees, as it were, *with* him, and gazes directly at the patient. A particularly striking image shows him examining a woman, who is, I infer, pregnant. She looks into her doctor's face while his hand rests on her belly. It is taken from beside and below his right side, it fills the entire page, and is soft rather than crisply focused like the image facing it (Berger and Mohr 1967: 66–7).

Beautiful in their own right as so many documentary photographs are, Mohr's images are nonetheless part of a polemical project. In this sense they engage with big questions about illness, suffering, healing, and the organization of medical care in ways that Hepworth's do not. They reveal views of medical practice, furthermore, that are quite historically specific and in this respect too they differ from the 'Hospital Drawings'. Hepworth's daughter was actually treated before the NHS came into effect, and the cost of her care placed a heavy burden on the family. Hepworth was working on the drawings between 1947 and 1949, but there is no sense of a political agenda here. Rather, her images appear out of time. Nonetheless, we perceive complex reciprocities between artists and medical practitioners in both cases. Such reciprocity is a theme that runs throughout this volume, and is dramatically present in the work of a leading British painter, John Bellany (born 1942), who mingled his art and medical experiences in a striking and intimate manner. He was treated by a doctor who did the same, which resulted in significant artistic work by them both.

Blended roles: John Bellany and Roy Calne

John Bellany was born in a Scottish fishing village, and has enjoyed a highly successful artistic career, with a major retrospective in Edinburgh in 2012 (Hartley 2012; McEwan 1994). In the 1980s he suffered from serious liver disease, eventually receiving a liver transplant at Addenbrooke's Hospital, Cambridge, from the pioneering transplant surgeon Roy Calne (born 1930), who has always painted. Bellany's work around the time of the transplant is notable by any standards. Calne's, which includes portraits of operations, patients and colleagues, has elicited wide interest. The manner in which they came together and influenced each other's lives and art is significant. Here we find once again that the texture and detail of the ways in which art and medicine blended are of fundamental importance. But new themes also emerge. The first is the centrality of religious imagery for understanding the images that both Calne and Bellany produced. The latter was brought up in a strict Christian atmosphere, and later engaged extensively with art-historical traditions, so it is not surprising that certain themes recur in Bellany's paintings. But the savagery with which suffering and pain, and motifs associated with the crucifixion, are depicted is truly arresting. This approach was established in his work long before his medical crisis. So too was the second theme – depicting oneself (for example Pointon 2013: ch. 5; Cumming 2009).

Bellany was preoccupied with self-portraiture: from the age of thirty, he painted himself every year on his birthday, and at other times too as the Addenbrooke's work reveals. He remained a figurative, and indeed monumental, painter through times when it was a less than fashionable form of expression. Yet many of his preoccupations were shared both by artists born a couple of decades later, who worked more conceptually and with less mainstream media, and more recently by patients, who are exploring the internet as a zone where experiences of disease can be represented. Bellany is a fine draughtsman and print maker as well as a painter. Drawing and painting were the core of his life, hence very quickly after his operation he returned to work, to the astonishment of those caring for him. We might say not only that it helped him to affirm his continued existence and identity as an artist – without a transplant he would have died fairly quickly – but that it assisted his recovery. There are few other examples where illness and its treatment were turned into art in such an immediate and visceral way. Given his style and approach, Bellany was also drawn to explore his experiences through figures, such as Prometheus, who had already figured extensively in Western art. Prometheus was punished for stealing fire from the gods by being chained to a rock and having his liver pecked at daily by an eagle – his torment was endless since the organ was regenerated each night. This episode from Greek mythology bears a complex relationship to Bellany's own story, and it is not hard to see why, as a theme with which artists of earlier generations had engaged, it attracted him (Hartley 2012: 82–3). Nor why the idea that he was a new Lazarus appealed to him (Hartley 2012: 77). According to St John's Gospel, Jesus brought Lazarus back to life four days after his death. Using a rather different idiom, he has referred to Calne as the man who gave him 'the elixir of life' (Calne 1991: 8, 11).

Bellany's work is full of such rich metaphors and potent symbols. It is 'medical' on at least two levels: first in the general sense that it addresses pain, suffering and death – for example, in the work produced after he visited Buchenwald, and second, in a more precise and intense sense around his own illness and return to life (Hartley 2012: 13, 16–17). It is impossible not to be struck by the repetition of certain themes, some of which strongly lend themselves to visual expression. I have already noted the shared interest in the hand between Hepworth and her surgeon collaborators. In 'My Hand, 15 May 1988', Bellany drew the bandages, plasters and the tube, his fingers and the cuff of his pyjamas in black chalk (Scottish National Gallery of Modern Art). It is extraordinarily poignant, and the more the viewer ruminates on the scene – a man barely two weeks after a life threatening operation lasting eight hours, lying in a hospital bed, and using one hand to depict the other, where his hands are central to his artistic life – the more moving it becomes. We can readily link this fragment with his Addenbrookes self-portraits in various poses. These show him in different ways; some are brightly coloured and others only in chalk or etched line, and with different levels of explicitness, from the face alone to searing images of slashed torso and stitches. But the part for the whole, the hand on the page has special power. Bellany's work hints at the challenges faced by the medical humanities if the visual arts are to be taken seriously. Such work invites sustained engagement that will go far beyond 'medicine', however generously defined, to include mythology, religion, the history of art in all media, and notions of the self.

But I have given only one part of the story. Roy Calne, who led the transplant team that treated Bellany, possessed an interest in art that started as a child. He integrated painting into his daily life, but did not wish to pursue it as a profession (Calne 1979, 1991; Patients and Colleagues 1999). One of his works is a dyptich, a form Bellany has used, which shows a modern version of Saints Cosmas and Damian, the patron saints of doctors, who are said to have transplanted a leg. Calne and Bellany depicted each other, while the National Portrait Gallery in London commissioned Bellany in 1992 to paint a double portrait of himself and Calne. Bellany is an artist, thus we might say that, like many of his colleagues, he works on subjects for a variety of reasons in which personal commitment, happenstance, and economic necessity play their parts. It is particularly likely that figurative artists engage with medical themes. But it is less obvious that contemporary medical practitioners would engage so intensely with the visual arts. It was a happy coincidence that Bellany was treated by a surgeon with an interest in art that chimed so harmoniously with his own. We still need to understand, however, why a medical practitioner devotes precious time and energy to producing artwork. From Calne's own accounts, I draw the sense that there is a different quality of engagement between people, a type of intimacy, which occurs when one of them is drawing another. There is certainly a desire to record, as in his depiction of the intensive care nurse, designed to reveal a particular kind of attention and care given to patients (Patients and Colleagues, 1999: 45). This tenderness is for Calne a significant component of medical care. Yet, to say the word 'tender' and to depict

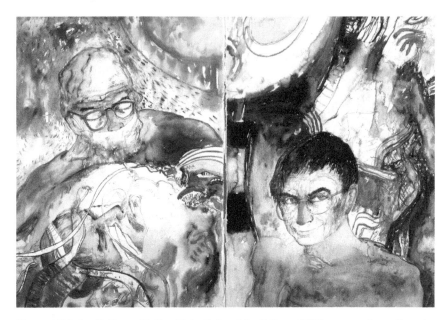

Figure 4.2 John Bellany, *Sir Roy Yorke Calne; John Bellany*, 1992, watercolour diptych, 76.8 × 113.2 cm

Source: © National Portrait Gallery, London

it visually are two entirely different operations. Then there are the issues of display. Calne has displayed his work not only in 'art' contexts but in 'medical' ones, for example on the walls of the hospital where he worked, which made highly personal images available to a community with ever-shifting boundaries for use in its own lived experiences. Such forms of display remind us of contemporary movements, both in Britain and else-where, to bring art to the hospital environment (Cork 2012).

I have been drawing attention to the complex transactions between words and images, while insisting that art works, designed to be responded to visually, including by appreciating the visual intelligence that produced them, function in a distinctive manner that scholars do well to appreciate (Jordanova 2012). Calne, for example, wrote medical books and articles, which are fundamentally different from the artwork he produced. It is only through meticulous description and analysis within a framework set up to do justice to visual materials, that the word-image relationship will be understood, and its specific characteristics in medical settings laid out. This is why we need both an overall approach to visual materials and detailed case studies, and for these two types of analysis to inform each other.

Up close and personal

Between 1978 and 1984, John Bellany taught painting at Goldsmiths College of Art, London, alongside a very different artist, Michael Craig-Martin (born 1941), who is often credited with playing a major role in nurturing the group of artists sometimes called the YBAs, which includes Damien Hirst (born 1965), Abigail Lane (born 1967), and Gavin Turk (born 1967) (Kent 1994; Cooper 2012). In turning to them we have to consider the ways in which artists, working in a range of media, used ideas and objects connected to medicine, rather than collaborating with medical practitioners, as Hepworth, Mohr and Bellany did. In order to set the YBAs in context, we need to consider the range of modes and media in which contemporary artists work. It is useful to return to the role of photography, and particularly self-portraiture (Clarke 1997: chs 6 and 7). Jo Spence, who died from breast cancer in 1992, exemplifies the ways in which photography, used autobiographically, can provide a powerful commentary on politics, generously defined. Using feminist ideas, and challenging the ways in which she was treated as a patient, Spence was able to construct a moving, tough-minded and highly influential set of images. It would sound bland to call her a 'documentary' photographer. She exposed herself, her scars, her own and her partner's bodies in order to offer a passionate commentary on her experiences. Frequently, her photographs are witty, as well as sharply critical, for example of orthodox medicine, which she came to reject. In *Putting Myself in the Picture* (1986), she presents not only her photographic career and her views on medicine, but her ideas about and experiences of taking photographs as a form of therapy, that is, as a means of understanding herself, reliving early experiences, and exploring new possibilities. Evidently, however we define that vexed term 'identity', it stood at the heart of Spence's photographic practice. There are, naturally enough, many ways of exploring identity visually, just as there are many points at which 'identity' intersects with 'medicine'. Spence's own body was her canvas. There are numerous examples of women artists in particular pursuing such themes, especially from the 1970s onwards, using personal experiences, and body parts, in their art (Parker and Pollock 1987; Meskimmon 1996).

Perhaps the most important example of this trend was the fiercely intelligent and wide-ranging artist Helen Chadwick, who frequently used her own body in her art, which deployed a number of media, from self-portrait photographs to multi-media installations, engaging in critical and thought-provoking ways with conventions of self-portraiture and ideas about women as artists. Chadwick was strikingly well read, as her library, now at the Henry Moore Institute in Leeds, reveals, and keen to discuss her ideas with scholars and writers, such as Marina Warner (for example Chadwick 1989). Thus, she used work in the history of medicine when it suited her, although 'medicine' is not the most obvious category to turn to when considering her art. But it is relevant, as it is to so many contemporary artists, in so far as they reflect on embodiment, femininity, sexuality, autobiography, death and taboos.

It is in this context that the YBAs are best approached, many of whom have had, it seems, little direct contact with, or knowledge of, medicine. A notable exception is Christine Borland, who has worked with doctors, surgeons, anatomists, medical educators and forensic specialists. Ideas have taken centre stage for the YBAs. The artist whose work touches most closely our concerns here is Marc Quinn, himself the son of a distinguished scientist. Three works stand out, one of which, *Alison Lapper Pregnant* (2005), has already been mentioned and constitutes one of the most powerful public statements about disability that it is possible to imagine.

Two of his earlier works also speak to 'medicine'. From the early 1990s, Quinn has repeatedly made a self-portrait using his own frozen blood, which is called simply 'Self'. One version was acquired in 2009 by London's National Portrait Gallery. It is in effect a double self-portrait, being made of material from his own body, his very lifeblood, and in being formed in the shape of his head and face. Nonetheless it is a work about ideas, even if it possesses an intensely physical presence. It consists of a life-size red head contained in a refrigeration unit, which has to be kept running all the time and is noisy. The Gallery's website suggests that it reminds viewers of the fragility of human existence. This places it in the tradition of *memento mori*: reminders that death comes to us all, and which sometimes feature skeletons or skulls (Pointon 2013: ch. 5). So, we may infer, Quinn is exploring the relationships between 'life', 'death', and 'self'; I wish to emphasize what complex abstractions these terms are.

There is another work by Quinn in the National Portrait Gallery, his portrait of Sir John Sulston (2001), the scientist who led the British team working on decoding the human genome. This controversial work consists of a heavy silvery frame (made of steel), with a yellowish oblong in the middle, and what look like flecks on it – a sample of the sitter's DNA in agar jelly. Manifestly, this portrait does not look like Sir John Sulston, of whom Quinn has also taken a photograph for the collection. Viewers cannot recognize him, although appropriate analysis of the DNA would presumably reveal his identity. Yet now it can readily be understood that in some sense a person's DNA is a 'portrait' of them, especially at a time when not just diseases, but many human traits are being explored through genetic research. The discovery that DNA was a double helix in structure and the decoding of the human genome are among the most dramatic scientific achievements of the period that this volume addresses; they have major implications for medicine and health care. Quinn's work thus speaks in intriguing ways to the medicine/art nexus, and it does so through complex abstract ideas, for example, through the notion of identity.

In the highly diverse art world of recent decades, it is helpful to distinguish between autobiographical uses of the body, for instance in the work

Figure 4.3 Marc Quinn, *Sir John Edward Sulston*, 2001, sample of the sitter's DNA in agar jelly mounted in stainless steel, 12.7 × 8.5 cm

Source: © National Portrait Gallery, London

of Chadwick, Spence, Quinn and many others, and the representation of sitters, such as Lapper, Sulston and Stephen Hawking (born 1941). Images of the famous disabled scientist, who has had motor neurone disease for decades – he was diagnosed in 1963 – are of particular interest in the present context. A portrait of Hawking was commissioned by the National Portrait Gallery in London in the 1980s as part of their commitment to include more scientists in the collection. It was completed before Hawking published *A Brief History of Time* (1988), which made him world famous. Since he uses a voice simulator, and his appearance is familiar from newspapers and television as well from portraits, his disability is prominent, and has arguably become inseparable from his scientific reputation. He is one of the most prominent disabled people of his time, a remarkable, widely

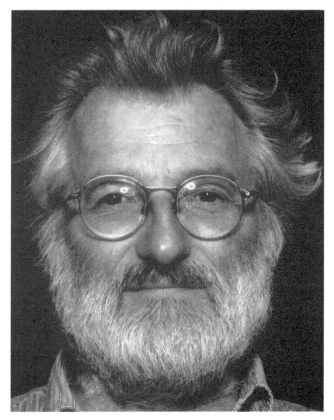

Figure 4.4 Marc Quinn, *Sir John Edward Sulston*, 2001, ultrastable pigment transfer print on polyester base laid on aluminium, 30.8 × 24.8 cm

Source: © National Portrait Gallery, London

lauded survivor. The artist selected by the National Portrait Gallery to depict him, Yolanda Sonnabend (born 1935), produced a popular, naturalistic and not especially radical image that makes no attempt to conceal his illness and its effects on his body. It shows him as young and vulnerable, with hunched shoulders and diminished body. It can be read as an assertion of the *undiminished* intellectual prowess of a disabled person, that is to say, it can readily be construed heroically, as a potent symbol of the value of a person, no matter what form their body takes. In a preparatory drawing, the simple, spare lines tracing Hawking's shoulders and hands reveal his disability with a poignant, understated elegance that touches us in the same way that Hepworth's 'Hospital Drawings' do. While it may well not have been intended as such, this piece of art possesses political efficacy for those concerned with disability rights and for those working to develop the field of disability studies. Like so many of the examples I discuss in this

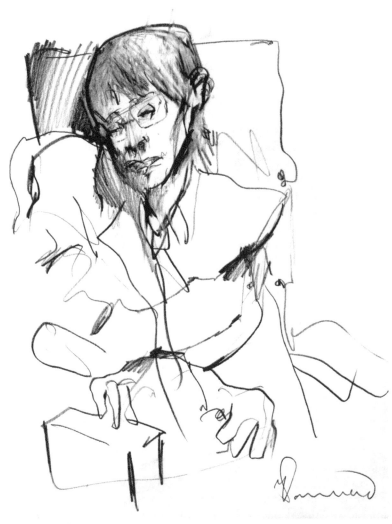

Figure 4.5 Yolanda Sonnabend, *Stephen William Hawking*, 1985, pencil,
   29.6 × 19.7 cm

Source: © Yolanda Sonnabend/National Portrait Gallery, London

chapter, it reveals how potent and politically important visual representations can be, and in a number of ways, although not necessarily by design.
The point is neatly demonstrated by Hawking's gift to the Gallery in 2006
of a portrait by Frederick Cuming (born 1930), which he had commissioned himself in the previous year, and in which his disability is
considerably less obvious. Thus, how individuals and groups represent
disability, their own and others, is evidently a delicate matter.

Display

So far, while I have mentioned some of the specific collections that house relevant works, I have paid little attention to forms of display. One way to bring this into focus is by considering recent exhibitions, which have explored the relationships between medicine and art by bringing many pieces into a single venue. By virtue of their subject matter, these have attracted considerable attention. For example, in 2006 Andrew Patrizio and Dawn Kemp curated an exhibition drawing upon resources in Scotland, called *Anatomy Acts,* and produced an accompanying book (Patrizio and Kemp 2006). Paying attention to such projects is one way of approaching 'medicine and the visual arts'. Patrizio and Kemp's subtitle is particularly revealing – *How We Come to Know Ourselves.* The premise is that we come to know ourselves through anatomy and its visual representation, and that this is a continuing quest with which contemporary artists remain engaged. Three were invited to participate in the exhibition, Christine Borland, Joel Fisher and Claude Heath. In this respect *Anatomy Acts* was similar to an earlier exhibition, *Spectacular Bodies,* at London's Hayward Gallery in 2000 and 2001, which also mixed historic art with medical artefacts and contemporary works, including by Borland and Marc Quinn (Kemp and Wallace 2000). Both exhibitions generated considerable interest for the ways they blended the medical and the artistic, the historical and the contemporary. In order to do so, a fairly loose definition of 'medical' was applied, and emphasis was given to representations of the human body, the terrain that medicine and art share. Since these phenomena are not new, we still need to gain a sense of what appears freshly relevant to audiences, to curators, to living artists and to historians. I have mentioned some of the shifts that we might turn to, which are particularly noticeable from the 1960s onwards. These are, we must admit, somewhat paradoxical. For example, on the one hand, the prestige of big science has grown hugely since the Second World War, and that is an international phenomenon. The current impact of genetics on medicine is simply vast. On the other hand, skepticism about medicine, also a global phenomenon, is widespread and profound. It is common to be critical of drug companies, the provision and withholding of treatment, the management of serious illness and dying, the competence of professionals and so on in ways that were hard to imagine in the earlier twentieth century. However, it is possible to say that it is precisely the existence of such tensions and paradoxes that provides spaces for the visual arts to flourish, especially in an environment where there are few limits on what can be represented.

As I have noted, some contemporary artists take particular pleasure in challenging norms and conventions, many of which concern body parts, sexuality and bodily functions. These are also 'medical' domains, both strictly interpreted in terms of expertise, and more loosely in pertaining to human beings, their well-being, and its absence. In these senses, the central focus is the human body; the shared domain for artists and audiences, medical personnel and patients. This, I take it, is what Patrizio and Kemp were alluding to when they devised their subtitle – *How We Come to Know Ourselves*. They invoked the insistent curiosity about bodies that many people feel, and are now able to pursue in relatively unfettered ways. It might be said that artists quite literally trade on this curiosity, using the privileges of their occupation to explore the limits of decency and voyeurism. Their capacity to do this is important because it allows thoughts, feelings, reactions and fears to be articulated in public, and thereby to be opened up for critical inspection. How can we think about boundaries creatively if they are not being challenged? But Patrizio and Kemp's phrase leads us in another direction – the injunction to 'know oneself' has often been repeated over the centuries. Knowing ourselves does not need to be interpreted in physical, that is to say, bodily terms. Indeed, in an environment heavily steeped in psychological therapies of one kind or another, advice and self-help books, the idea of knowing oneself through anatomy could be seen as rather odd. At the very least, it puts the relentless emphasis on representing the human body, with medical or quasi-medical visual allusions in a different, moralizing frame. Perhaps, then, we need to explore the medicalization of selfhood, the visualization of medicine, the somatization of sexuality, the rebellion against conventions surrounding the body, the sensational display of bodily phenomena and the commercialization of suffering, for example in misery memoirs, through the lens of 'medicine and the visual arts' – a hefty agenda for the medical humanities.

Cautionary coda

Here are some points to bear in mind in relation to the themes of this chapter, which hinge on images and objects, their contextualization and interpretation. I have selected the limited number of illustrations according to some rather specific criteria, of which cost and ease of availability are the most crucial. Successful works of art, like reproductions of them, are commodities within global markets. This has an impact upon which of them can be reproduced, under what conditions, and the cost. Scholars working on contemporary art have to take the operations of the market into account. Other humanities disciplines experience its effects much less directly. The response to provocative works, for instance, is rarely divorced from debates about their economic value, which in turn contributes, on the one hand, to the aura surrounding some artists, and on the other, to fierce controversies about the value – moral, political and aesthetic as well as economic – of avant-garde art. In recent times many high-profile artworks have challenged conventions and broken taboos, thus provocative representations of medicine and health, the body, sexuality and identity need to be understood in this context. And in this same context we find other phenomena: body fascism and eating disorders, narcissism and cosmetic surgery, aggressive advertising and reality television, for instance, which provide further layers through which the body in health and disease is mediated. My final conclusion then is that the topic, 'medicine and the visual arts' deserves not only a much fuller treatment from a medical humanities perspective than has been possible here, but one which fully integrates it into political, economic and social phenomena.

References

Addison, P. and Jones, H. (eds) (2005) *A Companion to Contemporary Britain 1939–2000*, Oxford: Blackwell.

Agee, J. and Evans, W. (1988 [1941]) *Let Us Now Praise Famous Men*, London: Pan Books.

Anderson, G. (2010) *Portraits, Patients and Psychiatrists*, London: Gemma Anderson.

Appiah, K. A. and Gates, H. L. (eds) (1995) *Identities*, Chicago; London: University of Chicago Press.

Archer, M. (2002) *Art Since 1960*, 2nd edn, London and New York: Thames & Hudson.

Balint, M. (1957) *The Doctor, His Patient and the Illness*, London: Pitman Medical Publishing Company.

Berger, J. and Mohr, J. (1967) *A Fortunate Man. The Story of a Country Doctor*, London: Allen Lane.

Calne, R. (1979) *A Gift of Life: Observations on Organ Transplantation*, Aylesbury: Medical and Technical Publishing Company.

Calne, R. (1991) *The Gift of Life: Recent Paintings by Sir Roy Calne*, Hebden Bridge: Sheeran Lock.

Chadwick, H. (1989) *Enfleshings*, London: Secker & Warburg, with an essay by Marina Warner.

Clarke, G. (1997) *The Photograph*, Oxford: Oxford University Press.

Clarke, P. (2004) *Hope and Glory: Britain 1900–2000*, 2nd edn, London: Penguin Books.

Cooper, J. (2012) *Growing Up: The Young British Artists at 50*, Munich, London; New York: Prestel.

Cooter, R. and Pickstone, J. (eds) (2003) *Companion to Medicine in the Twentieth Century*, London: Routledge.

Cork, R. (2012) *The Healing Presence of Art: a History of Western Art in Hospitals*, New Haven; London: Yale University Press.

Cumming, L. (2009) *A Face to the World: On Self-Portraits*, London: HarperCollins.

Fox, D. and Lawrence, C. (1988) *Photographing Medicine: Images and Power in Britain and America since 1840*, New York; Westport; Connecticut; London: Greenwood Press.

Gilroy, A. and McNeilly, G. (eds) (2000) *The Changing Shape of Art Therapy: New Developments in Theory and Practice*, London and Philadelphia: Jessica Kingsley Publishers.

Hartley, K. (2012) *John Bellany*, Edinburgh: National Galleries of Scotland.

Hawking, S. (1988) *A Brief History of Time: from the Big Bang to Black Holes*, London: Bantam Press.

Hepburn, N. (2012) *Barbara Hepworth: The Hospital Drawings*, London: Tate.

Hevey, D. (1992) *The Creatures Time Forgot. Photography and Disability Imagery*, London; New York: Routledge.

Hogan, S. (2001) *Healing Arts. The History of Art Therapy*, London; Philadelphia: Jessica Kingsley Publishers.

Hollowell, J. (ed.) (2003) *Britain since 1945*, Malden; Oxford; Melbourne: Blackwell Publishers.

Jackson, M., (ed.) (2011) *The Oxford Handbook of the History of Medicine*, Oxford: Oxford University Press.

Jordanova, L. (1992) 'The Hand', *Visual Anthropology Review*, 8: 2–7.

Jordanova, L. (2000) *Defining Features: Scientific and Medical Portraits 1660–2000*, London: National Portrait Gallery; Reaktion Books.

Jordanova, L. (2012) *The Look of the Past: Visual and Material Evidence in Historical Practice*, Cambridge: Cambridge University Press.

Kemp, M. and Wallace, M. (2000) *Spectacular Bodies. The Art and Science of the Human Body from Leonardo to Now*, Berkeley; Los Angeles; London: University of California Press.

Kent, S. (1994) *Shark Infested Waters: The Saatchi Collection of British Art in the 90s*, London: Zwemmer.

Keynes, G. (1966) *The Life of William Harvey*, Oxford: Clarendon Press.

Keynes, G. (1985 [1949]) *The Portraiture of William Harvey*, 2nd edn, London: Keynes Press, British Medical Association.

Marwick, A. (1998) *The Sixties: Cultural Revolution in Britain, France, Italy, and the United States, c 1958–c.1974*, Oxford: Oxford University Press.

McEwan, J. (1994) *John Bellany*, Edinburgh and London: Mainstream Publishing.

Meskimmon, M. (1996) *The Art of Reflection. Women Artists' Self-Portraiture in the Twentieth Century*, London: Scarlet Press.

Morgan, K. (2000) *Twentieth-Century Britain: A Very Short Introduction*, Oxford: Oxford University Press.

Parker, R. and Pollock, G. (eds) (1987) *Framing Feminism 1970–1985*, London: Pandora.

Patients and Colleagues (1999) *A Special Gift: An Appreciation of Sir Roy Calne*, Cambridge: Sheeran Lock.

Patrizio, A. and Kemp, D. (eds) (2006) *Anatomy Acts. How We Come to Know Ourselves*, Edinburgh: Birlinn Limited.

Pointon, M. (2013) *Portrayal and the Search for Identity*, London: Reaktion Books.

Rosenthal, N., Shone, R. *et al.* (1997), *Sensation: Young British Artists from the Saatchi Collection*, London: Thames & Hudson.

Schupbach, W. (1982) *The Paradox of Rembrandt's 'Anatomy of Dr Tulp'*, London: Wellcome Institute for the History of Medicine.

Spence, J. (1986) *Putting Myself in the Picture. A Political, Personal and Photographic Autobiography*, London: Camden Press.

5 Graphic medicine

The portrayal of illness in underground and autobiographical comics

Case study

Ian C. M. Williams

The medium of comics has been acclaimed over recent years as being worthy of study by scholars as a significant cultural product, both in a material sense and as a philosophy and practice (for example, Versaci 2007; Witek 1989; Hatfield 2005; Chute 2010). Due to the inseparability of the medium and its attendant culture, this chapter uses the collective singular form of 'comics' throughout to refer to both. 'Comics' holds particular value as a narrative form because the interplay between its hybrid elements – words and pictures – exceeds the sum of their parts to produce a uniquely cogent medium, capable of articulating complex and multilayered concepts. The myriad comics titles that appear each year include stories of disease or trauma known as 'graphic pathographies' (Green and Myers 2010: 574), many of which focus on problems that impact on society as a whole such as abortion, child abuse, mental illness, cancer and HIV/AIDS. Popular media will tend to reflect the concerns of the times in which they are produced, and in this chapter I shall examine the impact that medicine has had on comics, from the early years of the medium through to the development of the graphic novel. I will suggest that comics not only mirrors prevailing attitudes to, and advances in, healthcare, but also inform the way that illness and disease are culturally perceived, influencing what Deborah Lupton calls the 'iconography of illness, disease and death' (Lupton 2003: 75).

Visual knowledge plays an important part in popular and professional understanding of medicine, yet this mode of comprehension is generally undervalued in healthcare education, which places priority on textual learning and verbal communication. I shall focus on the way that the graphic medium facilitates a complex visual layering of subjective and objective experiences, bridging the gap between clinical facts and personal perception. I will pay particular attention to autobiographical comics, the progeny of the countercultural 'underground comics' of the 1960s and 1970s. This subversive genre fractured prevailing ideas of what could and should be shown with respect to the mind and body. It shifted the focus from the classic fictional hero to the flawed and neurotic self, inspiring subsequent generations of artists to articulate their corporeal experiences in words and pictures, a process that Elisabeth El Refaie refers to as 'pictorial embodiment' (El Refaie 2012: 8).

Origin stories: Comics, comix and medicine

Unreservedly contemporary, floppy pamphlets and newspaper strips were not designed for perpetuity and thus have always commented on the times that produced them. Sequential graphic images have existed for thousands of years but the arrangement of cartoons into a narrative sequence, and therefore the first steps into Western comic art, is usually credited to Rodolphe Töpffer. Published in 1837, and translated and republished in the US in 1842, *The Adventures of Mr Obadiah Oldbuck* was a comedic story using independent words and pictures. The development of comic strips in the UK and the US followed a roughly similar course: originally conceived as adult entertainment catering to the newly literate working classes, the cheaply produced pamphlets or national newspaper strips provided easily read entertainment and light relief. By the turn of the century, strip cartoons were in daily circulation in national newspapers, publishers having found that comic strips boosted sales (Weiner 2003: 1). In the UK during the first decade of the twentieth century children's supplements were found to be so popular that many comics altered their content – within weeks in some cases – to cater exclusively for children to whom the bright-coloured comics appealed (Sabin 1996: 27). The medium's commercial peak of the late-1930s to the late-1960s – occurring slightly later in the UK than the US – saw a noticeable interplay between the comics and movies featuring adaptations of Disney characters and Hollywood stars. The Second World War gave rise to a new breed of comic character – the 'superheroes' – and in the 1940s there was a blossoming of genres including romance, crime, horror, true adventure and science fiction.

Medical stories featuring doctors and nurses have proved popular in comics from the 1920s onward. The long running strip, *Rex Morgan, M.D.*, created in 1948 by psychiatrist Nicholas P. Dallis, maintained a readership for well over half a century and has been syndicated in over 300 US newspapers in 15 countries. Bert Hansen (2004) has studied the portrayal of notable medical figures in the true adventure subgenre. The quest for discoveries was portrayed as a form of heroism as valiant as that of the battlefield and, Hansen suggests, revealed much about ordinary people's notions of medicine and medical science (Hansen 2004: 162, 180). Graphic biographies of notable figures from medical, nursing and public health history were presented for the enjoyment of young readers. The stories featured compressed accounts of the lives and discoveries of Pasteur, Koch, Livingstone, Reed, Nightingale and many others.

However, the true adventure genre was not sustained much beyond the mid-1940s and, at a time of anti-communist witch-hunts and moral hysteria, concern over the increasingly violent content of comics mounted, particularly in the US. A climate of subversion, led by EC comics horror titles, eventually led to an anti-comics backlash that included book burning in school-yard bonfires in 1948 (Goulart 1986: 263). Frederic Wertham, a German–American psychiatrist who had worked with the criminally insane, tapped into the wave of popular feeling. Convinced that mass media had a deeply unsavoury influence on society, in 1954 he published *The Seduction of the Innocent*, blaming comics for youth disturbance, suicide and aggression. The medium was subjected to a US congressional inquiry, and to protect themselves from government legislation, the leading US comics companies produced the Comics Code, a convention to which content had to adhere in order for the title to be stocked in newsagents and grocery stores.

This moral panic was not confined to the US. In the UK and across Europe similar concerns were being expressed about the supposed flood of harmful material being imported from the States, or being reproduced this side of the Atlantic. The campaign against 'American Type' horror comics 'brought together such unlikely bedfellows as the Church of England, the National Union of Teachers and the Communist Party of Great Britain' (Chapman 2011: 46). Ironically, as Martin Barker explains in his study *A Haunt of Fears*, much of the early agitation was orchestrated by the Communist Party (Barker 1992 [1984]: 21). The Communist Party was actually more concerned about the influence of Americanization on British Society and the threat of McCarthyism than about the bloodthirsty content of the comics. Popular pressure moved the Conservative government to act, however, and Parliament passed The Children and Young Persons (Harmful Publications) Act in June 1955, which imposed a prison sentence and fines on anyone convicted of publication of material that fell foul of its legislation. This act is still in force today.

Anti-comics sentiment forced former purveyors of gore to look elsewhere for entertaining subject matter and doctors and nurses provided wholesome role models for young comic readers. Fiction based on real-life medical situations began to appear in EC comics' 'New Direction' magazines such as *MD* (1955) and *Psychoanalysis* (1955). *The Adventures of Young Dr Masters* (1964) proudly bore the Comics Code logo and told of the exciting exploits of the eponymous hero who climbs the skeleton of a building in construction to rescue an injured worker, performing an amputation while clinging to a girder 19 storeys up. Reading such comics now, it is easy to dismiss this sort of melodrama as worthless romantic cheese, aimed at a young audience, as evidenced by the 'teen career guide' which encouraged 'young girls' to consider nursing as a rewarding career. On closer inspection, however, *Young Dr Masters* does raise some interesting points. One such example is the conflict between the 'old' (humanist) style of family medicine, as practiced by Dr Masters senior, and the new 'scientific',

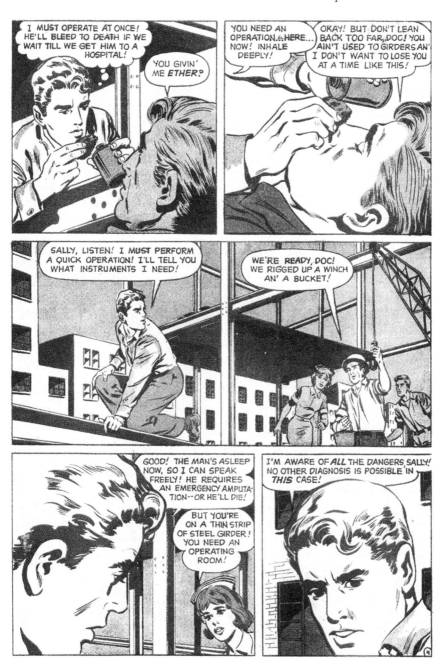

Figure 5.1 R. Bernstein and J. Rosenberger (1964: n.p.) *The Adventures of Young Dr Masters*, Cincinnati: Radio Comics

Source: Permission sought but no copyright holder traced

laboratory-based medicine practiced by his son, possibly an advocate of the 'clinical detachment' model promoted by Fox and Lief the previous year (1963).

Similar mawkish fare was being published on this side of the Atlantic. *Love on Ward B* (2008) is a compendium of reprinted comics from the 1960s featuring '[s]ix of the best hospital nurse picture library romances ever!' edited by Melissa Hyland. The originals aimed to provide romantic titillation to girls and young women. It would be difficult to argue that they are great literature but, as Hyland points out, in their time such comics may have had a small but definite role in shaping the nation's conception of what it was to be a nurse (or doctor) and what might be expected if one worked in a hospital. The nurses, portrayed in a generic illustrational style, are uniformly pretty, slim and 'man crazy' (Hyland [ed.] 2008: 139), while male patients, often the focus of the nurses' romantic aspirations, are ruggedly handsome. The nurses dream of meeting the perfect husband but are often disappointed by their swains, resigning themselves to forgo 'love and romance and devote themselves to their task of relieving pain, and helping those who needed them most' (Hyland [ed.] 2008: 70). Such stories provided a narrative of stability and hope. Dead patients, catastrophic mistakes and animals sacrificed in medical experiments were conveniently ignored. Hansen convincingly argues that values were less heterodox in those times, the public less bombarded by media and opinion before television was widely available, and radical cultural changes ensured that blind acceptance of medical power was soon to end (Hansen 2004: 167).

While superheroes flourished, authors began experimenting with comics aimed at older children, or adult readers. The Hippie movement, the opening of 'head shops', comic stores, independent publishers and small-scale reproduction technology meant comics could be distributed directly to the target audience, rather than through the mainstream publishing networks. The Comics Code could thus be effectively ignored. In the mid-1960s adult oriented 'underground comics', rechristened 'comix', delighted in graphic portrayals of sex, drug taking and violence. Imported with difficulty, or even bootlegged in the UK, these works spurred on UK comics artists to produce similar radical works (Sabin 1996: 92, 107).

Sabin traces the origins of the underground to three sources: Harvey Kurtzman's influential *MAD Magazine*; the politicized college magazines, which were more sophisticated than their UK 'rag mag' counterparts; and the radical reaction to Comics Code-era prohibition. Comix were 'perceptive reflections of the anti-war, anti-establishment fervour of the times', which 'arose at a critical time, when the convergence of political repres-sion, the protest movement, psychedelic drugs, and innovations in printing technology created the right mix for an impromptu and improvised art movement' (Rozenkranz 2002: 4).

Artists such as Robert Crumb, often regarded as the warped Godfather of underground comix, Gilbert Shelton and Art Spiegelman created memorable characters who were very different from the traditional comic book heroes of the comics code era: drug addicts, hustlers, stoned-out hippies and anthropomorphic animals who engaged in obscene acts. These underground artists were 'interested in self-expression above all, although they tended to conflate self-expression with breaking taboos' (Wolk 2007: 39). Crumb's obsession with the carnivalesque depiction of a certain female body type – huge buttocks and thighs below an exaggerated lumbar lordosis – and violent sexual fantasy has led to accusations of misogyny (El Refaie 2012: 80), but his supreme influence is seldom disavowed. Such work represented a gradual shift in focus away from the exploits of heroic archetypes and towards the 'self' as the subject, rejecting orderly script structures in favour of entertaining chronicles of misadventures, confessions and chaotic vignettes from the hip community.

Graphic autobiography

This fecund and subversive vibe gave rise to a work that has been hailed as signalling a new turn in the development of comics. As Jared Gardner points out, claims to 'firsts' are problematic (Gardner 2008: 7). However, the American cartoonist and 'neurotic visionary' Justin Green is often credited with inventing a new genre in 1972, when he chose to 'unburden his uncensored psychological troubles' onto the pages of *Binky Brown Meets the Holy Virgin Mary* – 'an astonishing self-flagellation of catholic guilt and obsessive-compulsive disorder' (Spiegelman 1995: 4). The protagonist Binky Brown (Green's alter ego) develops a compulsive neurosis as a child, and, having been brought up in a strict Catholic family, his obsessions take on a religious bent. He becomes tortured by intrusive carnal thoughts of the Holy Virgin and an ever-expanding web of associations, obsessions and compulsive ritual soon weighs down his world. It is hellish for him, but the way that Green ironically portrays himself is as hilarious as it is grotesque. In a way that might be cumbersome or unclear in prose narrative, Green is able to portray the effects of his disordered perceptions graphically. Ideas of blasphemy and bodily shame crystallize as 'pecker rays' radiating from his genitals or other phallic-shaped parts of his body that, like laser beams, maintain their power over vast distances, conferring spiritual contamination if directed at any representation of the Holy Virgin.

Green used the richness of the medium to give the invisible pecker rays a spatial form, portraying the intrusive images that plagued him and explaining visually how his very identity was splintered by shifting liminal fault lines in which the external and internal worlds grind against each other. Such imagery connects to the work of Adrielle Mitchell on graphic memoirs, who notes that 'planes of reality can coexist in the diegetic space of a comic – daily life, fantasy, spirit world, dream-space, myth, historical past, allegory, metaphor, metonym' (Mitchell 2010: 258). Green says that he made Binky Brown 'out of internal necessity' (Green 1995: 8) before he

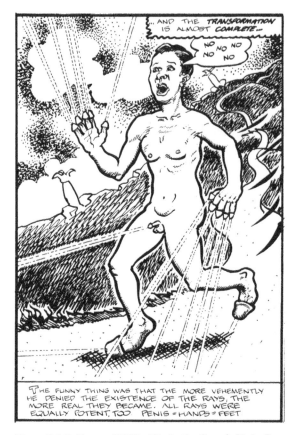

Figure 5.2 J. Green (1995: 42) *Justin Green's Binky Brown Sampler*, San Francisco: Last Gasp

Source: Reproduced with permission of author

knew he was suffering from obsessive-compulsive disorder. The comic could therefore be said to represent a portrayal of the condition in its purest form, unmediated by the 'official' language of psychiatry or medical terminology. Joseph Witek agrees with Gardner in rejecting the notion that the autobiographical genre arose de novo in Green's work, suggesting that autobiographical comics are related to earlier comics 'by the way that comics pages spatialize both physical and psychic experience whether the stories are self-narrated or not' (Witek 2011: 228).

Green's openness in illustrating his mental distress influenced younger artists such as Aline Kominsky-Crumb, helping her to find her own voice and use the medium to articulate her own psychological horizon in her 1972 piece 'Goldie: A Neurotic Woman' published in the first issue of *Wimmen's Comix* (reproduced in Kominsky-Crumb 2007: 126). In contrast to the idealized women of comics past, Kominsky-Crumb used a rough, untutored style to portray herself as abject and ugly, enslaved by her base desires and anxieties (Chute 2010: 29). In doing so, she paved the way for women cartoonists who adopted this hip medium to highlight matters of gender politics and social concerns producing a boom in comix by, and for, women (Sabin 1996: 104). Contentious concerns of the time were used as material. The landmark Supreme Court decision in *Roe v. Wade* (1973), which legislated on abortion, resulted in both the pro-choice comic *Abortion Eve* (1973) by Lyn Chevely and Joyce Farmer (writing under pseudonyms) and the pro-life comic *Who Killed Junior?* (1973) by the Christian group Right to Life. The latter comic portrayed the week-by-week development of 'Junior' who was a loveable cartoon baby living, apparently independently and without the need of an umbilical cord, inside a voluminous triangular shape – an abstract representation of the womb. At six weeks of gestation Junior is a fully formed cartoon baby and by the twelfth week he is shown running around the womb and articulating his own thoughts. The various methods of abortion are then shown – the distressed character is shown to be hacked apart or brutally burned to death using a salt solution. Thus the anonymous artist confers onto the character the attributes of cuteness, autonomy, thought and language, creating an emotive visual rhetoric to recruit the reader's sympathy.

In the 1970s a particular comic format came into its own: a full-length, square bound, serious comic book aimed at adults that has become known as the graphic novel. The graphic novel has proved to be 'comics' passport to recognition as a form of literature' (Hatfield 2005: ix) due to its ability to recruit readers from outside the usual demographic. Medical content in Western comics and graphic novels has tended to evolve along a radical, social realist line, showing little of the blind respect for the medical profession displayed by the comics of the 1950s and 1960s. It is likely that these highly subjective accounts will inform readers' perceptions of the condition described, as will the imagery used: the representation of the illness changes the illness experience of others (Gilman 1988: 2), altering their expectations and perceptions. Readers will therefore learn how to be ill from these stories, what signs to look for and even how to behave from the reality they perceive in the mimesis and diegesis of the graphic pathography. Such factors are crucially important to the theme of reciprocity that runs throughout this collection as, like the literary genre of pathography discussed in Anne Whitehead's chapter, graphic pathography both reflects and informs experiences of illness.

The iconography of disease

The spread of AIDS has had a significant impact on the relationship between arts and health in the late-twentieth century. Comics was no exception. From the 1980s onwards, the comics community played a significant role in heightening awareness of both the dangers of contracting HIV and of the plight of those living with or dying from AIDS. In correspondence with the author, comics artist David Hine recalled that:

> [T]his was a time of near-hysteria about AIDS and HIV. This was before the development of the antiretroviral treatments that have led to those who have access to the appropriate drugs living an almost normal life-span, albeit with all kinds of health issues. In the late 80s and early 90s it was a death sentence and indeed all the people we worked with at the time, who were infected, did die. That was a very sobering thought and gave an emotional impetus to our work.
>
> (Hine 7 December 2012)

The sight of friends, relatives and lovers dying from HIV galvanized the comics community into action. Benefit anthologies such as *Strip Aids* (1987) and *Strip Aids USA* (1988) were created to raise funds for charities and awareness of the problem. In 1991 the London-based Comics Company published *1+1*. This comic, financed by the Terrence Higgins Trust and the National AIDS Trust, featured work by Hine, Corinne Pearlman, Woodrow Phoenix and Myra Hancock. The comic resulted from a two-year collaboration of artists, drama workers and groups of young people during which time they tried 'to find out what information [they] needed to be putting out to young people and how to reach the people most at risk' (Hine 7 December 2012).

Hine's 'Dreaming of the 21st Century' in *1+1* (1991) features a hetero-sexual couple called Al and Gabi who are coming to terms with the fact that they have AIDS. Al, who contracted HIV from his occasional drug use when younger and unwittingly gave it to Gabi, dreams of New Year's Eve 1999 to the soundtrack of Prince's 1982 single, and wakes to the realization that both he and Gabi are unlikely to see the turn of the century. It is significant that Hine chose to portray a heterosexual, rather than a same-sex couple, a nod to the fact that drug users were also at risk and a reflection of the concern 'that the virus could move into the heterosexual community in a big way' (Hine 7 December 2012). He was also concerned about promul-gating stereotypes and making HIV a 'gay disease'. Indeed, visual imagery is important in the social construction of labels and stereotypes as well as in the formation of such cultural conceptions as normality, desirability, gender and disease (Gilman 1988: 4). These notions are internalized by patients shaping their experience of the condition (Gilman 1988: 2). As Hine says:

> I wanted to write a story that hit home to everyone who read the comic, straight couples as well as gays or drug users. This comic was going to be seen by a huge cross-section of young people and I wanted HIV/AIDS to be 'our problem' not 'their problem'.
>
> (Hine 7 December 2012)

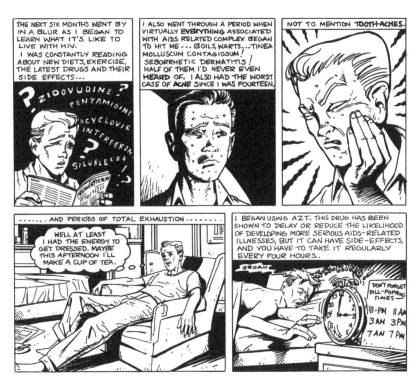

Figure 5.3 D. Hine (1991: 14) 'Dreaming of the 21st Century', in M. Hancock
   et al., *1+1*, London: The Comic Company: 9–16

Source: Reproduced with permission of author

This emphasis on the social conditions of the disease is important.
Autobiographical comics often achieve their power by emphasizing the
personal impact of a disease, inviting the reader to consider the individual
sufferer, as I will discuss shortly, thus evoking empathy and identification.
This strategy is not without problems. There is a risk of readers' empathy
turning into a vicarious suffering or, in a stigmatizing condition such as
HIV/AIDS, focus on the individual might actually serve to reinforce prejudice and dehumanize the sufferer, reinforcing the perceived link between
the disease and a specific community. Hine recalls that the comic was well
received at the time:

> I hope we contributed to the welcome change in attitude, at least here
> in the UK...Equally, the drama projects and meetings with young gay
> people were welcomed by them as a great opportunity to express their
> own anger, anxiety and hope for the future. I think all of us benefited
> from the experience.

(Hine 7 December 2012)

Iconographic representations of health, illness and disease have become more important in Western societies (Lupton 2003: 79). The imaging of diseased bodies also remains central to medical discourse for both diagnostic and educational purposes, informing and manipulating the way that healthcare professionals learn and think about disease. Traditionally, medical illustrators, health professionals or educationalists created most representations of illness, thus they also controlled the official visual discourse of disease. The makers of underground or autobiographical illness comics, by portraying their own concepts of the diseased body, could therefore be seen as seizing power away from the 'official' iconography that informs society's notion of an illness. It seems probable that professionals absorb images from popular culture in the same way as lay consumers and these images become synthesized into their working knowledge and self-perception, subtly informing the schemata that govern their attitudes, ethics and clinical knowledge. Of course comics can also be used to reinforce the official narratives, promulgating received ideas about the 'victims' of disease, or peddling controversial religious ideas as in the Christian Fundamentalist 'tracts' in comic form by Jack Chick. The most interesting works from the point of view of medical humanities, therefore, are often autobiographical, articulating the subjective experience and forging a new iconography. To publish a visual illness narrative is an act of constructive self-definition. The fashioning of the work, the intense examination, the literal re-viewing of events (Chute 2010: 2) and the continuous reiteration of the story might be expected to effect a change in the way that authors perceives themselves and remember the events described. El Refaie asserts that every time autobiographical comics artists draw themselves they are forced to engage with 'the sociocultural models that underpin body image, including categories of sex, gender, health and beauty' (El Refaie 2012: 73).

Comics has suffered its ups and downs in popularity since the early 1980s but the last decade has seen an impressive surge in interest in the medium, with autobiography becoming a major genre in the graphic novel format. Digital technology has revolutionized colouring and printing techniques, enabling small runs or desktop-produced comics and resulting in the rise of web-based comics. Medically themed comics made by both healthcare clients and professions or students are to be found online or sold as printed pamphlets at fairs and conventions. These strips, unpolished and unfiltered by commercial editing, could be said to represent the 'cutting edge' of comics. Although the vast majority will never see professional publication, these artists are producing new knowledge through the intellectual, emotional and manual act of somatic self-expression. They are monitoring, conceptualizing and digitizing their own bodies, which are reconstructed on paper or in pixels. Their work coincides with both a renewed academic interest in 'the body' – I will turn to the notion of 'embodiment' in graphic narratives towards the end of this chapter – and the emergence of the interdisciplinary arena that exists to both champion and critique the medium of comics studies as an exciting new space in the academy. Consequently, some of these self-published artists have found their work discussed at conferences or considered in scholarly journal articles. At the time of writing, it is still true that many academics who write about comics are academics who love comics, but it is also true that these scholarly fanboys and fangirls bring an essential element of academic rigour to comics criticism that distinguishes their work from popular histories of the medium or the elegiac essays that tend to preface comics anthologies. Serious criticism and theory about comics is in its emergence, as is the interdisciplinary study of comics from a healthcare perspective, although the quality and quantity of recent depictions of disease in graphic narrative still demands further scholarly attention.

The personal versus the universal

The interest in comic memoirs, particularly those that involve illness, has played a part in subverting traditional comics practices and the career paths of comics artists. Some practitioners with backgrounds in fine art or illustration have discovered that comics provide an ideal medium through which to express their stories. While caring for his terminally ill father, for example, Ross Mackintosh decided to make an 'alternative comic' about his experiences, even though he had little idea 'how to go about doing it' (Mackintosh 2011: 42–3). Although Mackintosh does not explain the inspiration behind his decision, one might suspect an awareness of graphic illness narratives played a part.

Seeds (2011) describes the final couple of months of Mackintosh's father's life. His fun-loving, pub-going, sport-loving but quietly philosophical 'Dad' died of disseminated prostate cancer in 2010. In stark contrast to nearly all graphic novels about cancer that originate from the US – in which significant themes seem to be the struggle with insurance companies to get treatment, and the lack of humanity of the healthcare staff – he praises the hospice care that his father received. Apart from one or two notable instances of poor communication or lack of tact, his father was treated with care and respect, and Mackintosh is grateful to the healthcare service.

The title of *Seeds* alludes to a metaphor that doctors have used in order to explain the dissemination of the cancer. In the story, the physical condition of Mackintosh's father declines rapidly following the diagnosis of lung metastases, and his family struggles to accept the diagnosis and forge a sense of normality over their day-to-day lives. Mackintosh concentrates on the grim little details of life as a terminal patient, such as the challenges in maintaining basic human functioning, the traumatic reality and horror of imminent death, the numbness felt when confronted with his father's corpse and the surreality of attending the funeral of a parent. One wonders, reading *Seeds*, about Mackintosh's experience of drawing his father's dead body – the decision-making process and visual devices employed in making his father's previously 'living' avatar look dead. The whole process of making the book could be seen as metaphor for the author's grief, bringing his father back to life in ink on paper and then finally laying him to rest.

In the introduction, Mackintosh describes his long-held feelings that he is observing his own life and the sensation of framing the unfolding events of his father's illness as a sequence of images, narrated by his new opinions. American comics artist Brian Fies, who wrote about his own family experience of terminal illness in *Mom's Cancer* (2006), says in his foreword to *Seeds*:

> Comics combine words and art to transcend the sum of their parts. Their lack of detail encourages readers to fill the void with details from their own lives and identify with abstract squiggles of ink. It's strange and wonderful: readers will tell a cartoonist, "My family and situation were nothing at all like yours but it's as if you were sitting in our home watching us!"
>
> (Fies in Mackintosh 2011: n.p.)

What Fies is referring to in the first sentence is the active participation of the reader, who operates as the accomplice of the author by filling in the gaps using his or her imagination. Comics is, suggests Scott McCloud, a medium of fragments that gives the sense of a continuous reading experience so seamless it actually 'feels like living' (McCloud 2006: 129). He calls the phenomenon of observing the parts, but perceiving a whole, 'closure' (McCloud 1993: 68). The strip is actually a sequence of static images, contained within panels, a 'staccato rhythm of unconnected moments' with gaps in between (McCloud 1993: 67). These gaps, which constitute an 'extra-diegetic space' (Lefèvre 2009: 160), are known as 'gutters', and it is here that McCloud proposes the 'magic and mystery' of comics takes place. In the second sentence of the above quote, Fies alludes to the reader's propensity for projecting their own experiences and viewpoint onto a character or characters. This identification may arise from various elements such as the author's portrayal of similar experiences to their own or perceived similarities in physical appearances, family structure or social background.

This active participation is very powerful and something that can be used to engage health professionals in training, providing a window into the subjective experience of illness and providing valuable insight which could shape attitudes. The value of comics for the study of medical narrative and imagery has lately been considered by Green and Myers (2010), Williams (2011) and Squier (2008). Scholars of the medical humanities, arts and literature are also beginning to investigate the potential of comics.

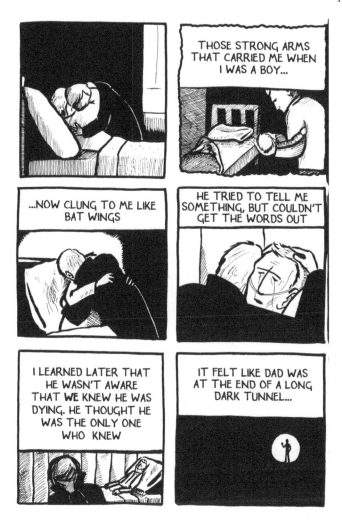

Figure 5.4 R. Mackintosh (2011: 56) *Seeds*, London: ComX

Source: Reproduced with permission of publisher

Green and Myers point out that although comics are not widely integrated into medical education, 'other fields have successfully used them to teach topics as diverse as professional ethics, creative writing…literature and physics' (Green and Myers 2010: 576). Reading comics is an excellent way to promote debate within discussion groups, particularly regarding communication issues and ethics, and making comics focuses the attention on the professional–patient relationship, self-reflection and analysis of one's own behaviours, habits and intentions. Graphic stories can also be used to teach observational skills (Green and Myers 2010: 576). Courses in Graphic Medicine for medical students have indeed been set up in Penn State Medical School, Hershey, Pennsylvania (Green and Myers 2010: 576) and Feinberg Medical School, Chicago, Illinois (Czerwiec 11 December 2012) in the US, and Brighton and Sussex Medical Schools (Al Jawad 19 October 2012) and my own course at Manchester Medical School here in the UK.

Embodiment in the graphic pathography

Student healthcare professionals, particularly medical students, are charged with absorbing large amounts of biomedical information regarding basic sciences and pathological processes. Although attention is paid to the psychological as well as the organic in current-day medical education, few medical students develop a deep understanding of mental illness by the time they qualify. The multilayered perceptual representations of graphic narrative are well suited to the portrayal of mental health problems, and comics memoirs about such topics continue to occur with increasing frequency. John Stuart Clark, the comics artist known as 'Brick', spent many years producing scathing political cartoons for pressure groups, trade unions and non-governmental organizations until a four-year bout of depression brought a sudden halt to his output. The result of his experience was the graphic novel *Depresso* (2010). This semi-autobiographical story follows Brick's graphic avatar, wry political cartoonist Tom Freeman, from the initial somatic symptoms of his depression, through suffering, failed treatment (both orthodox and alternative) to recovery, via myriad diversions, side stories and tales of travel.

In this rather angry book, Brick fires invective at many of the professionals who have crossed his path. Nevertheless, things start gently enough, with an interesting portrayal of the way that depression creeps up on the unsuspecting character. Brick is not enamoured of the medical profession and views the Western medical system as altogether less holistic than the practices of the east. The narrative is rather chaotic and jumpy, but there are some astute observations floating in the vitriol of *Depresso*, such as Tom's assertion that healthcare professionals carry a morbid fear of client suicide, and that their constant checking on their clients' status has more to do with their own anxiety than with patient well-being: 'do they want to know if I am well or safe?' he demands irritably (Brick 2010: 232).

The book displays a common dichotomy: castigating society for stigmatizing mental illness while professing Tom's own embarrassment at his own problems and labelling fellow sufferers as 'head cases', 'psychos', 'fruitcakes' or 'wackos'. However, one suspects that his use of such language must be at least partly ironic. His tales of finding himself at self-help groups – among people with whom he has little in common bar a diagnosis – evince a brutal veracity, and epitomize the plight of the individual who, saddled with an unsexy diagnosis, is torn between championing the cause of the sufferer and rebelling against his lot, uncomfortable with the identity thrust upon him.

Brick's hyper-expressive, cartoony style speaks of his background in short political strips or single panels. Using slick and masterly line-work he constructs striking visual metaphors to express his feelings of loss and sadness and the bewilderment and terror of depression. He pictures the depressive as entombed in wet, shrinking concrete, or shrunk to minute proportions, lying in a fetal position in bed (Brick 2010: 86).

Metaphor, a key quality of comics and an important way of conceptualizing illness (Lupton 2003: 54), is often used to articulate feelings and bodily sensations for which no adequate language exists. Comics artists are not alone in employing metaphor effectively to engage with or critique concerns related to health and medicine – for example, Fiona Hamilton's chapter within this collection highlights the importance of metaphor in poetry. However, the medium of comics presents a unique form of metaphor that is simultaneously visual and narrative. Comics' language is always characterized by a plurality of messages (Hatfield 2005: 36) through which difficult, ambivalent, chaotic or incomprehensible impressions, narratives or visions can be articulated. While verbal descriptors quickly become clichés through common usage, even hackneyed phrases can inform and entertain when playfully illustrated by the comics artist who can select from a number of rhetorical tropes – metaphor, metonymy, synecdoche, symbolism – as well as a panoply of pictorial elements to construct an arresting image (Mitchell 2010: 258).

Tom's suffering is expressed largely through the depiction of his own body. The vast majority of graphic stories are about people, broadly defined. These people take the form of human, humanoid or anthropomorphic characters, embodied and given 'life' on the page (Mitchell 2010: 11) in a seemingly concrete world constructed by the artist. Indeed, so important is the body in comics that Chute refers to the medium as a 'procedure of...embodiment' (Chute 2010: 193, original emphasis). In graphic works the author constructs a visual avatar that represents his or her own, ailing body and proceeds to show, as well as tell, the sequelea generated by the illness. As noted above, El Refaie (2012: 8) uses the term 'pictorial embodiment' to capture the different ways in which graphic memoirists' sense of self is linked with the act of visually representing their bodily identities. She draws upon the phenomenological work of Maurice Merleau-Ponty (1962) and Drew Leder (1990) to explain 'why the author's own body features most prominently and explicitly in autobiographical comics that deal with physical change or challenges of some sort' (El Refaie 2012: 61). It is at times of change (such as puberty), physical or mental illness or trauma that one is most likely to become 'aware' of one's body, which is normally characterized by its absence or 'disappearance' (that is a lack of awareness of the workings of one's own body). These times, these

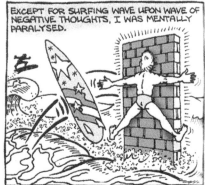

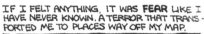

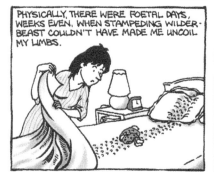

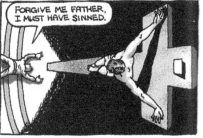

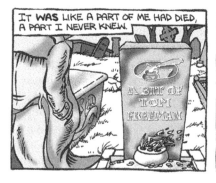

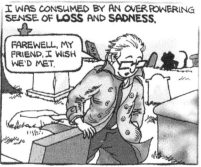

Figure 5.5 Brick (2010: 86) *Depresso*, London: Knockabout

Source: Reproduced with permission of author

'dys-appearances' (Leder 1990: 91), draw one's attention to the abnormal working of the body or to unwanted sensation such as pain. El Refaie suggests that a similar process occurs when one is required to represent oneself physically: 'Every act of self-portraiture entails a form of dys-appearance in the sense that one's body can no longer be taken for granted as an unconscious presence' (El Refaie 2012: 62).

The human body is the site of medical enquiry (Lupton 2003: 22) and stories of illness and disease are perennially popular subjects of both art and literature. It therefore should not, perhaps, come as much of a surprise that graphic pathographies have proven a popular means to engage with factors related to the body and embodiment. Comics serves as an important mode of expression for questions and concerns about the body, and for testing the boundaries of what can be asked and what can be shown. Artists such as Aline Kominsky-Crumb and Phoebe Gloeckner map out their own naked, viscerally sexual bodies on the page, exerting total control over how they present themselves. Gloeckner has a Masters degree in medical illustration and teaches at the University of Michigan. Her comics work in *A Child's Life and Other Stories* (2000) is painfully discomforting, a harrowing story of child abuse, neglect and drug abuse. While all disciplines of visual art can represent the body in complex and disturbing ways, presenting the viewer with statements or questions, comics has the added dimension of sequentiality and narrative text. It provides context and setting coupled with a temporality that is controlled by the reader, in a way that is not available to the filmgoer. The production of 'multiple drawn versions of the self entails an explicit engagement with physicality' (El Refaie 2012: 8), which gives an extra element to the narrative and raises questions about identity and self-perception. It is perhaps this repeated manual act of self-representation throughout the momentous work of making a graphic novel that results in the vivid intensity of some of these works, the reading of which really does 'feel like living' (McCloud 2006: 129). The relentless process of decision-making forces the artist to examine his or her fears, suffering, anger, disgust, disappointment and grief and distil the whole into a succinct series of sequential panels with which to transfer the narrative to the reader.

Conclusion

Graphic memoirs of illness and suffering constitute a significant source of alternative knowledge about the body, health and disease that can be mined by scholars and used to promote debate and reflection in healthcare education. Stories concerning disease and the portrayal of doctors and nurses have proved popular in the comics medium for the best part of a century, although it was only in the last quarter of the twentieth century that comics artists began to use the medium for self-expression and the representation of their own experiences. The underground comix movement tested the boundaries of what could be shown with regards to the body and created a new genre – the comic memoir. This genre has since become an important vehicle for the articulation of illness narratives and the experience of healthcare, as well as a medium for the 'pictorial embodiment' of ideas about the corporeal self. Comics has reflected the changing perception of medicine in society, from the blind faith in the heroic march of medicine of the first part of the twentieth century to the fractured disenchantment of the postmodern years, highlighting both the progress and flaws of the healthcare systems in highly personal narratives. In turn, these powerful works will not only inform popular conceptions of medicine, but also could actually alter the 'iconography of illness' and affect the way that individuals experience illness.

There are some major omissions in this chapter: I have not considered the influence of medicine on the massively popular superhero genre or on Japanese manga and have not commented on the stock figure of the 'mad doctor' or 'mad scientist' in horror comics and comedy comics. Nor have I covered the separate genre of educative comics that have operated for decades on the presumption that the hybrid nature and visual appeal of comics can be used to convey messages to demographics with presumed poor literacy levels although few studies have been published to back up these claims. Indeed, all these topics deserve their own studies, and will, no doubt receive them in time. Graphic Medicine is in its infancy, but there seems little doubt that comics has a role to play in medical humanities, and with the increasing popularity of the medium, this reflexive relationship will deepen and develop in years to come.

Acknowledgments

I would like to thank Dr Mita Mahato and Dr Roger Sabin for their helpful comments on the proofs of this essay, and acknowledge the work of Ethan Persoff who has, for many years, flagged up interesting work on his website 'Comics With Problems' which is where I found *Who Killed Junior?* and *Abortion Eve.*

References

Abilene Right-to-Life Committee (1973) *Who Killed Junior?,* Clovis, CA: Right to Life.
Barker, M. (1992 [1984]) *A Haunt of Fears: Strange History of the British Horror Comics Campaign,* Jackson, MS: University Press of Mississippi.
Bernstein, R. and Rosenberger, J. (1964) *The Adventures of Young Dr Masters,* St Louis: Radio Comics Inc.
Brick (2010) *Depresso,* London: Knockabout.
Chapman, J. (2011) *British Comics: A Cultural History,* London: Reaktion Books.
Chevely, L. and Farmer, J. (1973) *Abortion Eve,* Washington, DC: Nanny Goat Productions.
Chute, H. (2010) *Graphic Women: Life Narrative & Contemporary Comics,* New York: Columbia University Press.
El Refaie, E. (2012) *Autobiographical Comics: Life Writing in Pictures,* Jackson, MS: University Press of Mississippi.
Fies, B. (2006) *Mom's Cancer,* New York: Image.

Fox, R. and Lief, H. (1963) 'Training for "Detached Concern" ', in H. Lief (ed.) *The Psychological Basis of Medical Practice*, New York: Harper & Row.

Gardner, J. (2008) 'Autography's Biography, 1972–2007', *Biography*, 31: 1–26.

Gilman, S. (1988) *Disease and Representation: Images of Illness from Madness to AIDS*, New York: Cornell.

Gloeckner, P. (2000) *A Child's Life and Other Stories*, Berkeley, CA: Frog Ltd.

Goulart, R. (1986) *Ron Goulart's Great History of Comic Books / The Definitive Illustrated History from the 1890s to the 1980s*, McGraw-Hill: Contemporary.

Green, J. (ed.) (1995) *Justin Green's Binky Brown Sampler*, San Francisco, CA: Last Gasp.

Green, M. and Myers, K. (2010) 'Graphic Medicine: The Use of Comics in Medical Education and Patient Care', *British Medical Journal*, 340: 474–7.

Hansen, B. (2004) 'Medical History for the Masses: How American Comic Books Celebrated Heroes of Medicine in the 1940s', *Bulletin of the History of Medicine*, 78: 148–91.

Hancock, M., Hine, D., Pearlman, C. and Phoenix, W. (1991) *1+1*, London: The Comic Company.

Hatfield, C. (2005) *Alternative Comics – An Emerging Literature*, Jackson, MS: University Press of Mississippi.

Hine, D. (1991) 'Dreaming of the 21st Century', in M. Hancock *et al.*, *1+1*, London: The Comic Company: 9–16.

Hyland, M. (ed.) (2008) *Love on Ward B*, London: Prion.

Kominsky-Crumb, A. (2007) *Need More Love*, London: MQ Publications.

Lefèvre, P. (2009) 'The Construction of Space in Comics', in J. Heer and K. Worcester (eds) *A Comics Studies Reader*, Jackson, MS: University Press of Mississippi.

Leder, D. (1990) *The Absent Body*, Chicago, IL: University of Chicago Press.

Lupton, D. (2003) *Medicine as Culture: Illness, Disease and the Body in Western Societies*, 2nd edn, London: Sage.

Mackintosh, R. (2011) *Seeds*, London: ComX.

McCloud, S. (2006) *Making Comics: Storytelling Secrets of Comics, Manga and Graphic Novels*, New York: Harper Collins.

McCloud, S. (1993) *Understanding Comics: The Invisible Art*, New York: Harper Collins.

Merleau-Ponty, M. (1962) *Phenomenology of Perception*, trans. C. Smith, London: Routledge and Kegan Paul.

Melia, D. and Gracey-Whitman, L. (eds) (1987) *Strip Aids*, London: Willyprods/ Small Time Ink.

Mitchell, A. (2010) 'Distributed Identity: Networking Image Fragments in Graphic Memoirs', *Studies in Comics*, 1: 197–211.

Robbins, T., Sienkiewicz, W. and Triptow, R. (1988) *Strip Aids USA*, San Francisco, CA: Last Gasp.

Rozenkranz, P. (2002) *Rebel Visions*, Seattle: Fantagraphics.

Sabin, R. (1996) *Comics, Comix and Graphic Novels: A History of Comic Art*, London: Phaidon.

Spiegelman, A. (1995) 'Introduction', in J. Green (ed.), *Justin Green's Binky Brown*, Sampler, San Francisco, CA: Last Gasp.

Squier, S. (2008) 'So Long as They Grow Out of It: Comics, the Discourse of Developmental Normalcy, and Disability', *Journal of Medical Humanities*, 29: 71–88.

Töpffer, R. (1842) *The Adventures of Mr Obadiah Oldbuck*, New York: Wilson and Company.

Versaci, R. (2007) *This Book Contains Graphic Language: Comics as Literature*, London: Continuum.

Weiner, S. (2003) *Faster Than a Speeding Bullet: The Rise of the Graphic Novel*, New York: Nantier, Beal, Minoustchine.

Wertham, F. (1954) *Seduction of the Innocent*, New York: Rinehart & Company.

Williams, I. C. M. (2011) 'Graphic Medicine: Comics as Medical Narrative', *Medical Humanities*, 38: 21–7.

Witek, J. (2011) 'Justin Green: Autobiography Meets the Comics' in M. A. Chaney, *Graphic Subjects*, Madison, Wisconsin and London: University of Wisconsin Press.

Witek, J. (1989) *Comic Books as History: The Narrative Art of Jack Jackson, Art Spiegelman and Harvey Pekar*, Jackson, MI: University Press of Mississippi.

Wolk, D. (2007) *Reading Comics: How Graphic Novels Work and What They Mean*, Cambridge, MA: Da Capo.

6 Art in medical education

Practice and dialogue

Case study

Louise Younie

> I never made a painting as a work of art, it's all research.
>
> Pablo Picasso

Visual images have a long and interwoven history with medicine, from anatomical drawings such as those of Leonardo Da Vinci (1452–1519) to the use of textbook illustrations or photographs of disease, and radiological images of the internal structures of the body. There is a multitude of paintings that offer commentary on the doctor (Park and Park 2004) and medical practice more generally, as well as doctors who have picked up the brush themselves and engaged in painting (Weisz and Albury 2010). However, engagement with visual art as part of the learning process, to develop skills, explore practice or reflect on experience is a much more recent phenomenon. Visual art invites human meaning making through symbol, metaphor and imagery (Elliott 2011), often transcending time and culture (Schaff *et al.* 2011). Art celebrates existence and yet does not shy away from that which disturbs or is paradoxical (Elliott 2011). It is a means of responding to and exploring the world – both for the child with shapes and colours of all dimensions and for the professional artist seeking to critique or transform (Seeley and Reason 2008).

In this chapter I consider the contested penetration of the visual arts into the arena of medical education as part of the wider medical humanities (sometimes referred to as 'health humanities') movement. I review what the visual arts may have to offer educationally, particularly in the area of practice development, as well as the challenges of integration of visual art into the undergraduate curriculum.

Context for the visual arts in medical education

The term 'medical humanities' was coined in the 1960s in the US (Evans and Greaves 2010) yet half a century later there are still ongoing discussions as to its meaning and 'how they [the medical humanities] should be integrated into medical education' (Shapiro *et al.* 2009: 192). As Alan Bleakley *et al.* note, '[b]oth "medical" and "humanities" fail to capture the field, which goes wider than medicine to include healthcare and goes wider than the humanities to include the arts' (Bleakley *et al.* 2006: 206). The medical humanities have been variously seen as a 'list of disciplines' interwoven with medicine (Brody 2011: 1), a form of academic intellectual inquiry, a dimension of medical education or practitioner development (Evans 2008), as well as including the arts therapies, arts for health and visual arts on display (Hurwitz 2003). For the purposes of this chapter I consider visual arts within medical undergraduate education and include in that bracket sculpture, painting or drawing, photography and video art.

The field of medical humanities has been pioneered in American medical schools since the 1970s (Charon *et al.* 1995), becoming increasingly popular in the UK as well as internationally over the last 15–20 years (Lazarus and Rosslyn 2003). This can be seen in literature published in high-impact medical journals such as *The New England Journal of Medicine* or the *British Medical Journal* as well as medical education journals such as *Academic Medicine* and *Medical Education* (Kuper 2006). In the UK we saw the first publication of the journal *Medical Humanities* in 2000, and the formation of the Association of Medical Humanities (AMH) in 2002. In part, this introduction of the humanities to medical education in the UK was encouraged through the General Medical Council's (GMC) publication *Tomorrow's Doctors* (1993) (Evans 2008). Practically, the GMC document (updated 2009) introduced student selected components (SSCs) to the undergraduate curriculum, which provided opportunity for student choice and for educators to begin to engage small groups of students in exploratory ways with the arts (Macnaughton 1997). Fundamentally, in the original 1993 document, the GMC recognized the need to address attitudinal development and relational abilities in student professional development (Kirklin *et al.* 2000). This recognition may have been in response to multiple contemporary factors such as changing patient expectations, the movement towards patient-centred practice and a less paternalistic approach (Curry and Montgomery 2010), as well as a broader and more holistic conceptualization of health and well-being (Engel 1978).

There have been calls for a broadened medical curriculum on both sides of the Atlantic since the early-twentieth century. Raymond H. Curry and Kathryn Montgomery (2010) quote Francis W. Peabody from 1927, who noted the science overload in the curriculum and the need for primary attention to the patient. Six years after Peabody, Andrew Macphail wrote:

> When a student must be converted into a physiologist, a physicist, a chemist, a biologist, a pharmacologist, and an electrician, there is no time to make a physician of him. That consummation can only come after he has gone out in the world of sickness and suffering, unless

indeed his mind is so bemused, his instincts so dulled, his sympathy so blunted by the long process of education in those sciences, that he is forever excluded from the art of medicine.

(Macphail 1933: 395)

Mark Jackson (1996) quotes Macphail and further notes the remarks of the paediatrician Sir Robert Hutchinson from 1937, who lamented the cluttering up of 'the medical curriculum with all sorts of "ologies" ' and the wrong attitude at the bedside (Jackson 1996: 396). These quotes do not so much represent a polarization of arts/humanities and science (such polarization is strongly contested by Bleakley *et al.* 2006), instead highlighting the dominance of propositional knowledge acquired academically and the applied and practical knowledge needed when meeting with patients. Macphail (1933) suggested it was a going out into the 'world of sickness and suffering' that can 'make a physician' of someone, yet recognized this kind of development was not inevitable. The visual arts may have a role here in the extension of horizons of future doctors through creative-reflective engagement with clinical experience.

The first medical humanities modules to appear in the literature tended to be narrative or literary (Kuper 2006; Evans 2008). This may be due to the greater gap in thinking between the 'objective' intellectual knowing of biomedical science and an interpretive, embodied communication through visual art. A review of the literature by Pamela B. Schaff *et al.* (2011) found that the first art observation paper was by Jacqueline C. Dolev *et al.* (2001), which postulated that systematic observation of paintings might enhance student observational skills. A scattering of similar papers evaluated student learning through observation of art. They proposed that visual art could be used to aid development of visual observation skills, visual diagnostic thinking and pattern recognition (Dolev *et al.* 2001; Bardes *et al.* 2001; Klugman *et al.* 2011) or to encourage empathy, teamwork and communication skills through dialogue and discussion around the pieces (Reilly *et al.* 2005; Shapiro *et al.* 2006b). Such findings have parallels in the literature on the arts and medical practice more broadly, which has shown that mutual learning could take place through the pairing of different professions with experience in visual perception, such as visual artists, with consultants working in the specialties of dermatology, radiology and histopathology (Bleakley *et al.* 2003a; Bleakley *et al.* 2003b).

Another approach to the engagement of students with visual art is to invite them to explore their lived experiences and context through their own art practice. In the literature there are a few examples of student learning supported by artist-led electives (Willson 2006; Dumitriu 2009). The Glasgow artist, Christine Borland, invited medical students into the Glasgow School of Art to engage with art students in collaborative creative projects (Macnaughton 2009). There are also examples of artist–clinician collaborations (Gull 2005a; Weller 2002; Younie 2013), as well as educators inviting medical students to produce visual art as part of their course, whether clinical (Kumagai 2012; Younie 2009; LoFaso *et al.* 2010) or academic (Shapiro *et al.* 2006a; Thompson *et al.* 2010). Creation of visual art has been both the result of an individual reflective endeavour (Younie 2009) or part of a collaborative project with the final production of a joint creative text (Kumagai 2012).

To date, the purposes of medical student engagement with artistic creation have generally been related to personal and professional development through understanding themselves, others and their context afresh ('finding new eyes'). When visual art production has been part of clinical courses they have tended to focus on interpersonal dimensions such as developing student capacity to care for the chronically ill (LoFaso *et al.* 2010) and developing them as patient-centred clinicians (Kumagai 2012).

Applying the visual arts to my own teaching practice

My own work in this field, since 2003, is predominantly in the realm of interpersonal understanding and practitioner development. Course evolution with the arts has developed in a participatory fashion through listening and dialogue with students, artists and faculty as well as considering student texts and other courses (Thompson *et al.* 2010). I have borrowed the term 'arts-based inquiry' (Liamputtong and Rumbold 2008) to describe medical students' engagement with the arts and creative process as they reflect personally and professionally on their journey towards becoming clinicians. For instance, medical students have been invited to produce a creative-reflective text based on a patient home visit as part of their year one general practice clinical placement assessment (Younie 2009), or to engage with the creative arts through various SSCs coordinated and co-facilitated by myself as a clinician collaborating with a variety of artists working in healthcare (Younie 2013). These examples have all been grassroots emergent courses not requested by the establishment but introduced by the interested clinical practitioners seeking to extend students' ways of knowing.

My rationale for introducing the arts to medical education was a result of becoming a family physician (general practitioner GP) and meeting patients suffering not just in physical but also social, emotional and existential ways. I encountered the complexity of multiple perspectives, competing needs and time constraints. Although prepared with a medical toolkit, I had much to learn as a clinical practitioner wishing to be sensitive to patients' healing needs. An alternative toolkit was necessary to facilitate interpretation, understanding, presence, listening, silence and journeying with the patient. This toolkit draws on Schön's (1983) professional artistry (managing in situations of uncertainty, instability and conflict) and the concept of the therapeutic alliance (Brody 1999).

Through fostering different ways of thinking, seeing, knowing and communicating and the encouragement of personal engagement and expression, the arts may contribute to practice development, a neglected area of the curriculum (Shapiro *et al.* 2009). Practice development moves beyond propositional knowledge, to the way in which knowledge is applied in practice, which draws on professional craft knowledge and personal knowledge. Joy Higgs and Angie Titchen (2000) describe these three kinds of knowledge as core to practitioner knowing.

This chapter will now turn to examine the value of the visual arts in medical education in more specific terms: thinking through the language of the arts; looking and seeing; ways of knowing; and ways of communicating. In order to evaluate these four factors, the chapter examines published literature alongside evidence drawn from my own work with medical students.[1]

1. Thinking through the language of the arts

Elliot W. Eisner suggests that '[e]very task and each material with which we work both imposes constraints and provides opportunities for the development of mind' (Eisner 2002: 12). Producing a reflective text, whether verbal, visual or musical, requires the translation of an experience or emotion into the relevant form of language or sign system. Christine H. Leland and Jerome C. Harste describe 'arts, music, mathematics, drama...' as different sign systems 'which we have created to express meaning and to mediate our world' (Leland and Harste 1994: 339). These sign systems offer different possibilities and limitations in our cognitive and emotional work. As Beth Berghoff states:

> Music can express feelings we cannot put into words; language is a better medium for humor than math; yet math can represent concepts that are not easily represented in art, and so on.
>
> (Berghoff 1993: 218)

The visual arts offer engagement with pre-verbal and tacit ways of knowing (Seeley and Reason 2008), embracing imagery, metaphor and symbol as well as colour, texture and dimensions. Art, with its vocabulary of lines, colours, forms, spaces and structures is not only pre-verbal but may offer comprehension *beyond* that which words can express (Elliott 2011). Art can be used to grapple with the ineffable, to say what cannot be said, to respond to the emotional subjective realm, giving feeling form (Langer 1942). The following medical students' responses recount experiences of engaging with visual imagery in reflection:

> I spent a lot of time thinking about what colours represented the patient's mood.
>
> (Medical student 2011)

I...realized...you can depict both the patient's and your own emotions within the picture.

(Medical student 2010)

I thought I could convey what I wanted to say better in pictures than words.

(Medical student 2010)

Students are usually requested to combine their work with verbal or written reflective text; to put down some of their thoughts and reflections in response to the lived experience underlying the artwork as well as reflections on the process and product of their piece. Philosopher and educator Susanne K. Langer describes imagery and text as two fundamentally different ways of representing experience: 'presentational/aesthetic forms' that engage with wholes and tacit knowing, and 'discursive/propositional forms' that deal with parts and explicit knowledge (Langer 1942: 79–102). Intertextuality (Elliott 2011), or movement between communication systems such as art and written text, 'provides the opportunity for new perspectives on our knowing and, hence, for the expression of an expanded range of meanings' (Leland and Harste 1994: 340).

2. Looking and seeing

Creating visual art is a way of holding a mirror up to our experience, allowing us to revisit it, to speak about and learn from it (Elliott 2011). As Comte-Sponville notes, 'in art, humanity contemplates itself in the act of contemplating' (Comte-Sponville 2005: 100). Eisner suggests that the arts 'enable us to inspect more carefully our own ideas... [they] are means of exploring our own interior landscape... [and] help us discover the contours of our emotional selves' (Eisner 2002: 11). The arts can help us to slow down perception, learning how to savour qualities by taking the time to really look. The potential then is of seeing something new. One medical student wrote in her reflections after the SSC: '[w]e learn to see beyond clubbing and splinter haemorrhages to the story behind their withered hands, to the person and all their history'. In her close analysis of artists' practices, Brenda Elliott (2011) considers how artists use their art to explore burning questions and narratives with 'diligent persistence', actively reworking observations and insights. Further, the ability to be audience to one's own artwork allows the artist to provide a constant critical interpretive presence.

An important question to consider is to what extent students engage with learning through the process of producing a creative piece – do they reflect on an encounter and then produce an image, or does the actual production of the image shape how they reflect and consider their encounter? Some student quotes suggest the latter:

It [the creative piece] made me consider the patient more deeply as I had to think of how to display their issues visually.

(Medical student 2010)

I think the creative piece made me think more deeply about the patient's emotions.

(Medical student 2010)

However another student writes as if creative production and reflection are two separate processes:

Choosing a creative piece meant that you could become too focused on the aesthetics and not the story you are trying to convey.

(Medical student 2010)

Understanding the place of the visual text and the quality of aesthetics has caused some concerns for students and GP tutor markers alike. Development of clearer marking criteria that include the aesthetic dimension, as well as perception, reflection and impact was met with general approval from both parties. I developed these criteria alongside Dr Catherine Lamont-Robinson as clinician-artist pair, emergent through our engagement with student assignments. Affirmation of the criteria came from the ethnographic literature, where very similar evaluative criteria have been proposed (Richardson 2000) as well as seeking both student and GP tutor feedback on practical application of these criteria (Younie 2011).

3. Ways of knowing

The problem of medical education is expressed by George L. Engel who described the physician of the day – the 1970s – as having had 'the most thorough and scientific understanding of the disease for which the patient came for treatment, not the most thorough and scientific understanding of the patient who came for help' (Engel 1978: 173). Understanding disease and understanding personhood require different kinds of knowing. Understanding disease requires an intellectual knowing ('objective knowledge') about measurable facts thought to be universally true (Marcum 2008: 97–108). Understanding personhood ('subjective knowledge') (Marcum 2008: 108–18) and the inter- and intra-subjectivity inherent within a consultation is necessarily more complex and uncertain (Kuper 2007). 'Diagnostic and therapeutic power in clinicians', according to Eric J. Cassell, 'is directly proportionate to their ability to tolerate uncertainty... To seek certainty itself is ultimately to abandon the patient' (Cassell 2004: 220).

Elliott suggests that engagement with art calls upon us to 'accept enormous complexity, even uneasiness and anxiety' (Elliott 2011: 98). While

Shapiro *et al.* (2009) suggest that students may be uncomfortable with the lack of certainty and interpretive dimension of the humanities, my experience with students on the creative arts SSCs over the years has been that of embracing multiple perspectives. The following quote echoes what a number of the students write in their reflective journals during this course: 'I found it most liberating! It was interesting to see how everyone interpreted someone's piece of art, poetry or literature' (2005). Students adopting this perspective allows for a collaborative learning environment where the participants, including the facilitators, are learning from each other (Younie 2006).

Work is needed to help students to recognize, engage with and find a way of managing the complexity and uncertainty inherent in the 'swampy lowland' (Schön, 1983: 3) that they will face in their future clinical practice – the many situations of clinical uncertainty where professional artistry and good clinical judgment will be called upon. Although much significant learning takes place on the wards through clinician role-modelling, the visual arts afford students the opportunity for extended learning, to consider multiple voices, matters of interpretation and to seek to imaginatively explore the lived experience of another. Further, when faculty members are interested in students' lived experiences and perspectives, this may encourage a similar interest in, or provide a role model for, engagement with the patient's lived experience and perspective:

> By using creativity it allowed me to reflect upon my experiences with people in a much more personal, less scientific way.
>
> (Medical student 2010)

> I felt that the creative piece gave me the chance to give greater consideration to the personal experiences of patients…i.e. I was more inclined to think of the patients as people with individual lives.
>
> (Medical student 2010)

4. Ways of communicating – the ripple effect

According to Langer, 'visual forms offer their constituents not successively but simultaneously – grasped in one act of vision' (Langer 1942: 93). Her comment relates to the way in which visual representation offers medical students a potent way of communicating their experiences with patients both to healthcare professionals and to their peers. Since the introduction of the arts-based inquiry option within the year one GP placement, I have heard anecdotal evidence for the value of placing visual artwork in the GP surgery coffee room. Such artwork has stimulated dialogue across frontline healthcare professionals and has even shifted their perspectives over the course of one week, on participatory art and knowledge production within the undergraduate curriculum.

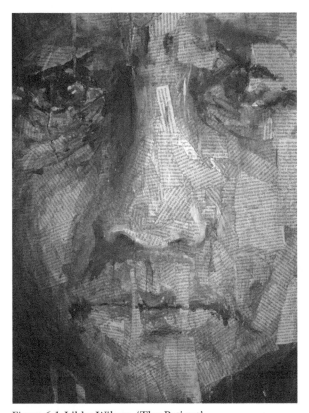

Figure 6.1 Libby Wilson, 'The Patient'
Source: Reproduced with permission of Libby Wilson

Despite some initial tentativeness among GP tutors, over the years they have increasingly embraced the use of visual arts in the medical curriculum (Younie 2011). Student artwork has even occasionally been shown to the patient in question by the GP. One example of this was a piece of work produced after meeting a patient with cancer.

The medical student in question, Libby Wilson, reflected on her work as follows:

> I decided to paint on a large canvas to represent the huge impact the cancer had on Mrs Smith's life.[2] I painted her face disappearing into copies of her crumpled medical notes as if in order to see her as a scientific being, you would have to look through her. I tried to portray Mrs Smith's fear, pain and exhaustion whilst fighting cancer. I crumpled and ripped the notes to represent people's fragility and purposely layered the text to give a sense of depth.

(Libby Wilson 2010)

The medium is the message. Libby embodies the fear and pain through the physical crumpling and ripping of paper. The work of layering the paper and the painting allows consideration of what lies beneath the medical presentation. The piece speaks for itself, evoking the audience to experience something of the felt sense that Libby experienced in her encounter. The family heard about the piece of artwork and wanted to see it, and having done so, asked for a photograph of the work to keep. This piece of art is also now on display in the GP's newly refurbished practice, which provides a potential space to communicate the medical student's perspective with that of the wider patient population.

Challenges to integration of the arts

Having presented ways in which students' engagements with visual art can stretch perception, insight and understanding, some of the challenges of integrating the arts into medical education need to be addressed. This section will address three of the main challenges to using the visual arts, and the medical humanities more generally, in medical education: integration, students' concerns and evaluation.

1. Integration

As noted by Shapiro *et al.*, 'the incorporation of medical humanities in medical training has not proceeded smoothly. By and large, medical humanities remain an intriguing sideline in the main project of medical education' (Shapiro *et al.* 2009: 193). This claim can be countered by medical schools that have positioned the medical humanities at the heart of their curricula, but they are noteworthy precisely because they are *exceptions*.[3]

More than a decade ago, Martyn Evans and David Greaves (1999) suggested that medical humanities needed to be more than bolt-on options for interested students, recommending fundamental integration of arts and sciences in the core philosophy of medical curricula. They proposed an integrative rather than additive approach, whereby an additive approach seeks to 'soften' future practitioners, the integrative looks to transform the knowledge base of medicine itself. While there are examples in the literature of such integrative thinking within the undergraduate medical curriculum (Bleakley *et al.* 2006), Ayelet Kuper and Marcel D'Eon are not alone in their position that 'becoming a doctor continues to entail, almost exclusively, the acquisition of large amounts of bioscientific knowledge' (Kuper and D'Eon 2011: 37).

Despite the progression of the arts as a bolt-on within the medical curriculum, we must ask why it has been so difficult to embed the humanities (Gull 2005b). Some point to student and faculty perspectives (Shapiro *et al.* 2009), others to the current dominating focus on a knowledge and skills competency approach to medical training (Gull 2005b;

Kuper 2006). Although it is logical that patients would like to encounter competent doctors, the competency approach can be criticized for building on a behaviourist framework, which breaks down work roles into discrete tasks and ignores both their interconnections and the underlying complexity of the real world (Leung 2002). Other factors for the lack of integration of the humanities, highlighted in the literature include the lack of clarity and purpose of the humanities in medical education (Shapiro *et al.* 2009) and the challenges of assessment and evaluation in this field (Kuper 2006).

2. Student-related concerns

Shapiro *et al.* (2009) raise a number of student-related issues with the humanities. This chapter has already discussed whether medical students feel anxious about uncertainty or embrace it through studying the arts. Shapiro *et al.* also consider the problem of the medical humanities being a domain outside the basic and clinical sciences. From my experience of working with medical students, I believe that problems occur when students cannot see how the arts might be relevant to their future roles. This is where clinician input might facilitate the application of arts-based learning to practice and is one of the reasons for my co-facilitation of the creative arts SSC mentioned above.

Another problem raised by Shapiro *et al.* is that of students resisting 'personal engagement as excessively intimate and intrusive' (Shapiro *et al.* 2009: 183). With a few exceptions this has not been my experience, either on the GP placement, during which students probably regulate the degree to which they will be open, or within my group-run SSC. Students repeatedly talk about the privilege of sharing more intimately with each other and within the SSC group. The following quotes illustrate such sentiments:

> It felt like quite a privilege to listen to people opening up and describing things that really touch and matter to them.
>
> (Medical student 2005)

> I was surprised how many of the group produced very emotional pieces. Maybe this was a reflection of the session, that the pieces of work we had observed were very meaningful.
>
> (Medical student 2005)

Through reflective, creative work students sometimes share personal vulnerability and are usually relieved at the group's resonance with what they might be feeling. As noted in one student's reflective journal after a medical humanities SSC at Barts and The London School of Medicine and Dentistry, in relation to Figure 6.2:

The photo I took to represent my time at med school so far was of a grape on a chessboard, surrounded by beautifully carved, hard, honed, black chess pieces lining up for battle. Whatever else I have learned or failed to learn, over the last week, I certainly feel more like a grape among grapes now. Shinier, more polished grapes, maybe, but at least I feel less like I must surely be on the whole wrong playing field.

(Stephanie Greenwald 2011)

This image of the grape among the chess pieces has allowed an idea to be expressed in metaphorical terms that likely would not have otherwise been spoken, the metaphors facilitating a shared understanding of a felt sense among the group. The photograph was one of a series constructed in response to being asked to photographically convey the lived experience of

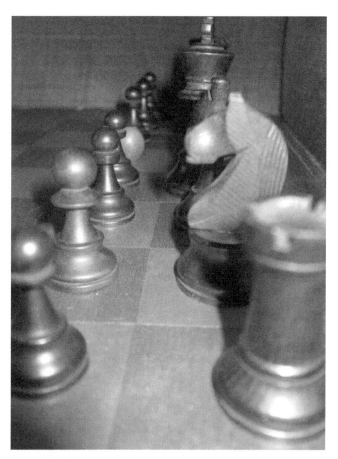

Figure 6.2 Stephanie Greenwald, 'The Grape'
Source: Reproduced with permission of Stephanie Greenwald

being a medical student. Most of the other images described, for example, the volume of learning, exam stress and the shared journeying with colleagues.

This general quality of shared dialogue may be due to students opting into this SSC, which means that SSCs are inherently unlikely to include deeply cynical students who might inhibit the depth of sharing of others (Younie 2006). Other factors may include the impact of the creative-reflective process itself as students learn about the therapeutic value of the arts for patients. Finally, dialogue takes place in a safe space where, for example, I as facilitator share my own vulnerability and uncertainties relating to my clinical practice. Having said this, there have been a couple of queries raised by male participants as to the degree of emotional expression, likening the session at times to a 'therapy group' (Younie 2006). These arose either within their reflective journal or the post-course focus group. Careful facilitation is therefore necessary while recognizing that a degree of discomfort may form part of learning to listen to the personal expression of others and finding boundaries for themselves as future doctors in whom patients will confide.

3. Purpose and evaluation

One of the biggest concerns facing the progression and development of medical humanities, or the engagement with visual arts in the undergraduate curriculum, is evaluation. Courses in the visual arts struggle to produce evidence that they reach Kirkpatrick (2006) evaluation levels 3 or 4, evaluation levels which equate to observed behaviour change or change in patient care and health outcomes. Paul Rodenhauser *et al.* (2004) recently found that over half of the 83 US medical schools who responded to their survey used the arts in medical education, including visual arts, film, performance arts, music and literature. However, Wershof Schwartz *et al.* (2009) suggest that the increased numbers of humanities courses delivered at medical schools does not correlate with a measured proven impact on doctors in training.

There are a variety of learning outcome evaluations found in the literature relating to visual art. These include visual observational skills (Dolev *et al.* 2001), visual literacy, team working, listening skills (Reilly *et al.* 2005), tolerance of ambiguity (Klugman *et al.* 2011) and development of empathy and awareness of multiple perspectives (Shapiro *et al.* 2006b). Methods of evaluation have included post-course questionnaires with Likert scales and/or open questions (LoFaso *et al.* 2010; Gull 2005a; Schaff *et al.* 2011), post-session interviews and instructor debriefings (Shapiro *et al.* 2006b), changes in self-reported evaluations such as using a tolerance of ambiguity scale (Klugman *et al.* 2011) and changes in ability to engage with and write about paintings (Klugman *et al.* 2011). None of these, however, fall into the higher Kirkpatrick (2006) levels of evaluation mentioned above. In fact, a recent review of the literature on effectiveness of arts-based interventions in medical education did not find any studies considering the effects of such education on behaviour (Perry *et al.* 2011).

This lack of evidence is disappointing, yet may relate to the complexity and challenge of evaluation. Jill Gordon (2005) reviews the significant challenges faced when trying to set up randomized controlled trials in this field, while Kuper (2006) suggests the challenge of evaluation of the humanities lies in not being able to problematize learning in the quantitative way often adopted by the medical education research community. Jane Macnaughton (2002) discusses the complexity of the educational outcomes we are attempting to investigate let alone quantify. Part of the problem lies in the difficulty of assessing attitudinal change or learning (Skelton *et al.* 2000; Macnaughton 2002) or subjective outcomes such as professionalism or self-care (Schwartz *et al.* 2009). Some of the learning lies in the important field of being rather than doing. Developing a more nuanced self-awareness, broadening horizons or offering a more interpretive space to patients are not easily measured quantitatively although, as Kuper (2006) suggests, more in-depth qualitative or ethnographic studies may be valuable here.

Schwartz *et al.* (2009) suggest that the research base is also affected by published studies often relating to small self-selecting groups of medical students, and a diversity in educational approaches with lack of consensus of desired outcomes. A number of issues are brought up here. Often, the delivery of medical humanities courses is still voluntary and depends on local initiatives. The educational research is thereby limited to what has been instituted in practice. Diversity in approaches and desired outcomes are inevitable, where modules are being developed in the available gaps in the curriculum according to capacity and interests of faculty. Local decision-making factors ranging from the economic and political to the individual and philosophical determine the nature of medical humanities initiatives alongside government recommendations. It is therefore difficult to perform an evaluation of visual arts courses within medical curricula that is suitable for all contexts. Furthermore, medical humanities courses are constantly in flux as they develop in response to student input and responses. Such innovation and diversity is useful in the development of the field, but limits our ability to pinpoint its nature and to measure its value. Also, predefined or too-rigid learning outcomes may limit the potential for practice-based transformative learning to occur.

Although more substantial integration may be desirable, we are faced with the chicken and the egg problem: greater integration needs more research and more research is not possible without greater integration. Part of the problem is that the medical humanities offer a fairly new discipline complex, perhaps better referred to as a field of study rather than a discipline (or even 'interdiscipline'), which needs to prove itself in the face of the prevailing medical orthodoxy.

Conclusion

In this chapter, I have reviewed the introduction and progression of the visual arts within medical education, drawing on the literature and my own educational experiences as well as students' and faculty members' perspectives. I have predominantly considered student engagement with the actual process of production of visual art creative-reflective texts as part of practitioner development. Visual art has been explored as a useful vehicle for taking a deeper look at ourselves and our practices, by engaging with metaphor and symbol. Whether this develops 'better' clinicians, in terms of nuance of understanding and interpersonal skills, still remains to be seen. However, it appears to be one way of providing a platform for considering students' lived experiences that, if used well, can extend their horizons. The challenge of producing research that proves any impact of working with the visual arts on clinical practice remains, yet as a preliminary position it could be hoped that extending students' understanding of themselves and the other might influence their practice as future doctors.

It is therefore argued that in order to develop our understanding of the field of visual arts (and the medical humanities in general) in medical education, further research is needed – both mixed-methods and longitudinal, and possibly cross-institutional. Longer-term follow-up is lacking in the literature and is needed in order to review ongoing learning and behaviour change. More in-depth qualitative research exploring tacit meanings constructed from students' experiences with art in medicine is needed (Kumagai 2012), for example, drawing on ethnography and more recently emerging narrative or arts-based inquiry methods (Knowles and Cole 2008) or heuristic and participatory designs (Moustakas 1990). It should be possible to produce more substantial research in this field. However, this would require teams with solid research methodology expertise as well as educational, clinical and artistic expertise. Social, economic and political factors will determine whether there is a collective will or the requisite resources to make such research a reality.

Acknowledgements

I would like to acknowledge Dr Catherine Lamont-Robinson for her contributions to this chapter and as a colleague in this arts-based inquiry work. I would also like to thank the medical students whose work and thoughts have contributed to this chapter as well as those who have engaged in this line of inquiry over the years.

Notes

1   Student artwork and names are used with permission.
2   The patient's name has been changed for confidentiality.

3   An exception in the UK has been Peninsula Medical School (Universities of Exeter and Plymouth), which developed a core, integrated medical humanities curriculum as well as a wide range of special study units.

References

Bardes, C. L., Gillers, D. and Herman, A. E. (2001) 'Learning to Look: Developing Clinical Observational Skills at an Art Museum', *Medical Education*, 35: 1157–61.

Berghoff, B. (1993) 'Moving Toward Aesthetic Literacy in the First Grade', in D. J. Lin and C. K. Kinzer (eds) *Examing Central Issues in Literacy Research, Theory, and Practice*, Chicago, IL: National Reading Conference.

Bleakley, A., Marshall, R. and Brömer, R. (2006) 'Toward an Aesthetic Medicine: Developing a Core Medical Humanities Undergraduate Curriculum', *Journal of Medical Humanities*, 27: 197–213.

Bleakley, A., Farrow, R., Gould, D. and Marshall, R. (2003a) 'Learning How to See: Doctors Making Judgements in the Visual Domain', *Journal of Workplace Learning*, 15: 301–6.

Bleakley, A., Farrow, R., Gould, D. and Marshall, R. (2003b) 'Making Sense of Clinical Reasoning: Judgement and the Evidence of the Senses', *Medical Education*, 37: 544–52.

Brody, H. (2011) 'Defining the Medical Humanities: Three Conceptions and Three Narratives', *Journal of Medical Humanities*, 32: 1–7.

Brody, N. (1999) 'The Doctor as Therapeutic Agent: A Placebo Effect Research Agenda', in A. Harrington (ed.) *The Placebo Effect: An Interdisciplinary Exploration*, Cambridge, MA: Harvard University Press.

Cassell, E. J. (2004) *The Nature of Suffering and the Goals of Medicine*, New York: Oxford University Press.

Charon, R., Trautmann Banks, J., Connelly, J. E., Hunsaker Hawkins, A., Montgomery Hunter, K., Hudson Jones, A., Montello, M. and Poirer, S. (1995) 'Literature and Medicine: Contributions to Clinical Practice', *Annals of Internal Medicine*, 122: 599–606.

Comte-Sponville, A. (2005) *The Little Book of Philosophy*, London: Vintage.

Curry, R. H. and Montgomery, K. (2010) 'Toward a Liberal Education in Medicine', *Academic Medicine*, 85: 283–7.

Dolev, J. C., Friedlaender, L. and Braverman, I. M. (2001) 'Use of Fine Art to Enhance Visual Diagnostic Skills', *JAMA: The Journal of the American Medical Association*, 286: 1020–1.

Dumitriu, A. (2009) 'Creative Communication for Medical Students: Using Installation and Performance Art to Communicate Ideas about Medicine', *The Academy Subject Centre for Medicine, Dentistry and Veterinary Medicine Newsletter*, 20: 23–5.

Eisner, E. W. (2002), *The Arts and the Creation of Mind*, New Haven and London: Yale University Press.

Elliott, B. (2011) 'Arts-Based and Narrative Inquiry in Liminal Experience Reveal Platforming as Basic Social Psychological Process', *The Arts in Psychotherapy*, 38: 96–103.

Engel, G. L. (1978) 'The Biopsychosocial Model and the Education of Health Professionals', *Annals of the New York Academy of Sciences*, 310: 169–81.

Evans, H. M. (2008) 'Affirming the Existential within Medicine: Medical

Humanities, Governance, and Imaginative Understanding', *Journal of Medical Humanities*, 29: 55–9.

Evans, H. M. and Greaves, D. A. (2010) 'Ten Years of Medical Humanities: A Decade in the Life of a Journal and a Discipline', *Medical Humanities*, 36: 66–8.

Evans, M. and Greaves, D. (1999) 'Exploring the Medical Humanities', *British Medical Journal*, 319: 1216.

General Medical Council (2009) *Tomorrow's Doctors*, London: GMC.

Gordon, J. (2005) 'Not Everything that Counts can be Counted', *Medical Education*, 39: 551–4.

Gull, S. (2005a) 'Life Drawing in Undergraduate Clinical Attachments', *The Academy Subject Centre for Medicine, Dentistry and Veterinary Medicine Newsletter*, 7: 8–9.

Gull, S. E. (2005b) 'Embedding the Humanities into Medical Education', *Medical Education*, 39: 235–6.

Higgs, J. and Titchen, A. (2000) 'Knowledge and Reasoning', in J. Higgs and M. Jones (eds) *Clinical Reasoning in the Health Professions*, Oxford: Butterworth-Heinemann.

Hurwitz, B. (2003) 'Medicine, the Arts and Humanities', *Clinical Medicine*, 3: 497–8.

Jackson, M. (1996) 'Medical Humanities in Medical Education', *Medical Education*, 30: 395–6.

Kirklin, D., Meakin, R., Singh, S. and Lloyd, M. (2000) 'Living With and Dying From Cancer: A Humanities Special Study Module', *Medical Humanities*, 26: 51–4.

Kirkpatrick, D. and Kirkpatrick, J. (2006) *Evaluating Training Programs*, San Francisco, CA: Berrett-Koehler Publishers.

Klugman, C. M., Peel, J. and Beckmann-Mendez, D. (2011) 'Art Rounds: Teaching Interprofessional Students Visual Thinking Strategies at One School', *Academic Medicine*, 86: 1266–71.

Knowles, G. and Cole, A. L. (eds) (2008) *Handbook of the Arts in Qualitative Research*, Thousand Oaks, CA: Sage.

Kumagai, A. K. (2012) 'Perspective: Acts of Interpretation: A Philosophical Approach to Using Creative Arts in Medical Education', *Academic Medicine*, 87: 1138–44.

Kuper, A. (2007) 'The Intersubjective and the Intrasubjective in the Patient–Physician Dyad: Implications for Medical Humanities Education', *Medical Humanities*, 33: 75–80.

Kuper, A. (2006) 'Literature and Medicine: A Problem of Assessment', *Academic Medicine*, 81: 128–37.

Kuper, A. and D'Eon, M. (2011) 'Rethinking the Basis of Medical Knowledge', *Medical Education*, 45: 36–43.

Langer, S. K. (1942) *Philosophy in a New Key: A Study in the Symbolism of Reason, Rite and Art*, Massachusetts: Oxford University Press.

Lazarus, P. A. and Rosslyn, F. M. (2003) 'The Arts in Medicine: Setting Up and Evaluating a New Special Study Module at Leicester Warwick Medical School', *Medical Education*, 37: 553–9.

Leland, C. H. and Harste, J. C. (1994) 'Multiple Ways of Knowing: Curriculum in a New Key', *Language Arts*, 71: 337–45.

Leung, W.-C. (2002) 'Learning in Practice. Competency Based Medical Training: Review', *British Medical Journal*, 325: 693–5.

Liamputtong, P. and Rumbold, J. (eds) (2008) *Knowing Differently: Arts-Based and Collaborative Research Methods*, New York: Nova Science Publishers.

Lofaso, V. M., Breckman, R., Capello, C. F., Demopoulos, B. and Adelman, R. D. (2010) 'Combining the Creative Arts and the House Call to Teach Medical

Students About Chronic Illness Care', *Journal of the American Geriatrics Society*, 58: 346–51.

Macnaughton, J. (2002) 'Research in Medical Humanities: Is It Time for a New Paradigm?', *Medical Education*, 36: 500–501.

Macnaughton, J. (2009) 'Flesh Revealed: Medicine, Art and Anatomy', in C. J. Saunders, U. Maude and J. Macnaughton (eds) *The Body and the Arts*, London: Palgrave.

Macnaughton, R. J. (1997) 'Special Study Modules: An Opportunity not to be Missed', *Medical Education*, 31: 49–51.

Macphail, A. (1933) 'The Source of Modern Medicine', *British Medical Journal*, 1: 443–7.

Marcum, J. A. (2008) *An Introductory Philosophy of Medicine; Humanizing Modern Medicine*, New York: Springer.

Moustakas, C. (1990) *Heuristic Research; Design, Methodology, and Applications*, Newbury Park, California: Sage.

Park, M. P. and Park, R. H. R. (2004) 'The Fine Art of Patient-Doctor Relationships', *British Medical Journal*, 329: 1475–80.

Perry, M., Maffulli, N., Willson, S. and Morrissey, D. (2011) 'The effectiveness of arts-based interventions in medical education: a literature review', *Medical Education*, 45: 141–148.

Reilly, J. M., Ring, J. and Duke, L. (2005) 'Visual Thinking Strategies: A New Role for Art in Medical Education', *Family Medicine*, 37: 250–2.

Richardson, L. (2000) 'Evaluating Ethnography', *Qualitative Inquiry*, 6: 253–5.

Rodenhauser, P., Strickland, M. and Gambala, C. (2004) 'Arts-Related Activities across U.S. Medical Schools: A Follow-Up Study', *Teaching and Learning in Medicine*, 16: 233–9.

Schaff, P. B., Isken, S. and Tager, R. M. (2011) 'From Contemporary Art to Core Clinical Skills: Observation, Interpretation, and Meaning-Making in a Complex Environment', *Academic Medicine*, 86: 1272–6.

Schön, D. A. (1983) *The Reflective Practitioner. How Professionals Think in Action*, New York: Basic Books.

Schwartz, A. W., Abramson, J. S., Wojnowich, I., Accordino, R., Ronan, E. J. and Rifkin, M. R. (2009) 'Evaluating the Impact of the Humanities in Medical Education', *Mount Sinai Journal of Medicine: A Journal of Translational and Personalized Medicine*, 76: 372–80.

Seeley, C. and Reason, P. (2008) 'Expressions of Energy: An Epistemology of Presentational Knowing', in P. Liamputtong and J. Rumbold (eds) *Knowing Differently: Arts-Based and Collaborative Research Methods*, New York: Nova Science Publishers.

Shapiro, J., Coulehan, J., Wear, D. and Montello, M. (2009) 'Medical Humanities and Their Discontents: Definitions, Critiques, and Implications', *Academic Medicine*, 84: 192–8.

Shapiro, J., Nguyen, V. P., Mourra, S., Ross, M., Thai, T. and Leonard, R. (2006a) 'The Use of Creative Projects in a Gross Anatomy Class', *Journal for Learning through the Arts*, 2: Article 20.

Shapiro, J., Rucker, L. and Beck, J. (2006b) 'Training the Clinical Eye and Mind: Using the Arts to Develop Medical Students' Observational and Pattern Recognition Skills', *Medical Education*, 40: 263–8.

Skelton, J. R., Macleod, J. A. A. and Thomas, C. P. (2000) 'Teaching Literature and

Medicine to Medical Students, Part II: Why Literature and Medicine?', *The Lancet*, 356: 2001–3.

Thompson, T., Lamont-Robinson, C. and Younie, L. (2010) ' "Compulsory Creativity": Rationales, Recipes, and Results in the Placement of Mandatory Creative Endeavour in a Medical Undergraduate Curriculum', *Medical Education Online*. Online. Available: www.med-ed-online.net/index.php/meo/article/view/5394 (accessed 9 December 2010).

Weisz, G. M. and Albury, W. R. (2010) 'The Medico-Artistic Phenomenon and its Implications for Medical Education', *Medical Hypotheses*, 74: 169–73.

Weller, K. (2002) 'Visualising the Body in Art and Medicine: A Visual Art Course for Medical Students at King's College Hospital in 1999', *Complementary Therapies in Nursing and Midwifery*, 8: 211–6.

Willson, S. (2006) 'Essay: What Can the Arts bring to Medical Training?', *The Lancet*, 368: 15–16.

Younie, L. (2006) 'A Qualitative Study of the Contribution Medical Humanities can bring to Medical Education', unpublished thesis, University of Bristol.

Younie, L. (2009) 'Developing Narrative Competence in Medical Students', *Medical Humanities*, 35: 54.

Younie, L. (2011) 'A Reflexive Journey through Arts-Based Inquiry in Medical Education', unpublished thesis, University of Bristol.

Younie, L. (2013) 'Introducing Arts-Based Inquiry into Medical Education: Exploring the Creative Arts in Health and Illness', in P. Mcintosh and D. Warren (eds) *Creativity in the Classroom: Case Studies in Using the Arts in Teaching and Learning in Higher Education*, Bristol: Intellect Publishers.

Section Three

Literature and writing

7 The medical humanities

A literary perspective

Overview

Anne Whitehead

Rita Charon, Professor of Clinical Medicine at Columbia University, has notably observed that it is neither possible nor desirable to define the relation between literature and medicine solely in relation to the emergence of the medical humanities as a recognizable field or discipline; rather, she argues, their connection 'is enduring because it is inherent' (Charon 2000: 24). Charon has played a leading role in creating the movement of narrative medicine, which is centrally concerned with opening up new approaches in medical education, and its core principles are encapsulated in her monograph *Narrative Medicine* (2006).[1] For her, the clinician's task is essentially one of narrative interpretation: the doctor is required to listen attentively to a complex and multi-faceted narrative, told in the patient case history, in the symptoms of the body, and in medical images and laboratory test results, all of which need to cohere into the formulation of a diagnosis and treatment plan.

Medical education should therefore aid the development of key narrative capabilities, defined by Charon as 'recognizing, absorbing, interpreting, and *being moved by* the stories of illness' (Charon 2006: 4; my emphasis). Moreover, for Charon, narrative should not only be read by the trainee practitioner but also written by her, in the form of a Parallel Chart that records what her patient endures. This, Charon explains, allows the medical student to '*enter* the worlds of [her] patients, if only imaginatively, and to see and interpret these worlds from the patients' point of view' (Charon 2006: 9; original emphasis). For Charon, then, narrative – whether read or written – is valued because it is productive of empathetic engagement with the patient.

Charon's work, which has proved highly influential in the rapidly burgeoning field of the medical humanities, comprises a compelling story about the literary, which is seen as an inherently narrative medium. It also shows the literary medium to be essentially humanizing, equipping students with 'compassion' (Charon 2006: 8), although Therese Jones rightly encourages caution about such assumptions in her introductory chapter within this volume. Charon's story, however, does not take into account historical and theoretical shifts in how literary narrative has been conceived. It also produces an account of the literary as enhancing what the medical practitioner already does. In the words of Martyn Evans and David Greaves, narrative is privileged because it can 'foste[r] clinicians' abilities to communicate with patients' (Evans and Greaves 1999: 1216). In what follows, it is my aim to reorient these two assumptions, which are embedded not only into Charon's work but also into a central strand of the field in the United States (US) and the United Kingdom (UK).

My argument will trace a brief history of how changing perceptions of narrative have shifted the relation between literature and medicine in the period since 1945, even as related changes in medicine have also inflected how the two terms intersect. While I do not seek to deny that there is an 'enduring' relation between literature and medicine, I contend that it is nevertheless important to historicize that relation. Within the scope of this chapter, this involves recognizing that the medical humanities coalesced as an identifiable field at a certain historical moment: in the 1970s in the US and, in a delayed response, in the 1990s in the UK. I argue in turn that we can productively distinguish the characteristic approach to literature that defines the medical humanities apart from earlier developments, which we can see as signs of what was to come, but that we should not retrospectively retrofit in relation to the contemporary moment. I also respond to the medical humanities from a specifically literary perspective, indicating aspects of literature that might enable the field to shift from what Evans and Greaves have termed 'an "additive" view, whereby an essentially unchanged biomedicine is softened in practice by the sensitised practitioner' towards 'an "integrated" view whereby the nature, goals, and knowledge base of clinical medicine itself' might be challenged and reshaped by its encounter with the humanities (Evans and Greaves 1999: 1216).

The first half of my chapter draws on Lars-Christer Hydén's work on illness and narrative to trace a postwar history of changing approaches to narrative, and their influence on how the relation between literature and medicine is conceived. Following Hydén, I distinguish between an early attention to the study of narrative 'in clinical practice' and in relation to the '*doctor's* experience', and a subsequent shift to interest in '*patients'* experience of suffering' (Hydén 1997: 51; my emphasis). I exemplify these trends through the studies of Michael Balint and John Berger in the 1950s and 1960s on the role of the general practitioner, and through the rise of the literary genre of pathography in the late 1980s and 1990s. In the second half of my chapter, I turn to the present to assess the main challenges and areas of potential within literature for the medical humanities. I examine first the arts in healthcare movement in relation to literature, particularly creative writing, and analyze the question of evidence as a central methodological concern within the field. I close by examining the current shift in the field towards the 'critical medical humanities', as discussed in Alan Bleakley's introductory chapter within this volume, asking what this might indicate in turn for its future direction and potential.

Postwar beginnings

In tracing the emergence of the medical humanities, Ronald A. Carson has argued that they are 'a product of the turbulent '60s, when authority and expertise were being questioned and traditional ways of doing things were being challenged' (Carson 2007: 322). Clinicians were particularly concerned about the increasing 'technologisation' of medicine and intensifying 'bureaucratic and market pressures' on clinical care, and they turned in response to the humanities as a source of reconnection (Carson 2007: 329). In what Hydén and Elliot G. Mishler have identified as a linguistic turn, attention was directed to 'the forms and functions of language in medical practice and training', and early research in this field, dating to the mid-1960s, focused in particular on the ways in which 'physicians may improve their communication skills so as to more effectively perform their clinical tasks: history taking, diagnosis, and treatment' (Hydén and Mishler 1999: 174). As Hydén further elaborates, in these early studies 'the illness narrative itself was a secondary concern'; of primary importance was whether doctors could, through illness narratives, 'become better able to attend to what their patients say' (Hydén 1997: 51–2).

In the British context, the pioneering work of Michael Balint at the Tavistock Clinic in London represents a significant early reorientation of the medical towards narrative. Balint trained as a psychoanalyst in his native Hungary, and developed there a belief that the psychoanalytic method could be utilized across a range of medical treatment settings. In London, Balint set up discussion groups in the early 1950s for doctors interested in importing a modified version of the 'talking cure' into general practice. In 1957, Balint published *The Doctor, His Patient and the Illness*, in which he introduced his novel ideas for the doctor's relationship with the patient. Analyzing the impulse towards diagnosis as often premature and as acting for the doctor's benefit, relieving him of 'the burden of either not knowing enough or of being unable to help' (Balint 1964 [1957]: 231), Balint advocates instead what he terms 'the long interview', in which the taking of a medical case history would be replaced by a more extended process of listening to the patient: '*if you ask questions you get answers – and hardly anything else.* What we try to foster is the growth in doctors of an ability to listen to the events as they develop in the doctor-patient relationship during the interview' (Balint 1964 [1957]: 288, 133; original emphasis). Balint's work, undertaken in the context of the nascent National Health Service in the UK, can be seen from the contemporary perspective to have provided an influential model of the 'good doctor' as an empathetic listener to the patient's narrative, and as a professional witness to the latter's suffering.

The publication in 1967 of John Berger's *A Fortunate Man*, itself deeply indebted to Balint's study, provides a powerful portrait of the role doctors play in their communities and of the doctor as compassionate witness.[2] Following John Sassall in the impoverished rural community of the Forest of Dean, we see him directly applying Balint's principles in his medical practice: 'In the evenings after supper he has long appointments lasting an hour with patients whom he believes he can help with psychotherapy. They suffer their crises with him' (Berger and Mohr 1997 [1967]: 124). Berger's analysis further reinforces Balint's model of medical practice. The process of diagnosis is one that 'includes doctor and patient', and that 'first recognize[s] the patient as a person' (Berger and Mohr 1997 [1967]: 74). Indeed, Sassall is positioned as a model of what we would now define as patient-centred care:

> He never separates an illness from the total personality of the patient – in this sense, he is the opposite of a specialist. He does not believe in maintaining his imaginative distance: he must come close enough to recognize the patient fully.
>
> (Berger and Mohr 1997 [1967]: 113)

In this process of recognition, Sassall does more for his patients than treat them when they are ill; he becomes for Berger 'an objective witness of their lives' (Berger and Mohr 1997 [1967]: 109). Entrusted by the community with their most intimate, and at times most anguished, moments, he keeps the record of these experiences and so acts as a repository of memory for the community in which he works.

There is much that seems familiar to the contemporary eye in Balint and Berger, and their model for medical practice can be read as a prototype of current ideals for whole-person care and empathetic treatment. Nevertheless, we can also distinguish their work as emerging from its own particular historical moment. Both studies reflect a social context in which general practitioners can expect a long-term relationship with their patients; this underpins not only Berger's identification of the doctor as 'clerk of...records' (Berger and Mohr 1997 [1967]: 109), but also Balint's economic model of the doctor–patient relationship as a 'mutual investment company', in which 'capital assets' are built up over an extensive period of repeated consultations and treatments (Balint 1964 [1957]: 251). In this sense, Balint and Berger both capture a world that is vanishing; the stable communities that they document are already in the process of transforming into the more mobile, fractured social environments of the present. As I have also indicated, the model of narrative that is reflected in their work is similarly evocative of the specific time in which they were writing, locating its interest primarily in relation to the doctor's rather than the patient's experience.

While both Balint's and Berger's studies position the good doctor as closely attentive to patient narrative, they notably embed the process of empathetic listening within a psychoanalytic framework. The value of the therapeutic model, however, remains a topic of debate within the current field of the medical humanities. Attention has shifted in narrative medicine from psychoanalytic to literary training over the last 50 years, with the assumption that engaging with literary texts enhances empathetic capacities and leads in turn to humane and compassionate action. In closing this section, I propose to briefly indicate some main critical responses to the literary model that Charon advances. For Geoffrey Hartman, the first doubtful proposition is that empathy can be taught as a skill, and that literature can be mobilized in this direction. Hartman accordingly questions: 'Short of pharmaceutical treatment, . . . can there be empathy management, as we now have pain management? And what role could the arts play, in the light of our notorious ability to compartmentalize feelings?' (Hartman 2004: 339). Recent literary studies have also called into question whether empathy felt for literary characters translates into real-world action on behalf of others. Suzanne Keen sceptically remarks in *Empathy and the Novel*:

> I ask whether the effort of imagining fictive lives . . . can train a reader's sympathetic imagining of real others in her actual world, and I inquire how we might be able to tell if it happened. . . . I wonder whether the expenditure of shared feeling on fictional characters might not waste what little attention we have for others on nonexistent entities, or at best reveal that addicted readers are simply endowed with empathetic dispositions.
>
> (Keen 2007: xxv)

In a similar vein, Bert Keizer questions in the medical context whether reading a novel would enhance a doctor's empathy, and what its effect on medical practice might be:

> The idea that certain fictional approaches to illness would somehow improve a person's power of empathy is, I think, unfounded. . . . Fiction may tell a reader what it is like to be crazy, alcoholic, depressed, constipated, paralytic, epileptic, asthmatic, sleepless, frantic, exhausted, addicted, mad, demented or scared. It is unclear to me how this telling would contain a lesson in cases when the reader is a doctor.
>
> (Keizer 2003: n.p.)

Neither critic denies that as readers we can develop an empathetic identification with fictional characters; indeed, this is often a powerful effect of the literary. Rather, the question that they raise is precisely how this response is related to broader social action, whether this comprises altruistic deeds on behalf of others or improved medical care. For my own purposes, a central problem with Charon's narrative medicine, and its harnessing of the literary to empathetic training, is that it also implies a merely additive role for literature. It assumes, in the words of Jane Macnaughton, that literature 'helps doctors do what they are already doing in a more humane, empathic way', while leaving 'untouched' the assumptions, methodologies and practices of medicine itself (Macnaughton 2011: 928).

The rise of pathography

I have so far argued that in British medicine, the 1950s and 1960s were characterized by a predominant interest in narrative as it connected to the doctor's role in the clinical encounter, and by a methodological turn to language and psychoanalysis. We can, however, discern a decisive shift in the conception of narrative in the 1980s and 1990s. More recent accounts of narrative focus on its function in helping us to know and understand our social world, and on its constitutive relation to identity. The publication of Arthur Kleinman's *The Illness Narratives* (1988) acted, in Hydén's view, to give this particular conception of narrative currency within the medical sphere: '[f]or Kleinman the narrative is the form in which patients shape and give voice to their suffering' (Hydén 1997: 51). If illness is a profoundly disruptive experience, narrating the story of that illness can act as a means to give it meaning, to reconstruct the patient's identity and sense of relation to the world. Moreover, Kleinman drew attention to the patient's narrative as one of *suffering*; as Hydén elaborates, narrative becomes a vehicle not only to 'articulate suffering', but also to voice the illness experience 'apart from how illnesses are conceived and represented in biomedicine' (Hydén 1997: 51). These decades also witnessed the predominance of postmodern theory within the academy, and the widespread influence of ideas such as Jean-François Lyotard's (1984) account of the collapse of grand narratives, which were seen as no longer adequate to explain our knowledge and experience. Hydén observes that this translated in the medical context into 'doubts about the possibility of biomedicine to cure ills and relieve suffering' (Hydén 1997: 49). The way was thereby paved for illness narratives to challenge the voice of medicine, and for authority to shift from the doctor's expertise to the patient's experience. Further support for the newfound resistance of patient narratives to a perceived 'medical colonialism' (Tallis 2004: 2) arose from feminist and queer theory, and from the emerging field of disability studies.

The literary genre of pathography – autobiographical accounts of illness, or memoirs by partners, children or caregivers of those suffering from illness – is, as Roger Luckhurst has noted, 'a distinctly contemporary form' (Luckhurst 2008: 128). Coming to prominence with the AIDS crisis of the late 1980s and early 1990s, it subsequently burgeoned to encompass other illness narratives. In the UK, it found particular expression in the 1990s in 'newspaper columns devoted to the progress of an illness' (Luckhurst 2008: 130). The rise of pathography can clearly be related to the shifts in the conception of narrative analyzed above. It acted at once to focus attention on patient narrative and experience, to critique scientific biomedicine's concentration on disease rather than illness, and to protest the perceived distance and disengagement of medical professionals as well as broader institutional flaws and inequities. There are, nevertheless, other important aspects to pathography that are not encompassed in this description. John Wiltshire has astutely observed that pathography 'has a broader agenda than simply, like the postcolonial subject, to "write back" to the conquering imperialism of biomedicine' (Wiltshire 2000: 412–13). Rather, he focuses attention back on the pathography as illness narrative, noting that 'the raw material of pathography is illness, usually devastating or mortal illness', which involves 'the evacuation or stripping of meaning from both person and event' (Wiltshire 2000: 412–13).

Pathography differs from ordinary (auto)biography because its subject is not chosen: the pathographer often writes reluctantly and out of necessity. For the writer, then, the illness narrative is produced '[u]nder duress' and is shaped by 'contingency' (Wiltshire 2000: 414). For readers of pathographies, the narratives offer access to the dramas and dilemmas of life and death, which 'in our secular state we have now few other means of apprehending' (Wiltshire 2000: 15). For both writer and reader, then, pathography functions as the site of a limit experience, an encounter with (possible) death that engages powerful questions of consciousness, agency, and identity. Although Wiltshire notes that the narrative imperative of many pathographies 'is to make sense of this' in a 'proces[s] of meaning-creation' (Wiltshire 2000: 412–13), it is also the case that pathographies often falter, fail in, or actively resist this endeavour at mastery.

Jackie Stacey's *Teratologies: A Cultural Study of Cancer* (1997) is a (self-) reflective contribution to a genre of pathography that was already well developed. It is, as Franziska Gygax has observed, 'both an autobiographical illness narrative and a theoretical exploration of the cultural constructions of cancer' (2009: 291). A British academic specializing in women's studies and cultural studies, Stacey consciously writes her cancer narrative in the tradition of US feminists Audre Lorde (1980) and Eve Sedgwick (1993), emphasizing that the personal is also the political; that the retelling of her own experience necessarily opens out to broader cultural concerns or, as she phrases it, 'the meanings attributed to cancer in today's changing health cultures' (Stacey 1997: 25). Stacey opens her narrative by declaring, like Wiltshire, that what most patient accounts of cancer share in common is an impulse towards mastery, the imparting of knowledge snatched from the brink of collapse:

> If the person with cancer has lived to tell the tale, the story is often of a heroic struggle against adversity. Pitting life against death and drawing on all possible resources, the patient moves from victim to survivor and 'triumphs over the tragedy' that has unexpectedly threatened their

life.... The person who has faced death and yet still lives, who has recognised the inevitability of human mortality, now benefits from a new-found wisdom. Accepting the fragility of life itself, the cancer survivor sees things others are not brave enough to face (or so the story goes).

(Stacey 1997: 1)

Arthur W. Frank promulgated a particularly influential version of the 'story' that Stacey recounts in his typology of illness narratives, *The Wounded Storyteller* (1995). Here, Frank classified illness narratives into three categories – 'restitution', 'chaos', and 'quest' – which are also suggestive of a journey towards mastery in the patient. Hydén accordingly notes that the problem with Frank's model is that it advances 'a meta-narrative of illness: from "chaos" to "quest" ' (Hydén 1997: 54).

Against the closure and certainties that dominate the patient cancer stories that she turns to in her own illness, Stacey's narrative holds onto the 'chaos' experienced in illness. She places the desire for mastery that she encounters in illness narratives alongside the same impulse that she finds at work in both scientific medicine and self-help practices. In particular, Stacey makes clear that the prevailing rhetoric of control stands in painful opposition to the multiple, often contradictory, theories of cancer with which the sick person is confronted. Individual responsibility for health can be empowering, she acknowledges, but it can equally be overpowering, resulting in the patient's feeling confused and overwhelmed. Against the multiple narratives of certainty that surround cancer, which encompass the patient, the medical clinician, and the self-help manual, the theoretical sections of Stacey's book become, in the eloquent words of Gygax, 'exercises in searching and challenging, charged with uncertainty rather than mastery' (Gygax 2009: 298). Stacey's conclusion positions 'mystery' in opposition to 'mastery', and confronts biomedicine with the need to tolerate mystery as something other than 'an object to be known'; to more fully encounter that which resists meaning, and which is not predictable in outcome (Stacey 1997: 238). In her own autopathography, therefore, Stacey (re)orients theory away from definite answers and towards questioning; she thereby confronts contemporary medicine with a powerful contradiction between the rhetoric of (self-)mastery that it preaches, and the uncertainty if not outright confusion that can result in practice.

In what follows, I propose that Stacey's study is indicative of a possible route towards a more integrated approach to the literary in the medical humanities. First, the *form* of Stacey's study, which mixes autobiography and theory, indicates the potential for the field to engage with an expanded notion of literary genre, encompassing more fragmentary or mixed-media narrative modes. Hartman takes up this point, noting: 'more could be done in the medical humanities with different aspects of literature, not only its narrative component' (Hartman 2004: 342). Within this volume, we can turn to Ian Williams' analysis of the graphic pathography, as well as the broader attention paid to art, music, and drama alongside literature, as productive examples of this kind of work. Stacey's dwelling upon, and within, the more chaotic and contingent aspects of her experience is also suggestive that there are dimensions of illness that do not readily conform to conventional narrative modes. In mixing literary modes, Stacey indicates that her cancer experience is elusive to expression; that a single literary form can go so far, but then a switch to an alternative genre is required. Returning to Hartman, he argues that the medical humanities should 'be sensitive also to nonnarrative, apparently inconsequential or lyrical moments, surprises in the narrator's mood and mode' (Hartman 2004: 343). Against a predominant emphasis on realist fiction and autobiography, Hartman indicates that we could productively also incorporate more poetic and experimental genres, as well as attending carefully to moments of narrative disjunction and discontinuity. Rather than subscribing to a dominant impulse towards meaning and control, we might then also benefit from what the literary can reveal to us about what it means to live in a condition of *un*certainty.

Stacey's compelling critique of the impulse towards mastery across illness narratives and medical/alternative therapies also indicates that, in addressing what the literary can tell us about how we are potentially undone by illness, we might also reorient medicine itself. Kathryn Montgomery has recently examined the extent to which medicine is a discourse of mastery. In spite of its reliance on 'a well-stocked fund of scientific knowledge and its use of technology', Montgomery argues, medicine is 'not itself a science' but rather 'a practice: the care of sick people' (Montgomery 2006: 3). Montgomery's reorientation of medicine towards treatment places emphasis on how general rules – scientific principles or clinical guidelines – apply to the particular patient. In other words, medicine's core activity is one of 'interpretive practice', which renders it a 'still uncertain quest' and one characterized above all by 'contingency' (Montgomery 2006: 4–5). A more expansive sense of the literary might, then, potentially also open up a more integrated approach to literature in the medical humanities; one which enables us to address medicine's own inherent uncertainties, and the skills of interpretative reading that it accordingly requires of its practitioners.

Emerging at the same time as the medical humanities in the UK, the genre of pathography can be seen to share many of the same concerns: to refocus attention on the patient narrative, to voice experiences that are too often occluded from the medical account, and at times to challenge and contest biomedical practices. It is unsurprising, then, that the medical humanities have readily incorporated pathography into teaching curricula. Paul Crawford and Charley Baker accordingly privilege pathography over fictional narrative for medical professionals because of its focus on 'actual experiences as opposed to created, imagined experience' (Crawford and Baker 2009: 247). They are particularly concerned with psychiatric training and pathographies of mental illness can, they argue, provide insight into 'the traumatising experience of mental illness' and help the trainee practitioner to 'get a sense of what it might be like to be depressed, addicted to drugs or disrupted by psychosis' (Crawford and Baker 2009: 253–4). If the medical humanities have embraced the genre of pathography, then, it is valued primarily as a vehicle to mobilize the practitioner's empathetic understanding. I have suggested in this section, however, that pathography can be, and do, more than this. It can lead us beyond conventional narrative forms to more experimental, mixed-media modes and genres.

I do not wish to claim that these kinds of texts are a privileged mode for representing illness, which circulates across all forms of cultural production. There is, nevertheless, arguably something about such works – and about attending to disruptive and disconnected moments in more conventional accounts – that can open up important aspects of the patient experience. Pathography can also signal the ways in which illness often challenges – and reveals as illusory – discourses of mastery, whether they emerge from the patient, the doctor, or the self-help manual. In so doing, it signals a more integrated role for the literary in the medical humanities, which would be centrally concerned with the literary and the medical as inherently contingent modes. Shared affinities between the medical and the literary operate not only at an emotional level (how doctors feel), but also at an interpretive level (how doctors think). Rather than harnessing literature to an existing agenda, in which empathy is treated as yet another skill for doctors to master, we might therefore productively connect clinical diagnosis and literary reading as necessarily uncertain, yet essential, modes of interpretative practice.

Arts in healthcare

I have so far examined major shifts in the conception of narrative prior to, and coincident with, the emergence of the medical humanities in the early 1990s, in order to trace the roots of the medical humanities from a specifically literary perspective. The establishment of the medical humanities as an identifiable field of study dates in the UK from the 1990s, however, and in the remainder of my chapter I accordingly turn to the 1990s and 2000s with the aim of outlining what I see as the main challenges for, and areas of potential within, the current field. In this section, I focus on the arts in healthcare movement. Fiona Hamilton further explores this movement within this volume, bringing a practitioner's perspective to bear on her literature and medicine case study. My own discussion identifies the arts in healthcare movement as one of significant potential, but also as a strand of the medical humanities that reveals one of its most formidable challenges. My closing section then goes on to examine the current shift towards a critical medical humanities, and to ask how that development might potentially (re)shape the present field of study.

The medical humanities are broadly understood to encompass the burgeoning arts in healthcare movement, and the naming of the disciplinary field – its inherent privileging of medicine over health, and of the humanities over the arts – has accordingly become a vital subject of contention and debate. The arts in health movement has recently moved in the UK from what Macnaughton *et al.* describe as 'a small, local and poorly resourced movement fuelled by deeply committed artists, involved health-care professionals, and participants' (Macnaughton *et al.* 2005: 337) to a more diverse field, operating in a variety of healthcare contexts and with newly emergent areas of specialist expertise. Indeed, such has been the reported success of arts in healthcare initiatives that the Department of Health report to review arts in health in 2007 found that: 'arts and health initiatives are delivering real and measurable benefits across a wide range of priority areas for health' (Crown, 2007).

With regard to literature specifically, arts in health initiatives are focused on creative writing workshops delivered across a wide range of healthcare settings and to professionals as well as patients. There has also been significant activity around shared reading, emerging from the initiatives of the Reader Organisation in Liverpool, that have now spread nationwide. In spite of numerous endorsements of the field, however, a major challenge remains in defining exactly how the success of such initiatives might be measured or evaluated, and according to what criteria. In assessing arts in healthcare projects, Macnaughton *et al.* explain that practitioners typically accept it as unrealistic 'to aim at directly measurable health gain', because this usually entails 'locating some numerically assessable physical change' (Macnaughton *et al.* 2005: 335). Part of the problem, they point out, is that the success of arts in health projects is typically based in a diverse range of factors, which encompass not only the arts activity itself, but also the relationships between all of those involved in the project, how it is delivered, and the environment within which it is performed. To access evidence of all of these gains, practitioners often 'fall back on the voluntary testimony of participants themselves, which can readily be dismissed as "soft"' (Macnaughton *et al.* 2005: 336). The arts in health movement seems, therefore, to be caught in an intractable situation, which Macnaughton *et al.* summarize as follows:

> Unless [the arts in health movement] produces an appropriate evidence base for its work it will not gain access to better sources of funding from the health sector, and because it does not have access to sufficient funding it is struggling to work up this evidence base. The bind tightens when arts and health projects attempt to approach evaluation of their work in a way that satisfies the health sector's view of what constitutes appropriate evidence.
>
> (Macnaughton *et al.* 2005: 338)

In confronting this double bind, Macnaughton *et al.* recommend that the field adopt a robust approach, which would involve 'stak[ing] its claim to the research context in which it is operating' rather than 'trying to appease potential funding bodies by forcing the field into the straitjacket of a medical model of research' (Macnaughton *et al.* 2005: 338).

While I agree that it is vital to define and defend what is distinctive about research in the arts and humanities, I am also wary of a potential disciplinary entrenchment that further reinforces the divide between arts and sciences. If personal accounts and qualitative research studies are insufficient to convince funding bodies of the success of arts initiatives, creative and collaborative thinking is needed from both the humanities and medicine in order to formulate innovative criteria of evaluation. One area in which such conversations are currently taking place is the new brain-imaging technologies. These offer the potential to measure what happens in the brain when, for example, people write, read out, or respond to a poem, and therefore begin to bridge arts and humanities research and medical paradigms of evidence. At the same time, it is important that the conversation on brain imaging does not become one-sided, with scholars in the humanities simply absorbing medical technologies into their own research practice and accepting at face value the rhetoric of proof that surrounds them. This is a technology, after all, that produces images or representations that should themselves be interrogated aesthetically, culturally, socially, and historically, and with critical attention to how such images are read (Daston and Galison 1992). It is not only, then, that arts in health can play an additive role in medicine, enhancing healthcare environments and service provision; the arts and humanities can also intervene critically, as Sander L. Gilman has recently suggested, engaging with medical representations 'not to show their duplicity or truth but to reveal their function in their historical context' (Gilman 2011: 73). Here again, it seems, a more integrated potential for the humanities in relation to medicine might potentially be located.

This section has used the example of the arts in health movement in order to identify a major challenge posed to the medical humanities by questions of value, evidence, proof, and measurability. While endorsing the call by Macnaughton *et al.* for the arts and humanities to defend their own practices and methodologies, I also suggest that the medical humanities might offer a fruitful context for both the humanities and medicine to articulate what it is that they do, and to rethink how their respective areas of expertise might most productively intersect. In the following section, I examine the rise of the critical medical humanities in particular as a key forum for the furthering of such an agenda, focusing on its turn away from the treatment dynamic of practitioner-patient, around which our discussion has so far been focused, and towards a redefinition of the human in both individual and social terms. I will identify in my discussion two main works of recent British fiction that can be productively linked to the critical medical humanities, namely Kazuo Ishiguro's *Never Let Me Go* (2005) and Ian McEwan's *Saturday* (2005).

The rise of the critical medical humanities

In this section, I seek to propose an alternative mode by which the literary might be positioned in relation to contemporary medicine, by focusing on the emergence of the critical medical humanities. As the field shifts, its focus is moving away from the education of the medical practitioner and towards a more critical, analytical, and politicized account not only of the human, but also of a notably technologized biomedicine. In doing so, the field is establishing itself within a multi-disciplinary base, bringing to its engagement with the medical insights drawn from disciplines as diverse as philosophy, narrative and film theory, critical neuroscience, and medical anthropology. A first implication of this work that can be noted, then, is that it challenges thinking along disciplinary lines; a broad interdisciplinary perspective is needed, which in turn calls into question whether we can still speak of a specifically 'literary' perspective on the medical humanities. In what follows, I nevertheless analyze the critical medical humanities through examination of Kazuo Ishiguro's *Never Let Me Go* and Ian McEwan's *Saturday*, with a focus on biomedicine and the brain sciences. However, my discussion of the field has wider implications. It is also applicable to Patricia Norvillo-Corvalán's chapter within this section, which shows how the literary reinterpretation of myths has been used for the purposes of cultural and political critique. Within this critical analytical model, the medical humanities are not conceptualized in purely humanizing or humanistic terms.

I turn first to Patricia Waugh's astute analysis of what current literature might have to offer to science. In surveying contemporary fiction, Waugh notes that new developments in science have significantly invigorated the novel genre: 'the vocabularies, images and ideas' of recent scientific discoveries have, she argues, 'stimulated an important... "fantastic" turn in literature itself' (Waugh 1997: 158). What, then, might literary fiction offer to science in return? Waugh herself offers a decisive answer to this question, by positioning imaginative fiction as an important site for the exploration of ideas and for rethinking the familiar:

> Possible worlds, the radically heterogeneous, the other, can most effectively disturb our settled modes of thought and unconscious prejudices when they are embodied, fleshed out, made available for recognition and empathy. Only when given such form can they linger on, continuing to disturb the familiar, leaving unresolved the implications of that disturbance.
>
> (Waugh 1997: 158)

It is notable, then, that if Waugh turns specifically to the narrative form of the novel, it is not to conventionally realist texts that she looks, but to more experimental, imaginative, and fantastical works of fiction.

Written in 1997, Waugh's observations predate the publication of Ishiguro's *Never Let Me Go* by almost a decade. Nevertheless, her description is remarkably evocative in relation to Ishiguro's depiction of an alternative England of the 1990s, which uncannily mirrors our own reality in order to provoke unsettling questions concerning both the nature of the human, and contemporary scientific biomedicine and the institutions of care. It is, to adopt Waugh's terminology, through 'fleshing out' his 'possible world' with Kathy H. and the other clones that Ishiguro achieves the remarkable effects of the novel, as these embodied presences do indeed 'linger on' for readers after the novel's close, haunting and disturbing 'familiar' and 'settled' modes of thought. A particular strength of the novel form, in this context, lies in its capacity to enable us to encounter, through extended interior narrative, another mind and the world as it is constituted by that mind. As we read Kathy H's narrative, we are at once immersed in her story-world and distanced from it through defamiliarization, which works effectively in turn to give us compassion for her at the same time as we question critically the nature and limits of the human. This capacity of the novel to draw us in through recognition, while at the same time causing us to rethink our inherent assumptions, has been powerfully explored and articulated by contemporary narratological critics such as David Herman (2002, 2011) and Alan Palmer (2008), whose work on the narrative representation of consciousness, and in particular on the interaction of the fictional mind and the reader's mind, has proved valuable in reorienting the relation between medicine and literature.

In relation to contemporary biomedicine, Gabriele Griffin has noted that *Never Let Me Go* coalesces 'a number of different but interrelated biotechnological developments – cloning, organ harvesting, designer babies – into one set of fictional preoccupations' (Griffin 2009: 649). Rather than reflecting biotechnology faithfully, however, Ishiguro's novel deliberately marks its own departure from science. Griffin observes that this is achieved in the first instance through an explicit disinterest in how the science of cloning actually works; although Kathy and the other students relate various theories about their 'possibles' – the people from whom they have been cloned – these remain only stories, and the novel notably avoids the technical vocabulary that is usually associated with the science-fiction genre. More than this, however, Griffin observes that Ishiguro consciously embeds into his fiction 'a gap . . . between biotechnological developments and their representation' (Griffin 2009: 649). Thus, even as science begins to move towards the engineering of human tissue, rendering obsolete the need to rely on complete organs for transplantation, Ishiguro sets out in the opposite direction, imagining the cloning of people. The space that is thereby opened up enables Ishiguro to focus his reader's attention not on the actuality of biomedical practice, but on the moral and ethical matters that it raises; in other words, his fiction provides a site for reflecting on, rather than for simply mirroring, contemporary scientific developments.

While Griffin's emphasis is on Ishiguro's engagement with biomedicine, I have argued elsewhere that he deploys the same strategy of defamiliarization to reflect on contemporary institutions of care (Whitehead 2011). The run-down and underfunded recovery centres that the donors of Ishiguro's novel inhabit represent a bleak reworking of the contemporary British landscape of privatized care homes and centres, which, in the words of Tony Judt, have 'reduced the quality of service to the minimum in order to increase profits and dividends' (Judt 2010: 114). The word which is placed under most pressure in the novel, and which takes on sinister overtones from the very opening page, is 'carer'. In *Never Let Me Go*, the reader learns that this seemingly innocuous word conceals the terrible reality that, within this alternative England, children are cloned, raised in isolation from other children, and on reaching adulthood have their organs harvested in a series of operations in order to treat human diseases. Again, although this clearly does not reflect historical actuality, we can recognize in it not only an established international trade in organ harvesting but also the scandal-hit care institutions of the UK, in which the word 'care' has too often concealed hidden histories of cruelty and abuse. Ishiguro's novel therefore holds up an uncanny, distorted mirror to British medical practices and institutions, providing readers with a space for reflection on a bureaucratized materialism that shadows our own reality and that exists in contiguity – if not in continuity – with our own social and political world. In this sense, then, *Never Let Me Go* intersects with and illuminates the more politicized dimensions of the critical medical humanities, which are concerned with how new medical technologies can negatively transform landscapes and processes of treatment, as well as commodifying the relation of care itself.

Ian McEwan's *Saturday* offers an alternative, although complementary, insight into the current field of the medical humanities. Although in many ways a straightforwardly realist novel, McEwan's narrative of a day in the life of Henry Perowne has nevertheless been defined by critics as experimental in standing at the forefront of the burgeoning genre of the neuronovel. Laura Salisbury has accordingly noted that if the novel has traditionally concerned itself with 'the penetration of another consciousness', McEwan's recent fiction has 'repeatedly offered up scientised reconfigurations of this moment of aesthetic sensibility' (Salisbury 2010: 884); while Dominic Head, commenting specifically on McEwan's reworking of the modernist stream of consciousness novel – the spanning of a day nods both to James Joyce's *Ulysses* (1922) and to Virginia Woolf's *Mrs Dalloway* (1925) – observes that the novelist is 'trying to produce, perhaps, a diagnostic "slice of mind" novel – working towards the literary equivalent of a computed tomography (CT) scan – rather than a modernist "slice of life" novel' (Head 2007: 192). What is immediately apparent, then, is that McEwan holds up for inspection the role and remit of the contemporary novel, suggesting that it can and should be responsive to changing scientific views of consciousness and cognition; literature, in other words, is inseparable from other disciplines, which thereby intersect with and inform each other.

My comments so far have suggested that McEwan is responsive to developments in cognitive science, seeking ways in which to embed them into narrative discourse. Yet, in line with the impetus of the critical medical humanities, critics have also indicated that there is a more reciprocal relation between the novel and neuroscience than this implies. Thus, Jonah Lehrer has positioned *Saturday* as the genesis of a new cultural movement, 'a new fourth culture, one that seeks to discover relationships *between* the humanities and the sciences' (Lehrer 2007: 196; original emphasis), while Susan Green affirms that the novel reflects 'the new momentum between the sciences and the humanities giving rise to the interdisciplinary study of the mind – cognitive science' (Green 2010: 58). If these claims are valid, then *Saturday* assumes particular significance in relation to a further strand of the critical medical humanities, which brings contemporary neuroscience into dialogue with a renewed turn to phenomenology in the work of philosophers such as Shaun Gallagher (2005) and Dan Zahavi (2008), together with narratological explorations of how we understand and interact with fictional minds by critics such as Herman, Palmer, and Monika Fludernik (1996).

Although it is beyond the scope of this chapter to produce an extended reading of *Saturday*, it might nevertheless be worth pausing over the novel's opening lines to ponder what they suggest about contemporary literature's 'penetration of another consciousness', to borrow Salisbury's phrase:

> Some hours before dawn Henry Perowne, a neurosurgeon, wakes to find himself already in motion, pushing back the covers from a sitting position, and then rising to his feet. It's not clear to him when exactly he became conscious, nor does it seem relevant. He's never done such a thing before, but he isn't alarmed or even faintly surprised, for the movement is easy, and pleasurable in his limbs, and his legs and back feel unusually strong. He stands there, naked by the bed – he always sleeps naked – feeling his full height, aware of his wife's patient breathing and of the wintry bedroom air on his skin. That too is a pleasurable sensation. His bedside clock shows three forty. He has no idea what he's doing out of bed: he has no need to relieve himself, nor is he disturbed by a dream or some element of the day before, or even by the state of the world. It's as if, standing there, he's materialised out of nothing, fully formed, unencumbered.
>
> (McEwan 2005: 3)

I noted in the previous section that the new brain-imaging technologies are proving fertile ground for the intersection of medicine and the humanities. In the opening sentence of his novel, McEwan establishes this connection as his neurosurgeon protagonist reflects on his own coming to consciousness. Returning to Head, we can say that McEwan is offering us 'the literary equivalent of a CT scan' (Head 2007: 192); if the scan can show us cognitive activity, however, the novel explores what it feels like – it gives us a crucial subjective dimension. In so doing, the passage notably takes on an unmistakable phenomenological aspect: firstly, Perowne's mind is necessarily embodied, so that any narrative of his cognition has to take into account, more or less consciously, his physical and sensory experiences; secondly, conscious or cognitive experience here follows the physical, or in the words of Gallagher, 'the body anticipates and sets the stage for consciousness' (Gallagher 2005: 2); and finally, embodied cognition entails that consciousness leads out to engagement with the world and with others: it is not, in other words, a solipsistic experience. The novel's opening also clearly gestures towards the narratalogical – Perowne's coming to consciousness is also the coming into being of his fictional mind. He has indeed, in this sense, 'materialised out of nothing, fully formed' for the reader on the page; but the reader is also left to question throughout the novel the precise form that is taken by this act of 'materialisation'. The following questions are accordingly central to McEwan's recent work of fiction: How exactly do we interact with the mind of Perowne? To what extent do we immerse ourselves in his storyworld? What is at stake in entering another's consciousness through the act of reading? In this sense, then, we can position *Saturday* as a novel that is highly resonant with the critical medical humanities, not least in its self-reflexive intermingling of narrative, scientific, and philosophical accounts of consciousness and cognition.

This section has offered an approach to the literary which stands in deliberate contrast to the mode of reading often regarded as characteristic of the medical humanities. I have focused on two novels, both of which demonstrate aspects of formal experimentation. My discussion of Ishiguro's *Never Let Me Go* draws on Waugh to emphasize that more fantastic works of fiction can allow space, in her terms, for 'cognitive estrangement without the burden of scientific proof' (Waugh 1997: 159). I have suggested that within the alternative worlds embodied in imaginative fiction, ideas are rendered strange in ways that can open up space for reflection and critique, or can even potentially, to return to Waugh, 'actually create that for which there was previously no concept or idea' (Waugh 1997: 159). In Ishiguro, this space of reflection opens up questions, central to the critical medical humanities, concerning the nature and limits of the human, as well as the material and political effects of biomedical technologization. My reading of McEwan's *Saturday* indicated a further area of current research, namely the interdisciplinary study of the theory of mind. Not only does this work enrich the form of the novel itself, but the act of reading – our pleasurable interaction with fictional minds – can also stimulate in turn important questions of cognition and of empathy.

Conclusion

In this chapter I have argued that the first wave of the medical humanities, here encapsulated by Charon's narrative medicine, has developed a distinctive but restricted approach to literature, both in terms of the canon of texts – predominantly realist fiction and autobiography – that it integrates into teaching curricula; and in its hermeneutic approach, which espouses a somewhat traditional attitude to the humanities as humanizing, and emphasizes a model of reader empathy leading directly to compassionate action. I have sought to open up a number of approaches by which this conception of the literary might usefully be expanded, although it is intended that my suggestions should be read as indicative rather than exhaustive in nature. Following Hartman, I have indicated that mixed media, fragmentary, and experimental texts also provide a productive mode for examining how experiences of illness and pain might be represented in literary form. I have proposed that literature can fruitfully intersect with medicine in opening up the uncertain and contingent; in this sense, drawing on Montgomery, it might help to reorient medical practice itself away from the rhetoric of scientific certainty and towards interpretive reading and thinking. Turning to more recent developments in the field, I focused first on the arts in healthcare movement, which has launched a range of Creative Writing initiatives across a variety of institutional settings, and has been widely recognized as beneficial to health and well-being. However, initiatives have notably struggled to provide an evidence base to measure value in a way that is acceptable to funding bodies, and I have argued that both creative and collaborative thinking is needed in this area. I ended by examining the second wave of the medical humanities, namely the critical medical humanities, which are explicitly concerned to move away from a focus on questions of practitioner pedagogy and training, and to situate themselves instead in a more critical and analytical relation to medicine. If this development in the field is indicative of its future direction, then we will see a more politicized, a more theorized, and a more radically interdisciplinary field coming into view.

In closing, I turn to Gilman's recent diagnosis of the current state of the humanities. In these straitened financial times, he argues, both creative and constructive thinking are required within the academy. 'We need to think more intensely', he observes, 'how our wider theoretical expertise can, indeed must, mesh with alternative forms for the presentation of humanities knowledge and experience'. Gilman contends that the potential for such thinking already exists, albeit 'still in a tentative way', in the field of the medical humanities (Gilman 2004: 387). Gilman's rapid sketch of the field provides an accurate summary of its priorities in the first wave of activity; he notes that it has embraced narrative 'as an inherent compo-nent of pedagogy', that the 'act of reading' has become a mode through which 'young physicians are trained', and that it has claimed 'the tools of interpretation' as 'inherent to the [medical] profession itself' (2004: 386). My chapter has sought to build on these 'tentative' beginnings, and to iden-tify potential areas for future work, although this has necessarily entailed moving beyond the literary to some degree. To some extent, I share Gilman's optimistic sense of what might be possible over the next decade or so. 'Times of stress', he points out, 'should enable us to rethink in ways that times of excess do not'. He crucially adds, however: 'Here the role of the humanities should be paramount' (Gilman 2004: 389). To date, the medical humanities have tended to be dominated by the needs and priori-ties of medicine itself. It remains to be seen whether a more truly collaborative enterprise can grow out of the activity in the critical medical humanities, creating a field that expands beyond the more immediate concerns of training and pedagogy to explore the multiple and complex ways in which medicine and the humanities might interact critically and analytically with one another.

Acknowledgments

I would like to acknowledge here the colleagues at the Universities of Newcastle and Durham with whom I am working in the area of the critical medical humanities: Sarah Atkinson, Jane Macnaughton, Jennifer Richards, Patricia Waugh, and Angela Woods. The usual caveat naturally applies: that the views expressed here and the responsibility for any errors or misstatements are entirely my own.

Notes

1   Although I have started my narrative with Charon, the texts which first paid extended attention to narrative medicine were, in the US, Montgomery Hunter (1991) and in the UK Greenhalgh and Hurwitz (1998).
2   This connection is not purely literary. On the visual aspects of Balint, Berger and Mohr, see Ludmilla Jordanova's chapter within this volume.

References

Balint, M. (1964 [1957]) *The Doctor, His Patient and the Illness*, 2nd edn, Edinburgh and London: Churchill Livingstone.
Berger, J. and Mohr, J. (1997 [1967]) *A Fortunate Man: The Story of a Country Doctor*, New York: Vintage.
Carson, R. A. (2007) 'Engaged Humanities: Moral Work in the Precincts of Medicine', *Perspectives in Biology and Medicine*, 50: 321–33.
Crawford, P. and Baker, C. (2009) 'Literature and Madness: Fiction for Students and Professionals', *Journal of Medical Humanities*, 30: 237–51.

Charon, R. (2006) *Narrative Medicine: Honoring the Stories of Illness*, Oxford and New York: Oxford University Press.

Charon, R. (2000) 'Literature and Medicine: Origins and Destinies', *Academic Medicine*, 75: 23–7.

Crown (2007) 'Report of the Review of the Arts and Working Health Group', Department of Health, 4 April. Online. Available: http://webarchive.national archives.gov.uk/20130107105354/ http://www.dh.gov.uk/en/Publicationsand statistics/Publications/PublicationsPolicyAndGuidance/DH_073590 (accessed on 18 May 2013).

Daston, L. and Galison, P. (1992) 'The Image of Objectivity', *Representations*, 40: 81–128.

Evans, M. and Greaves, D. (1999) 'Exploring the Medical Humanities', *British Medical Journal*, 319: 1216.

Fludernik, M. (1996) *Towards a 'Natural' Narratology*, London and New York: Routledge.

Frank, A. W. (1995) *The Wounded Storyteller: Body, Illness, and Ethics*, Chicago, IL: Chicago University Press.

Gallagher, S. (2005) *How the Body Shapes the Mind*, Oxford: Clarendon Press.

Gilman, S. L. (2004) 'Collaboration, the Economy, and the Future of the Humanities', *Critical Inquiry*, 30: 384–90.

Gilman, S. L. (2011) 'Representing Health and Illness: Thoughts for the 21st Century', *Journal of Medical Humanities*, 32: 69–75.

Green, S. (2010) 'Consciousness and Ian McEwan's *Saturday*: "What Henry Knows" ', *English Studies*, 91: 58–73.

Greenhalgh, T. and Hurwitz, B. (eds) (1998) *Narrative Based Medicine: Dialogue and Discourse in Clinical Practice*, London: BMJ Press.

Griffin, G. (2009) 'Science and the Cultural Imaginary: The Case of Kazuo Ishiguro's *Never Let Me Go*', *Textual Practice*, 23: 645–63.

Gygax, F. (2009) 'Life Writing and Illness', *Prose Studies*, 31: 291–99.

Hartman, G. (2004) 'Narrative and Beyond', *Literature and Medicine*, 23: 334 –45.

Head, D. (2007) *Ian McEwan*, Manchester: Manchester University Press.

Herman, D. (2002) *Story Logic: Problems and Possibilities of Narrative*, Lincoln and London: University of Nebraska Press.

Herman, D. (ed.) (2011) *The Emergence of Mind: Representations of Consciousness in Narrative Discourse in English*, Lincoln and London: University of Nebraska Press.

Hydén, L.-C. (1997) 'Illness and Narrative', *Sociology of Health and Illness*, 19: 48–69.

Hydén, L.-C. and Mishler, E. G. (1999) 'Language and Medicine', *Annual Review of Applied Linguistics*, 19: 174–92.

Ishiguro, K. (2005) *Never Let Me Go*, London: Faber.

Judt, T. (2010) *Ill Fares the Land*, New York: Penguin.

Keen, S. (2007) *Empathy and the Novel*, Oxford and New York: Oxford University Press.

Keizer, B. (2003) 'Tales of Empathy', *Threepenny Review*, 94: unpaginated.

Kleinman, A. (1988) *The Illness Narratives: Suffering, Healing, and the Human Condition*, New York: Basic Books.

Lehrer, J. (2007) *Proust Was a Neuroscientist*, Edinburgh: Canongate.

Lorde, A. (1980) *The Cancer Journals*, San Francisco, CA: Aunt Lute Books.

Luckhurst, R. (2008) *The Trauma Question*, London and New York: Routledge.

Lyotard, J.-F. (1984) *The Postmodern Condition*, Manchester: Manchester University Press.

Macnaughton, J. (2011) 'Medical Humanities' Challenge to Medicine', *Journal of Evaluation in Clinical Practice*, 17: 927–32.

Macnaughton, J., White, M. and Stacy, R. (2005) 'Researching the Benefits of Arts in Health', *Health Education*, 105: 332–39.

McEwan, I. (2005) *Saturday*, London: Jonathan Cape.

Montgomery, K. (2006) *How Doctors Think: Clinical Judgment and the Practice of Medicine*, Oxford: Oxford University Press.

Montgomery Hunter, K. (1991) *Doctors' Stories: The Narrative Structure of Medical Knowledge*, Princeton, NJ: Princeton University Press.

Palmer, A. (2008) *Fictional Minds*, Lincoln and London: University of Nebraska Press.

Salisbury, L. (2010) 'Narration and Neurology: Ian McEwan's Mother Tongue', *Textual Practice*, 24: 883–912.

Sedgwick, E. (1993) *Tendencies*, Durham, NC: Duke University Press.

Stacey, J. (1997) *Teratologies: A Cultural Study of Cancer*, London and New York: Routledge.

Tallis, R. (2004) *Hippocratic Oaths: Medicine and Its Discontents*, London: Atlantic Books.

Waugh, P. (1997) 'The New Prometheans: Literature, Criticism, and Science in the Modern and Postmodern Condition', *European Journal of English Studies*, 1: 139–64.

Whitehead, A. (2011) 'Writing with Care: Kazuo Ishiguro's *Never Let Me Go*', *Contemporary Literature*, 52: 54–83.

Wiltshire, J. (2000) 'Biography, Pathography, and the Recovery of Meaning', *The Cambridge Quarterly*, 29: 409–22.

Zahavi, D. (2008) *Subjectivity and Selfhood: Investigating the First-Person Perspective*, Cambridge, MA: MIT.

8 Reinterpreting the wound of Philoctetes

Literature and medicine

Case study

Patricia Novillo-Corvalán

This chapter explores the contemporary relevance of the foundational myth of Philoctetes, in Britain and beyond. It shows how the twentieth-century reception of this myth can provide valuable insights into the ways in which different practices – from Ancient Greek medicine to postwar medicine to the Afro-Caribbean Obeah healing tradition – can help to alleviate chronic pain, comfort the patient, and offer the promise of a cure within the historical and social contexts in which they operate. As one of the greatest archetypes of physical disability in literature, the story of the wounded Philoctetes (in its Ancient Greek and more recent versions) is of increasing importance to the emerging field of the medical humanities, a point that I develop in the opening part of this chapter. This is followed by a twofold reassessment of the myth. In the first section, I examine the legacy of Asclepian temple medicine through a close reading of Sophocles' *Philoctetes* within the cultural, medical, and religious context of fifth-century Greece. In the second section, I map a cross-cultural terrain across Britain, Ireland, and Saint Lucia, particularly focusing on literary appropriations of Philoctetes by the poets Seamus Heaney and Derek Walcott. At the same time, this creative engagement with the topos of the archetypal figure of the wounded and long-suffering hero raises important questions that will be addressed throughout the chapter. Why have contemporary writers participated in the retelling of a story of illness and disability? How have they engaged with their own medical and cultural traditions in their rewritings of Sophocles? And, finally, what can these newer versions of Philoctetes add to our understanding of chronic pain, and the way in which different societies cure and comfort the sick?

Rethinking Philoctetes for the medical humanities

The myth of the Greek hero Philoctetes stands as one of the earliest depictions of physiological illness to have merited literary treatment. The greatest Attic tragedians – Aeschylus, Sophocles, and Euripides – produced their own versions of the myth, although only Sophocles'

Philoctetes has survived (produced in 409 BCE). According to the version by Sophocles, Philoctetes was bitten on the foot by a snake on his way to Troy, as he unwittingly trespassed into the sacred shrine of the goddess Chryse. The wound became infected, emitted a foul odour, and caused Philoctetes to experience generalized seizures. The Greek army mercilessly abandoned him on the deserted island of Lemnos, partly because Philoctetes' divinely inflicted wound stood as a sign of the wrath of the gods, but mainly because his fellow warriors could not tolerate his awful stench and agonizing cries of pain. The accursed hero endured his enforced exile and incurable wound, surviving with the aid of the supernatural bow of Heracles, which he inherited as a reward for helping him light a funeral pyre. After a decade of misery and solitude, the Greek army recalls Philoctetes because a prophecy revealed that the Trojan War could not be won without the famous archer and his legendary bow. Thus, Philoctetes is eventually led back to the besieged Troy, where the sons of Asclepius, the physicians Machaon and Podalirius, experts on treating wounds, heal his foot.

It should be pointed out, however, that compared with other tragedies by Sophocles – mainly the Theban cycle – *Philoctetes* remains a marginal work, having failed to attract the stage performances or the amount of critical scrutiny that has been assiduously devoted to *Oedipus Rex* or *Antigone*, not least Freud's appropriation of the former as the paradigmatic myth for the field of psychoanalysis. Yet this long overdue literary neglect has been readdressed and reconsidered in the second half of the twentieth century, as writers and critics across the world rediscovered the significance of Sophocles' tragedy about physical pain by producing a proliferation of translations, rewritings, and adaptations of the wounded Greek hero. The revival of the myth of Philoctetes as a contemporary story of suffering is largely indebted to Edmund Wilson's seminal essay 'The Wound and the Bow' (1941), in which he insightfully explores the interplay between illness and creativity, genius and disease, and art and healing that lies at the heart of the legend.[1] Wilson diagnoses Philoctetes as 'the victim of a malodorous disease which renders him abhorrent to society', on the one hand, and as 'the master of a superhuman art which everybody has to respect and which the normal man finds he needs', on the other (Wilson 1941: 294). For Wilson, therefore, the crux of the drama lies precisely in the conception of a disabled hero with a unique gift, thus turning Philoctetes into a symbol for both personal and social healing. Just as the sons of Asclepius will cure Philoctetes' wound, so the diseased archer and his divine bow will cure the ailing body politic.

Moreover, a number of contemporary critics working at the interface between literature and medicine have followed in Wilson's footsteps by similarly exploring the contemporary significance of the tragedy. In her much-acclaimed study *The Body in Pain* (1985), Elaine Scarry repeatedly evokes the figure of the wounded Greek hero, elevating Philoctetes as one of the most powerful representations of the sick body on stage, especially since Sophocles' play empowers 'the nature of the human body, the wound in that body, the pain in that wound' (Scarry 1985: 10). In *The Culture of Pain* (1991), a study that offers a comprehensive examination of the representation of pain in literature and culture, David B. Morris puts forward another significant examination of the myth. Morris continues and develops Scarry's discussion of the cultural meaning of pain, upholding Sophocles' *Philoctetes* as an ancient work 'ripe for rediscovery in the postmodern era of chronic illness' (Morris 1991: 249). Morris insists that the play is primarily 'a tragedy of pain', stressing that its significance lies in the fact that it encourages readers and audiences to reflect on the meaning and experience of pain, particularly since 'pain is always historical – always reshaped by a particular time, place, culture, and individual psyche' (Morris 1991: 6). It may then be argued that if Sophocles' *Antigone* is the political tragedy par excellence, then *Philoctetes* is the exemplar tragedy about the human body in pain; a story of illness that depicts a character afflicted with a chronic disease and the dramatic manifestation of his suffering.

The spectre of the lame Philoctetes also conjured up a corpus of postwar literary works spanning several continents and belonging to the genres of poetry, prose, and drama. These include, but are not restricted to, Heiner Müller's *Philoctetes* (1968), J. K. Baxter's *The Sore-Footed Man* (1971), Derek Walcott's *Omeros* (1990), Seamus Heaney's *The Cure at Troy* (performed 1990, published 1991), Alfonso Sastre's *Too Late for Philoctetes* (1990) and Mark Merlis's *An Arrow's Flight* (1998). On an allegorical level, moreover, in the majority of these works the image of Philoctetes is pitted against the backdrop of a larger historical malaise, whether the Greek hero is used as a foil to embody a social critique of the legacy of slavery and colonization in the Caribbean island of Saint Lucia; the conflict of The Troubles in Northern Ireland and the unremitting search for peace and reconciliation; or the production of a political version of the tragedy that stages the repressive regime of the former German Democratic Republic.

The story of Philoctetes reflects on the relationship between illness, storytelling, and healing, thus offering an ancient myth that shares the major concerns of the rising genre of narrative medicine. 'I use the term *narrative medicine*', declares Rita Charon, 'to mean medicine practiced with these narrative skills of recognising, absorbing, interpreting, and being moved by the stories of illness' (Charon 2006: 4). *Philoctetes* can then be seen as a paradigmatic 'illness narrative' that is in tune with the current rise in interest in patients' stories, particularly what Anne Hunsaker Hawkins refers to as 'the myths, attitudes, and beliefs of our culture that a sick person uses to come to terms with illness' (Hawkins 1999: 4). Such illness narratives are discussed extensively in Anne Whitehead's overview chapter for this section and, as Ian Williams shows in his chapter on graphic pathography, have engaged with a number of art forms beyond the purely literary. Indeed, as I show in this chapter, reinterpretations of the myth of Philoctetes have included plays in which the art of writing overlaps with the art of performance. The myth of Philoctetes thus provides an important case study of the intersections between history, pathography, narrative medicine, and different art forms – although I focus here on its literary aspects.

The recovery and reinterpretation of the myth of Philoctetes as a story that conveys a powerful narrative of pain, including the various ways in which pain can be modulated, the manner in which the sufferer is relieved from it, the possible remedies for the affliction, and the role that the community plays in the healing of the individual, are all factors that remain at the heart of the medical humanities. Narrative medicine, as Whitehead shows in her overview chapter within this volume, has shifted its attention 'from psychoanalytic to literary training over the last 50 years, with the assumption that engaging with literary texts enhances empathetic capacities and leads in turn to humane and compassionate action' (Whitehead in this volume: 111). This vital shift to 'literary training' is particularly noticeable in the implementation of literature courses in a number of medical schools across the UK and the USA, enabling future health practitioners to gain crucial narrative and interpretive skills. According to Anne Hunsaker Hawkins and Marilyn McEntyre, 'literary skills enable physicians to think both critically and empathetically about moral issues in medicine' (Hawkins and McEntyre 2000: 5).

Furthermore, in the last decade the Philoctetes myth has served as an instructive platform for the discussion of chronic pain, the physician–patient relationship, and the physiological and psychological recovery of military personnel. For example, the Institute for the Medical Humanities, University of Texas Medical Branch in Galveston, staged a performance of the play as part of their graduate programme in January 2008, thus introducing their students to an engaging mythical story aimed to enhance their future relationship with patients and their understanding of the complexities of pain. The Philoctetes Center in New York, co-directed by Francis Levy (fiction writer) and Edward Nersessian (Clinical Professor of Psychiatry at Weill Cornell Medical College), held a round-table discussion moderated by Dr Lyuba Konopasek (Weill Cornell Medical College in Qatar) that discussed the doctor–patient relationship in *Philoctetes* in December 2007. The aim of this event was to improve clinical practice through a close examination of the 'special bond that forms between a young, inexperienced soldier and a suffering veteran' (Konopasek 2013), particularly how the younger Neoptolemus is increasingly moved by Philoctetes' plight as he compassionately listens to his woeful tale of pain and isolation. Finally, the Vincent's Trauma and Wellness Center, New York, holds therapy programmes that utilize Sophocles' war plays (*Philoctetes* and *Ajax*) to rehabilitate soldiers suffering from post-traumatic stress disorder. A similar type of public health project has been undertaken by the 'Theatre of War: Outside the Wire', New York, which also stages Sophocles' war plays to comfort and aid in the psychological recovery of servicemen, veterans, and their families.

Ancient Greek medicine and the cult of Asclepius

Sophocles' reworking of the myth focuses on the recall of Philoctetes in Lemnos by the crafty Odysseus and the young Neoptolemus (the son of Achilles also known as Pyrrhus). The tension of the drama lies in the inherent moral conflict between the law of the gods (divine oracle) and the unscrupulous plans of humans (Odysseus' trickery); the ethical struggle between private conscience (Neoptolemus) and public duty (the fall of Troy); and the interrelationship between the illness of the individual (Philoctetes' wound) and the metaphorical malaise of the body politic (the corruption of the Greek army).

The dramatic effect of the tragedy is complexly conveyed around these opposing Sophoclean tensions, which are finally resolved with the supernatural intervention of Heracles by means of the plot device of *deus ex machina*. Heracles commands Philoctetes to go to Troy willingly, where, by killing Paris with his infallible arrows he will be rewarded with immortal glory (*timē*) and, equally importantly, an Asclepiad will cure his wound. Still, beneath these ethical dilemmas and the inexorable will of the gods, lies the injured and ostracized Philoctetes whose chronic pain and suffering remains at the heart of the tragedy. In the *Poetics* Aristotle declares 'Sophocles said that he portrayed people as they should be, Euripides as they are' (Aristotle 1996 [*c.* 330 BCE]: 43). It may be the case that in most of Sophocles' tragedies characters are portrayed as they 'ought to be', yet what is particularly striking about *Philoctetes* is the unmitigated clinical and realistic treatment of the subject of illness, thus making it Sophocles' most Euripidean play, not least in the tragedian's odd embracing of the *deus ex machina*. The visceral quality of the drama is conveyed through language and representation, chiefly in the undiluted dramatization of the wailing and sick Philoctetes whose tragic role arises from the suffering and distress punctuating the action, in which he unapologetically moans, screams, howls, yells, agonizes, faints, and even sleeps. Inevitably, this realistic and graphic portrayal of the pain and torment of the tragic figure arouses the pity and sympathy from the audience. 'In the *Philoctetes* of Sophocles', Hegel reminds us, 'a physical malady is the cause of the collision' (Hegel 1962: 115), while Terry Eagleton states that 'we feel sympathy for Philoctetes because he is in agonizing pain from his pus-swollen foot' and because he bears his pain without 'a shred of stoicism' (Eagleton 2003: xiv, 31). R. P. Winnington-Ingram also stresses the unsparing pain of Philoctetes by asserting that 'his foot takes on an existence independent of himself' (Winnington-Ingram 1980: 291).

As a tragedy whose subject matter is pain and healing, *Philoctetes* is intimately connected with the origins of Greek medicine through the figure of the divine healer Asclepius (Latin *Aescula'pius*), regarded today as the father of modern medicine. In ancient medicine, the art of healing was considered a 'craft' inherently associated with the Olympian deity Apollo, god of poetry, healing, and prophecy. Yet Apollo's chief attribute as the patron of medicine was later eclipsed by the influential cult of his own son Asclepius, who inherits the healing properties of his divine father, and is enshrined in the Greek pantheon as the legendary founder of the art of medicine. The archetypal rod of Asclepius, with its intertwined sacred snake, is intrinsically related to the sacred rites of healing and purification. Indeed, the image of the coiled serpent symbolizes the curative potential of medicine through its powers of regeneration by cyclically shrugging off its skin. According to J. Schouten, the rod-and-serpent iconography of Asclepius is 'used indiscriminately to symbolise medicine', thus becoming a recognizable emblem of the medical profession (Schouten 1967: 230).

The healing powers of Asclepius became famously associated with ancient temple medicine, a treatment based on the process of incubation through which patients suffering from a wide range of physical afflictions were cured as they slept in an Asclepiad sanctuary. Patients allegedly received an epiphany from the god, thus regaining a miraculous state of health – or a prescribed cure (*iama*) – upon awakening from these sanative and prophetic dream-visions (see Hartigan 2005; Schouten 1967; Kerényi 1959; Longrigg 2001). It has been speculated that the arrival of Asclepius in Athens was closely linked to the devastation caused by the great plague of Attica that struck the Athenian population in the early years of the Peloponnesian War.[2] The deadly epidemic triggered the importation of the Asclepian cult to Athens, widely contributing to the reverence of the divine healer by the Athenian citizens, and to the subsequent erection of numerous sanctuaries devoted to the god throughout Ancient Greece. The establishment of the cult in Athens, furthermore, is closely tied up with the heroic and distinguished life and career of Sophocles, who allegedly played an important role in its introduction (Scodel 2005: 233). As Andrew Connolly puts it, 'Sophocles gave lodging to the cultic snake or statue of Asclepius [...] and in recognition for these services as the so-called "Receiver" of Asclepius he was heroized after his death under the name Dexion' (Connolly 1998: 1).

If Asclepian temple medicine offered the promise of a miraculous cure, so at the end of Sophocles' play, Philoctetes is assured that an Asclepiad in Troy will heal his gangrenous foot. It then becomes clear that Sophocles uses Greek medicine as a 'vigorous topic of public debate' (Nutton 2004: 52), in an attempt to engage his Athenian audience with the vital religious cult that had been recently adopted in the city, and in which he had been personally and religiously involved. Thus, Sophocles' *Philoctetes* foregrounds the complex interplay between tragedy, myth, and medicine as integral aspects of a religious institution in which drama held a clearly defined civic and cultural function in fifth-century Athens. And since Attic tragedy emerged as a spring festival performed in honour of the god Dionysus, in *Philoctetes,* Sophocles is complexly gesturing towards the meeting between the Dionysian and the Asclepian cults – the art of tragedy and the art of medicine. The connection between Dionysus and Asclepius also stems from the crucial fact that the theatre of Dionysus and the Asclepian sanctuary were located on the southern slope of the Acropolis within a few metres from each other. 'In Athens this relation between the spheres of Asklepios and Dionysos', states C. Kerényi, 'is reflected by the proximity of the Asklepieion to the theater of Dionysos and in nearby Marathon by the situation of the tomb of the *heros iatros* [Asclepius] beside the sanctuary of Dionysos' (Kerényi 1959: 73). Therefore Sophocles deliberately constructs *Philoctetes* as a tragic drama caught between the worship of the newly imported healing deity and the traditional celebration of the god of wine and fertility in the Dionysian festival. Hartigan makes the pertinent suggestion that the adjacency of the Asklepieion to the theatre of Dionysus signals the therapeutic properties of tragedy as a curative experience, proposing that the ancient Greeks may have believed that 'drama could assist the healing process' (Hartigan 2005: 176). At the same time, the medicinal aspect of tragedy is, of course, integrally linked to the elusive Aristotelian notion of 'catharsis' that lies at the heart of the theatrical experience through the purification, or purgation, of the emotions. Both deities are ultimately associated with the process of healing, whether via ecstasy, unbridled emotions, and suffering (Dionysus) or via temple medicine, the regenerative powers of the Asclepian serpent, and medical treatment based on herbal remedies and temple medicine (Asclepius).

Yet the atypical 'happy ending' of *Philoctetes,* which culminates in reconciliation and promises the cure of the individual and the body politic, flies in the face of Aristotle's precept advocating that the perfect tragedy ought to involve a change '*from* good fortune *to* bad fortune' (1996: 21), even if he admits that the reverse outcome 'from bad fortune to good fortune' is also possible. As C. M. Bowra puts it, 'Aristotle recognises a kind of tragedy in which the change of fortune is from bad to good, but he is not much interested in it and says elsewhere that in the perfect plot the change should be from happiness to misery' (Bowra 1944: 261). Nonetheless, *Philoctetes* shows that the complexity, effectiveness, and seriousness of the drama are not entirely determined by, nor reliant upon, a tragic death and an impending disaster. The conciliatory ending of *Philoctetes* is accomplished not just by the resolution of the plot, but also mainly by the promise of a cure in which Philoctetes 'can accept physical healing' (Easterling 1983: 225). Indeed, the Asclepian restoration of health (*hygieia*) and the removal of disease (*nosos*), as well as Philoctetes' future reintegration into public life, stand in stark contrast to, say, Oedipus' poignant act of self-mutilation, Jocasta's desperate suicide, and the hardships of exile. The end of *Philoctetes* opens not an interrogation but an affirmation, solace and healing over grief and disaster, and reconciliation over the irreversible loss of life: 'You will find doctors there, to heal your wound;/You will be chosen champion of the Greeks' (Sophocles 1990: 225) proclaims Heracles as he is gloriously lowered onto the stage by the *mēchanē* theatrical device.

Thus the Sophoclean happy ending struck a chord with contemporary writers eager to talk back to *Philoctetes*, as they adapted their responses to the specific demands of their own historical circumstances and literary conventions. Heaney's version of Sophocles' *Philoctetes*, aptly titled *The Cure at Troy*, foregrounds the promissory dimension of the Attic tragedy, while Walcott's *Omeros* stages the cure of Philoctetes' Caribbean namesake, the 'foam-haired Philoctete' (Walcott 1990: 9) whose swollen foot – which stands as a metaphor for the wounds of colonization – is finally healed by an Obeah woman. In the next section I demonstrate that Heaney's and Walcott's versions of Philoctetes emphasize the importance of empathy, dialogue, and hope as the best antidotes to alleviate the wounds of the individual and the body politic.

Modernizing Philoctetes in the twentieth century and beyond

In *Amid Our Troubles: Irish Versions of Greek Tragedy* (2002), Marianne McDonald draws attention to the complex relationship between Attic tragedy and the Irish theatrical tradition: 'In the twentieth century, there seem to be more translations and versions of Greek tragedy that have come from Ireland than from any other country in the English-speaking world. In many ways Ireland was and is constructing its identity through the representations offered by Greek tragedy' (McDonald 2002: 37). In a larger way, it may also be claimed that Greek mythology more broadly has cast a powerful spell on the Irish writer's imagination. This Hellenizing creative impulse takes centre stage in James Joyce's *Ulysses* (1922), as Joyce circulates Homer's *Odyssey* through the renewed currents of the Hibernian Sea, combining in one stroke homage and parody, reverence and irreverence (Novillo-Corvalán 2009: 148). Joyce indulges in an exercise of transmutation, converting the '*Epi oinopa ponton*' (the wine-dark sea) of the Greek original into 'a new art colour for our Irish poets: snotgreen' (2002 [1922]: 4). Ironically, the modernization of ancient sources became a dominant trope adopted by the nationalist impetus of the Celtic Renaissance, as the patriotically driven William Butler Yeats put on the Dublin stage *Cathleen ni Houlihan* (1899) – a female heroine who stands as an allegory for Hibernia – and one of the most recognisable dramatic personages of Greek theatre, *Oedipus King* (written 1916, performed 1926, published 1928). Nonetheless, Yeats built a different level of signification into the Theban play that erected a new ideological structure upon the historical edifice of Greek tragedy. While endorsing Sophocles' use of theatre as a vehicle for public debate, Yeats simultaneously incorporates a contemporary meaning pertinent to the political climate of Ireland in the wake of the war of independence. For example, J. Michael Walton has appropriately drawn attention to Yeats's symbolically laden phrase 'we were amid our troubles' arguing that 'a Dublin audience, hearing such a phrase in 1926, would be hard put not to look for subtext when listening to the rest of this "version"' (Walton 2002: 10). This highly idiosyncratic Yeatsian adaption of *Oedipus* offered to an Irish audience a fresh dramatization of a Greek tragedy in which archaic and anachronistic elements were complexly compounded with an Irish inflection and poetic sensibility so as to strengthen its contemporary appeal.

It may be argued, then, that Heaney aspired to do for *Philoctetes* what Yeats had done for *Oedipus King*. Prompted by the traumatic political upheavals of Irish history, both poets transposed two of the greatest archetypes of Sophoclean drama to twentieth-century Ireland, deftly superimposing multiple layers of meaning upon the cryptic riddle of the Sphinx and the murder of Laius (Yeats), and to the wound of Philoctetes and his conciliatory return to Troy (Heaney). On the whole, their dramatic adaptations became a blueprint for a historical vision that is succinctly captured in oft-quoted phrases that transcended the original context of their plays. Walton is right to point out that 'Yeats's phrase "Amid our Troubles" spreads its tail like a peacock', since its resonance has become pervasive throughout Irish culture (Walton 2002: 32), while Hugh Denard states that Heaney's peace-making expression 'so hope for a great sea-change on the far side of revenge' (Heaney 1991: 77) projects a vision of 'a radical reconciliatory future for Northern Ireland' (Denard 2000: 17).

The Irish literary tradition appropriates archetypal figures from Greek tragedy and the notion of theatre as a cultural institution that embodies the prevalent norms and beliefs of a particular society. Derek Walcott similarly privileges an aesthetic that transplants characters from the world of Ancient Greece onto his native Caribbean island of Saint Lucia. For one thing, Walcott's kinship with Irish literature simultaneously embraces Stephen Dedalus' dictum that history 'is a nightmare from which I am trying to awake' (Joyce 2002: 28)[3] and Heaney's optimistic sensibility and altruistic belief in hope and a 'great sea-change'. For both Laureates, therefore, the chronic wound of Philoctetes becomes a poetic and dramatic vehicle for tackling social concerns in an ethical and idealistic attempt to forge a larger historical commentary that seeks to heal their respective communities of their traumatic past.

At the same time, the recognizable classical (and later romantic, as illustrated in Wordsworth's sonnet 'When Philoctetes in the Lemnian Isle' [1827]), topos of the remote island offers a location at once harsh and idyllic that depicts the fundamental tensions between social conflict and personal survival. This topos is strongly invoked by Sophocles, Heaney, and Walcott within the regional landscapes of Lemnos, Ireland, and Saint Lucia, respectively. For Walcott, the protean mutability of the Philoctetes myth is reinvented as a complex symbol for the cultural richness of Saint

Lucia and the darker waters of colonialism in a radically altered *epi oinopa ponton*. In this manner, 'Homer' becomes *Omeros,* a cultural legacy stripped of a capital 'H' and turned from the singular monologic 'Homer' to the plural dialogic '*Omer(os)*', suitably representing the cultural diversity of colonized peoples whose hybridity is characteristic of an in-between identity that results from the merging of multiple worlds, languages, and races (Novillo-Corvalán 2007: 159). Therefore the canonical figure of Homer acquires a new literary and creolized cultural meaning within a Caribbean landscape:

> I said, "*Omeros,*"
> And *O* was the conch-shell's invocation, *mer* was
> both mother and sea in our Antillean patois,
> *os*, a grey bone, and the white surf as it crashes
> and spreads its sibilant collar on a lace shore.
> Omeros was the crunch of dry leaves, and the washes
> that echoed from a cave-mouth when the tide has ebbed
>
> (Walcott 1990: 14)

The emphasis upon the polyvalence of the French word 'mer' in the local Saint Lucian patois, signifying both 'mother' and 'sea', is celebrated throughout *Omeros.* The shape-changing qualities of myth are also reflected in the symbolic name of the island of Saint Lucia, otherwise known as the 'Helen of the Caribbean'. This mythical designation juxtaposes the Homeric quarrel between Greeks and Trojans over Argive Helen, and the historical disputes between Britain and France over the sovereignty of the island. At the same time, Walcott declares that Christopher Columbus had named the island 'after the blind saint [Saint Lucy]' (Walcott 1993: 24). According to Christian hagiography, Saint Lucy plucked out her beautiful eyes because they proved attractive to a male admirer. This vow of chastity also enabled the martyr to renounce all earthly possessions in her total devotion to God (Novillo-Corvalán 2007: 158). Pérez Fernández remarks that 'her blindness stands for the inward, transcendental vision that the Western literary tradition has accorded to this condition' (Pérez Fernández 2001: 61). Hippolyte Delehaye insightfully refers to the iconography of the saint who is 'sometimes represented carrying two eyes on a plate, to remind people that she is invoked for the cure of eye troubles' (Delehaye 1998: 31). The motif of blindness, moreover, is related to Sophocles' use of dramatic irony in *Oedipus Rex*: the metaphorically blind Oedipus is paradoxically able to *see* and understand his opaque destiny after tragically stabbing his eyes with the gold brooches from Yocasta's robe. 'Tragedies such as *Oedipus* and *Lear* do show a kind of progress toward self-knowledge', writes George Steiner, 'but it is achieved at the price of ruin' (Steiner 1961: 169).

Meanwhile, Walcott's Philoctete is a local fisherman who bears a wound from a rusty anchor, which acquires a larger allegorical meaning as the epic develops and becomes a metaphor for the suffering of the Saint Lucian people. 'Names, relationships and situations familiar from Homer', asserts Lorna Hardwick, 'also bring with them reminders of enforced diaspora and a plantation culture which replaced the African names of its slaves with classical ones' (Hardwick 2006: 356). The wound of the individual becomes a microcosm that illustrates the larger wounds of the body politic, whether the corrupt social structures are embedded in Thebes, Troy, Ireland, or Saint Lucia.

Still, both Heaney's and Walcott's versions of *Philoctetes* operate at multiple levels of meaning and are not strictly intended as allegorical representations of political and historical events. Like Sophocles, both writers locate the experience of chronic pain at the centre of their stories of illness, foregrounding a pathological perspective of the myth that also examines the effects of pain, suffering, and isolation. Even Heaney is cautious about the inherent limitations of politically motivated allegories, openly disclaiming 'Philoctetes is not meant to be understood as a trimly allegorical representation of hardline Unionism. He is first and foremost a character in the Greek play [...] the wounded one whose identity has become dependent upon the wound' (Heaney 2002: 175). Heaney offers an unmitigated version of Philoctetes' suffering, fluently transposing the visceral quality of the play in a dramatization that abounds in onomatopoeic and alliterative word formations that seek to convey sounds and expressions traditionally associated with pain. 'Realism was the dominant mode when it came to his foot and spasms', writes Heaney in his 'Production Notes' (Heaney 2002: 179). Therefore his Philoctetes agonisingly struts and frets across the stage, abruptly bursting into pain: 'Ahhhhhhhhh. Ahhhhhhhhh. Hohohohohoh' (Heaney 1991: 39), thus allowing Neoptolemus, the Chorus, and the audience to get an insight into the nature of his affliction. Heaney is at his most Joycean in championing the protean expressibility of the English language – even at the deceptively basic level of syllabic and consonantal rearrangement – like the whistling of a train in Molly Bloom's unpunctuated soliloquy: 'frseeeeeeeeefronnnng' (Joyce 2002: 621). Heaney's unrestrained literary construction of pain acquires even more force due to the performative dimension of the actor's body on stage.

Whereas Sophocles' *Philoctetes* repeatedly makes references to the ubiquitous figure of Asclepius, Heaney and Walcott resituate their allusions to the Greek deity within the medical and religious practices of their respective cultures and traditions. In this way, references to healing are closely bound to the flora and fauna of each island, including allusions to the curative powers of autochthonous herbs. For example, Sophocles' Philoctetes provides a commentary of Ancient herbal medicine, as the wounded archer seeks anaesthetic relief in the palliative properties of a local herb: 'One thing above all: a herb I have found/To poultice the wound and ease the pain' (Sophocles 1990: 194). Not for nothing does Apollo, as the ancient god of healing and father of Asclepius, proudly boast in Ovid's *Metamorphoses* of possessing 'the power of every herb' (Ovid 1998: 16). And it is instructive to draw attention, furthermore, to E. D. Phillips' observation that a scholium on Pindar's *Pythian Ode I* offers a detailed description of Philoctetes' cure by an Asclepiad whose medicinal craft is strongly rooted in the knowledge of herbal medicine: 'While he [Philoctetes] was asleep, Machaon cut away the gangrenous flesh from the festering ulcer, poured wine over it, and sprinkled on the wound a herb that Asclepius had obtained from Chiron' (Phillips 1973: 17). This mythological allusion to the wise centaur Chiron – a highly respected legendary healer skilled in the arts of medicine and tutor to Achilles and Asclepius – draws attention to the porous boundaries between medicine and religion. This type of medico-mythical healing practice is also interconnected to the health-giving properties of the Asclepian snake and its powers of regeneration. Commenting on the prominent symbolism of the snake, Mitchell-Boyask stresses the important fact that 'a snake will be involved in both the attack on Philoctetes and his cure [since] a deity and a serpent wounded Philoctetes, so will a deity and a serpent heal Philoctetes' (Mitchell-Boyask 2007: 97–8).

In *Omeros* Walcott accentuates the shift from Ancient Greek medicine to the syncretic Caribbean Obeah healing tradition that conflates African beliefs with Christian practices. If in Asclepian temple medicine the sleeping patient is healed through a dream vision, offering a cure that may be accompanied by rites, incantations, and curative herbs, in *Omeros* the ancient sacred temple has been replaced by the Saint Lucian 'No Pain Café', a local bar/shop for the community and a sanctuary for spiritual and bodily afflictions presided by Ma Kilman, a female Obeah practitioner. Loretta Collins states 'Obeah is an Afro-Caribbean practice that utilizes herbal remedies, possession by ancestral spirits or African-based deities, and diagnosis or divination through trancework' (Collins 1995: 147). These ritualistic and visionary practices highlight the powerful role that an Obeah practitioner exerts within the identity of a particular community, on one level, and the construction of healing traditions as an antidote of, and critique to, European colonialism and Western medicine and rationality, on another. Ma Kilman's centrality in the text as a spiritual motherly figure endowed with the arts of divination, sorcery, and healing is indicated in her composite depiction as:

> A *gardeuse*, sybil, obeah-woman
> webbed with a spider's knowledge of an after-life
> in her cracked lenses. She took Holy Communion
> with Maud sometimes, but there was an old African
> doubt that paused before taking the wafer's white leaf
>
> (Walcott 1990: 58)

While Walcott foregrounds the resistance to, and inevitable absorption of, Christianity within Caribbean culture, Heaney liberally sprinkles his version of Philoctetes with references to Irish culture and religion. In his 'Production Notes' he suggests that *The Cure at Troy* seeks to overlay upon the Ancient Greek religion the faith-healing associations of Irish Roman Catholicism and its deeply ingrained belief in the occurrence of miracles and supernatural phenomena: '*Cure* is backlit ever so faintly in Irish usage (or should I say Irish Catholic?) by a sense of miracle. Lourdes and all that. Warts cleared up at holy wells' (Heaney 2002: 172). The *New Testament*, for example, features the well-known miracles performed by Jesus, including the miraculous healing of a blind man in the Gospel according to John:

> He [Jesus] spat on the ground and made clay with the saliva; and He anointed the eyes of the blind man with the clay. And He said to him, "Go, wash in the pool of Siloam". So he went and washed, and came back seeing.
>
> (Anon 1982: John 9: 6–7)

In his *Philoctetes*, therefore, Heaney brings together the cult of Asclepius and the Christian faith in the performance of miracles, imparting an optimistic vision that becomes the underlying message of the drama: 'Believe in miracles/And cures and healing wells' (1991: 77). In so doing, Heaney is also underscoring the relationship between theatre, healing, and divine intervention that is at the heart of Sophocles' tragedy, while also demonstrating that the play can be modernized to articulate social commentaries about Northern Ireland's 'troubled' history. Yet it merits mentioning that the Irish poet also takes several liberties with the original in an attempt to readdress the gender politics of the Greek play that featured an all-male cast. Heaney dismantles the strict masculinist ethos of the Sophoclean drama with the inclusion of a tripartite female Chorus figure played by actresses who simultaneously stand for, and replace, the divine character of Heracles. This powerful female choric figure, to whom Heaney assigns entire new lines in the drama, also incarnates subtle hints of Shakespeare's emblematic weird sisters in *Macbeth*, thus adding an element of magic and sorcery into the play that goes hand-in-hand with Walcott's similar embodiment of the practice of Obeah in the figure of Ma Kilman. 'I suggested three women for the Chorus', writes Heaney, 'in order to give a sense that the action was being invigilated by the three Fates, the Weird sisters or whoever – this was the mythical dimension to the decision' (Heaney 2002: 172).

Just as Sophocles' Philoctetes seeks soothing relief from a local herb, so Walcott's Ma Kilman treats his Caribbean counterpart with a special botanical ointment that consists of 'a flask of white acajou, and a jar of yellow Vaseline' (Walcott 1990: 18). The cashew seed belongs to the botanical family *anacardiaceae*, native to the Brazilian litoral, and variously known in the Americas as 'acajou', 'acajú', and 'cajuí'. The oil extracted from the plant is 'used for dermal afflictions' and can be also applied to 'inflammatory disorders' as well as to 'expel worms; active ulcers, corns, warts' (Mors 2000: 7). Ma Kilman utilizes this botanical remedy for its temporary analgesic and anti-inflammatory effects, just as the medicinal plant that Philoctetes extracted from the Lemnian region offered analogous properties.

Her final curing of Philoctetes with a medicinal bath operates on two interrelated levels, as her use of curative plants works in symbiosis with the casting of spells through a trance-like experience. For example, in chapter XLVII Ma Kilman is depicted in a mystical state that atavistically reconnects her with the spirits of her African ancestors. The cure of the fisherman is enacted within a larger ritualistic ceremony that seeks to cleanse the wounds of history. Collins remarks that 'Philoctetes's medicinal bath [...] generates a community-wide healing, a new connection to the African tribal warrior and freedom from the painful memory of the "coffles" ' (Collins 1995: 244). Thus, in her trance-like state Ma Kilman gathers herbs, aromatic plants, and water that will at last heal the 'sutured wound that Philoctete was given by the sea' (Walcott 1990: 242). Walcott also deliberately conflates the acts of Obeah ritual possession with the divinations of the ancient Sibyl of Cumae in Virgil's *Aeneid*, the famous prophetess who ambiguously inscribes oracles on leaves in her dark cave, and advises the pious Aeneas on his voyage to the underworld: 'the spidery sibyl/hanging in a sack from the cave at Cumae' (Walcott 1990: 245). Like the Sibyl in the *Aeneid* who 'flung herself widely into the cave-mouth' (Virgil 1996 [*c.* 19 BCE]: 169), Walcott's Obeah is possessed by spiritual forces within a state of uncontrolled divine possession. In fusing the ecstatic trances of the Saint Lucian Obeah with the Cumaean Sibyl, Walcott is deliberately going back full circle as he interlaces African-Caribbean practices with the Apollonian powers of prophecy and healing. It is worth remembering that Apollo transmitted the oracles of the ancient priestess, thus indicating that Walcott's connection with Attic tragedy, via the creation of a 'New World' Philoctete, is further enriched by the larger epic tradition of Homer and Virgil that envelops the poem.

Conclusion: Philoctetes, his lives, and afterlives

In his essay 'The Task of the Translator' (1923) Walter Benjamin undermines traditional approaches to translation by proposing that the original owes its survival to the translation. The latter, he claims, endows the former with an 'afterlife' that extends and enriches its lifespan, thus fulfilling its potential as it migrates across history, culture, and language. For Benjamin, 'all great texts contain their potential translation between the lines' (Benjamin 2001 [1923]: 22). In other words, literary works aspire to be translated and transformed, to voyage from one culture to another in order to become renewed within a process of both mutability and stability, as each culture is able to perceive new elements that previous ones had been unable to discover. This chapter has charted the migration of Philoctetes from Ancient Greece to the late-twentieth century. It has thus validated the Benjaminian claim of the underlying layers of meaning inherent in the tragedy that have been uncovered by successive generations of readers, writers, audiences, and now health practitioners. Interestingly, Sophocles', Heaney's, and Walcott's versions of the legend uphold the motif of pain and suffering as the cornerstone of the tragic drama, yet all three writers provide a different diagnosis and cure for the wounded Philoctetes, reminding us that healing practices are culturally and historically dependent. The metaphorization of Philoctetes as an emblematic figure of suffering is therefore predicated upon the particular context out of which his pain is being reinterpreted, thus refracting a wide spectrum of health concerns and social commentaries. For the medical humanities, then, the myth of Philoctetes provides a valuable narrative of illness and a story of personal integrity in the face of agonizing pain and distress, appealing to health practitioners through its ability to comment on the complex meanings of pain, and the importance of empathy in the physician–patient relationship. The Philoctetes myth also foregrounds the relationship between literature and medicine, particularly the way in which both disciplines have the potential to inform and enrich each other. Finally, the mythical story of Philoctetes – his pain, endurance, isolation, and creativity, and the final promise of healing – has provided writers past and present with a template upon which to diagnose social and individual illnesses. The myth has also allowed writers to anatomize different ways of relieving pain and supporting chronically ill patients. Ultimately, the optimistic ending of Philoctetes explains why the unremitting search for a cure in the history of medicine still matters.

Notes

1   For a comprehensive assessment of the European reception of Sophocles' *Philoctetes* see Budelmann (2007).
2   For a view that supports the theory that the importation of the cult of Asclepius is closely linked to the Attic plague, see Garland (1992: 130–2). Wickkiser, meanwhile, argues that, 'it is much more likely that a constellation of factors motivated Asklepios' importation to Athens' (2009: 58) and not just the outbreak of the plague.
3   See Pollard (2001) for an insightful examination of the literary relationship between Walcott and Joyce.

References

Anon (1982) *Holy Bible: The New King James Version*, Nashville: Thomas Nelson Publishers.
Aristotle (1996 [*c.* 330 BCE]) *Poetics*, trans. M. Heath, London: Penguin.
Baxter, J. K. (1971) *The Sore-Footed Man and the Temptations of Oedipus*, Auckland: Heinemann.

Benjamin, W. (2001 [1923]) 'The Task of the Translator', in L. Venuti (ed.) *The Translation Studies Reader*, London and New York: Routledge.

Bowra, C. M. (1944) *Sophoclean Tragedy*, Oxford: Clarendon Press.

Budelmann, F. (2007) 'The Reception of Sophocles' Representation of Physical Pain', *American Journal of Philology*, 128: 443–68.

Charon, R. (2006) *Narrative Medicine: Honoring the Stories of Illness*, Oxford: Oxford University Press.

Collins, L. (1995) ' "We Shall All Heal": Ma Kilman, the Obeah Woman, as Mother-Healer in Derek Walcott's *Omeros*', *Literature and Medicine*, 14: 146–62.

Connolly, A. (1998) 'Was Sophocles Heroised as Dexion?', *Journal of Hellenic Studies* 118: 1–21.

Delehaye, H. (1998 [1955]) *The Legends of the Saints*, trans. D. Attwater. Dublin: Four Courts Press.

Denard, H. (2000) 'Seamus Heaney, Colonialism, and the Cure: Sophoclean Re-Visions', *A Journal of Performance and Art*, 22: 1–ß18.

Eagleton, T. (2003) *Sweet Violence: The Idea of the Tragic*, London: Blackwell.

Easterling, P. E. (1983) 'Philoctetes and Modern Criticism', in E. Segal (ed.) *Oxford Readings in Greek Tragedy*, Oxford: Oxford University Press.

Garland, R. S. J. (1992) *Introducing New Gods: The Politics of Athenian Religion*, London: Duckworth.

Hardwick, L. (2006) ' "Shards and Suckers": Contemporary Receptions of Homer', in R. Fowler (ed.) *The Cambridge Companion to Homer*, Cambridge: Cambridge University Press.

Hartigan, K. (2005) 'Drama and Healing: Ancient and Modern', in H. King (ed.) *Health in Antiquity*, London and New York: Routledge.

Hawkins, A. H. (1999) *Reconstructing Illness: Studies in Pathography*, 2nd edn, West Lafayette, IN: Purdue University Press.

Hawkins, A. H. and McEntyre, M. C. (2000) 'Introduction: Teaching Literature and Medicine: A Retrospective and a Rationale', in A. H. Hawkins and M. C. McEntyre (eds) *Teaching Literature and Medicine*, New York: The Modern Language Association.

Heaney, S. (2002) '*The Cure at Troy*: Production Notes in No Particular Order', in M. McDonald and J. M. Walton (eds) *Amid Our Troubles: Irish Versions of Greek Tragedy*, London: Methuen.

Heaney, S. (1991) *The Cure at Troy: A Version of Sophocles' Philoctetes*, New York: Farrar, Straus and Giroux.

Hegel, G. W. F. (1962) *Hegel on Tragedy*, A. Paolucci and H. Paolucci (eds) New York: Harper.

Joyce, J. (ed. H. W. Gabler) (2002 [1922]) *Ulysses*, London: The Bodley Head.

Kerényi, C. (1959) *Asklepios: Archetypal Image of the Physician's Existence*, trans. R. Manheim, New York: Pantheon Books.

Konopasek, L. (2013) 'Roundtable, Doctor/Patients Relationships'. Online. Available: http://philoctetes.org/event/doctor_patient_relationships (accessed 6 January 2013).

Longrigg, J. (2001) *Greek Medicine: From the Heroic to the Hellenistic Age*, London: Duckworth.

McDonald, M. (2002) 'The Irish and Greek Tragedy', in M. McDonald and J. M. Walton (eds) *Amid Our Troubles: Irish Versions of Greek Tragedy*, London: Methuen.

Merlis, M. (1998) *An Arrow's Flight*, New York: St. Martin's Press.

Mitchell-Boyask, R. (2007) 'The Athenian Asklepieion and the End of the "Philoctetes"', *Transactions of the American Philological Association*, 137: 85–114.

Morris, D. B. (1991) *The Culture of Pain*, Berkeley: The University of California Press.

Mors, W. B., Toledo Rizzini, C. and Alvares Pereira, N. (ed. R. A. DeFilipps) (2000) *Medicinal Plants of Brazil*, Michigan: Reference Publications.

Müller, H. (2011 [1968]) *Three Plays: Philoctetes, The Horatian, Mauser*, trans. Nathaniel McBride, London: Seagull Books.

Novillo-Corvalán, P. (2009) 'The Theatre of Marina Carr: A Latin American Reading, Interview, and Translation', *Irish Migration Studies in Latin America*, 7: 145–53.

Novillo-Corvalán, P. (2007) 'Literary Migrations: Homer's Journey through Joyce's Ireland and Walcott's Saint Lucia', *Irish Migration Studies in Latin America*, 5: 157–62.

Nutton, V. (2004) *Ancient Medicine*, London and New York: Routledge.

Ovid (1998 [AD 8]) *Metamorphoses*, trans. A. D. Melville, Oxford: Oxford University Press.

Pérez Fernández, J. M. (2001) '*Terza Rima*, the Sea and History in *Omeros*' in J. L. Martínez-Dueñas Espejo and J. M. Pérez Fernández (eds) *Approaches to the Poetics of Derek Walcott*, Lewiston: Edwin Mellen Press.

Phillips, E. D. (1973) *Greek Medicine*, London: Thames and Hudson.

Pollard, C. W. (2001) 'Travelling with Joyce: Derek Walcott's Discrepant Cosmopolitan Modernism', *Twentieth Century Literature*, 47: 197–216.

Sastre, A. (1990) *Demasiado tarde para Filoctetes* [*Too Late for Philoctetes*], Bilbao: Hiru.

Scarry, E. (1985) *The Body in Pain: The Making and Unmaking of the World*, Oxford: Oxford University Press.

Schouten, J. (1967) *The Rod and the Serpent of Asklepios: Symbol of Medicine*, trans. M. E. Hollander, Elsevier Publishing: Amsterdam

Scodel, R. (2005) 'Sophoclean Tragedy', in J. Gregory (ed.) *A Companion to Greek Tragedy*, London: Blackwell.

Sophocles (1990) *Plays Two: Ajax, Women of Trachis, Electra, Philoctetes*, London: Methuen.

Steiner, G. (1961) *The Death of Tragedy*, London: Faber and Faber.

Virgil (trans. Robert Fitzgerald) (1996 [*c.* 19 BCE]) *The Aeneid*, London: Harvill Press.

Walcott, D. (1993) 'Leaving School' in R. D. Hammer (ed.) *Critical Perspectives on Derek Walcott*, New York: Three Continents Press.

Walcott, D. (1990) *Omeros*, London: Faber and Faber.

Walton, M. J. (2002) 'Hit or Myth: The Greeks and Irish Drama', in M. McDonald and J. M. Walton (eds) *Amid Our Troubles: Irish Versions of Greek Tragedy*, London: Methuen.

Wickkiser, B. (2009) 'Banishing Plague: Asklepios, Athens, and the Great Plague Reconsidered', in J. T. Jenson, G. Hinge, P. Schultz and B. Wickkiser (eds) *Aspects of Ancient Greek Cult: Context, Ritual and Iconography*, Aarhus: Aarhus University Press.

Wilson, E. (1941) *The Wound and the Bow: Seven Studies in Literature*, Cambridge, MA: Houghton Mifflin.

Winnington-Ingram, R. P. (1980) *Sophocles: An Interpretation*, Cambridge: Cambridge University Press.

9 The heart of the matter

Creating meaning in health and medicine through writing

Case study

Fiona Hamilton

Literature has an ingenious capacity to articulate human beings' 'vulnerable complexity', to borrow words from poet John O'Donohue (1999: 14), and it is the desire to understand this complexity that energizes narrative approaches to medicine. This chapter examines the interface between medicine and literary arts through the case study of 'expressive and reflective writing' (ERW), as a practice offered to patients in clinical settings. I describe and engage with a range of writing techniques from a practitioner's point of view and examine the practice's historical development and its identity in relation to clinical and other therapeutic modes. The notion of 'the patient's point of view' will be considered throughout, particularly in terms of how is it articulated, interpreted, heard and responded to. Patients' perspectives in this chapter are represented through their own writing and comments, in addition to published works of fiction and poetry in which the rôles of writer, patient and doctor overlap. While acknowledging that these identities and their attendant narratives are interdependent and that they change, for the purposes of this chapter I will consider them as discrete entities. I consider how ERW provokes a challenge to biomedical definitions of *health* and *therapeutic* and how this facilitated literary art can contribute to these aims by expanding definitions, opening up creative and discursive spaces in clinical settings and allowing patients opportunities to be experts in their own stories.

Scrutiny of stories, words, and writing process highlight a range of discourses that operate within the arenas of health and illness. Doctors with an interest in medical humanities are particularly aware of the complexities of communication and interpretation. Oncologist Sam Guglani remarks:

> [T]here is so much that can be done to my patients – drugs, radiotherapy, surgery, referrals, drains and biopsies, to name only a few. As well as distilling the possible technical algorithms, judgments are required about what ought to be done for patients. And further, within these two charged poles of the possible, patients must be engaged in a way that encompasses and communicates this complex arena. This is

within the context, of course, of our frequently divergent expectations and fears.

(Guglani 2011: 4)

The question of 'what is best for the patient' provokes emotional responses from both patient and doctor. The decision involves sophisticated interpretive skills encompassing the personal and the clinical as well as contextual considerations, such as the doctor's working environment, region, country and political system at any given date. The task of balancing these factors while incorporating new elements brought by an individual patient could well be described as an art in itself. Guglani continues: 'my engagement with a patient's experience is infused utterly with the stuff of humanity, in all its confused, irrational and emotive weight'.

Two contrasting identities are suggested by Guglani's analysis: medicine as a scientifically based practice, and medicine as a practice dealing with the messiness and diversity of human lives. Words and symbols are crucially involved in these intersecting elements, both in clinical consultations and as units of meaning in an overall semiology guiding and framing medical practice. A push and pull of cultures is evident: 'medicine establishes itself in large part within the discourse of "science"... yet its history forces continuous deconstruction of that position' (Crawford 1993: 42). Questions thus arise about whether we should consider the two as distinct camps or instead view them as intertwined. This tussle has been increasingly evident in articulations of and attitudes to the 'patient's voice' in the post-war period. A range of new theoretical perspectives has challenged the assumptions of fixed rationalist terms, particularly post-structuralism as exemplified by Michel Foucault's questioning of objective and pure clinical terms throughout *The Birth of the Clinic* (1963). Yet despite these complications, a clear 'scientific' discourse of medicine serves a variety of purposes. T. Hugh Crawford states that 'this absolute clarity could enable ownership – the doctor's diagnosis and the truth of the named disease. At the same time, admittance to that discourse is rigorously controlled, so members readily recognize each other and interlopers are kept at bay' (Crawford 1993: 82). Patients, as well as doctors, benefit from believing in doctors' authority based on science; patients usually prefer diagnoses to be efficient and accurate. An article in the *British Medical Journal* critiques the idea that 'the right treatment choice is a matter of science alone', as it notes how the adoption of the role of 'expert' by the doctor can relieve the patient of some anxiety and responsibility but also that this obscures some of the complex factors involved in making best diagnoses (Mulley *et al.* 8 November 2012). However, the extent to which patients want 'scientific' diagnoses should not be overstated. Other studies show that many patients prefer honesty over false claims to 'expertise' and can tolerate uncertainty if it is within this context (Brashers 2001: 477). Communication between patient and doctor is thus important, but not consistent in the clinical encounter, as patient expectations about the language and desirability of medical 'expertise' are heterogeneous.

To this point I have indicated that language is a crucial part of identifying, treating and experiencing illness and supporting health (Hamilton 2012). I now wish to turn to the case study of ERW, which offers expressive and interpretive options to participants (whether patients or doctors). In this chapter I primarily examine ERW as a process for patients seeking therapeutic resources and consider how this activity relates to the published literature giving 'the patient's point of view'.

Expressive and reflective writing: What, when, where?

ERW is a generic term for writing practices where creative process and personal expression and reflection are prioritized over writing as a finished product or artefact. ERW has applications in healthcare, social care, prisons, businesses, education, residential care homes and other settings. Where there is no clinically identifiable illness, the focus is often personal development or well-being, or the healthy functioning of an organization or team. ERW may be facilitated or take non-facilitated or self-facilitated forms, for example in journaling, whose styles and techniques have been described by Progoff (1992), Adams (1990) and Thompson (2010). While an exposition of theories underpinning ERW is not within the scope of this chapter, it is worth noting three potentially therapeutic aspects of this form of writing: firstly, ERW has the capacity to alleviate effects of trauma and afford new ways of thinking about experience; secondly, the creative process provides opportunities for self-actualization; thirdly, ERW can contribute to holistic and self-supporting healthcare. This chapter later returns to debates about the extent to which writing is therapeutic, but it is worth outlining these theories at the outset. ERW's 'therapeutic' effect, I suggest, operates both by affording mental and emotional resources to participants and by implicitly permitting a patient-centred critique of biomedical definitions of health, allowing opportunities for meaning-making that institutional clinical practice frequently, and unconsciously, precludes or restricts.

In the UK, writing projects with therapeutic aims have developed a strong presence in diverse settings. A significant moment for medical interest in arts was when the UK's Chief Medical Officer Sir Kenneth Calman, following a meeting with the Minister of Health in 1996, invited representatives from arts, medical and therapeutic fields to discuss incorporating them into the National Health Service (NHS), leading to the Windsor I Conference in 1998. Current and recent projects based in the NHS include Bristol Writing for Health, ArtLift in Gloucestershire, Year of Writing in Cumbria and The Biscuit Tin in Inverness. Yet writing practices with patients have not achieved a comparable position in mainstream

healthcare in the UK as art and music, which acquired identities as therapies in the 1970s and 1980s.

The roots of ERW can be identified in overlapping literary and psycho-
logical interests in the post-war period. In North America, the work of
Adler, Jung, Arieti and Reik in particular were influential from the 1960s.
Psychiatrists such as Roger Lauer in Maryland devised writing interventions
and in 1963 the poet Eli Greifer published a pamphlet entitled *Principles of
Poetry Therapy*. The Association of Poetry Therapy was formed in 1969 to
represent and support practitioners and promote excellence in the field.
In the US 'poetry therapy' and 'bibliotherapy', 'the intentional use of
poetry and other forms of literature for healing and personal growth',
achieved professional recognition through certification by the National
Federation for Biblio/Poetry Therapy (established 1980). Such certification requires 'poetry therapists' to have extensive prior training in a mental
health field such as counselling, social work or psychology, or through
medical training, in order to work in clinical settings. Arts-trained practitioners can qualify as 'poetry facilitators' to work in 'developmental
settings'. If they work in clinical settings they must do this under the supervision of a qualified mental health professional. In 1987 the *Journal of Poetry
Therapy* was launched in the US with Nicholas Mazza, a Professor of Social
Work, as its editor. Human rights and feminist movements such as the
Women's Health Movement also created a space for the voices of stigma-
tized and marginalized groups.

The emergence of ERW in Britain, in the 1980s and 1990s, was particularly concerned with training for writer-facilitators, albeit less formalized
than in the music therapy movement discussed in Helen Odell-Miller's
chapter within this volume. The Poetry Society commissioned an internal
report on matters of 'health, healing and personal development' to examine what training, advocacy and support might be suitable for
writer-facilitators, many of whom had embarked on work with diverse
groups and subsequently felt a need to acquire skills in groupwork and
managing emotional problems. The organization Lapidus was formed in
the same year and continues as a networking and information organization
and publisher of *Lapidus Journal*. It has developed guidelines and an ethical code for writer-facilitators of ERW. Although training opportunities
have grown in recent years – for example, Metanoia Institute and
Middlesex University established an MSc programme in Creative Writing
for Therapeutic Purposes in 2011 – there is no formal accreditation procedure for practitioners of ERW or poetry therapy in the UK.

Possible reasons for this disparity may be that either ERW has trouble
articulating its own identity clearly or that professional training and
accreditation within the field are in development. Within ERW, 'therapeutic creative writing', 'therapeutic writing' and 'writing for well-being'
are frequently used terms and 'reflective practice' is sometimes separately
identified. While there is not space here to comment on each of these

terms, my own practice combines creative process with attention to mental processes and physical symptoms in attempting to enable participants to articulate what is important to them. A major principle is that stories – and reflexive awareness of these – can play an important role in health, especially but not exclusively mental health, not least because they enable meaning-making options for individuals in relation to pre-existing frames of meaning. While I do argue for therapeutic effects, I also see problems in formalizing ERW into a 'therapy', particularly where definitions of therapy draw heavily on medical paradigms rather than artistic-literary ones.

Another obstacle to ERW's progression within statutorily governed environments of healthcare is the widespread awareness that literature and the writing process, like medicine, can have potential iatrogenic outcomes as well as produce positive effects. An association between mental illness and creativity regularly expressed in popular media simplifies the 'mad genius controversy' investigated by Becker (1978) and others and tends to stimulate caution among those wary of creative process. However, scientific evidence as to whether writing eased or provoked the suffering of writers such as John Clare, Sylvia Plath and Virginia Woolf has not emerged. In ERW, facilitator competencies and attention to working conditions are crucial to ensure best practice and minimize potential harmful effects (Flint, Hamilton and Williamson 2004). In therapeutic writing training, students learn how to use appropriate stimuli, facilitate creative process and hold a space so that diverse responses can be explored.

The patient's voice

The 'patient's voice' has become increasingly central to healthcare, poetry therapy and ERW in the last 40 years. In the late-twentieth century, poetry therapy and ERW on both sides of the Atlantic were influenced by broader culture trends. These trends included the interest in narratives that came with the linguistic turn of the 1970s and 1980s and a related renewed cultural focus on marginalized voices. In the 1980s, the arts in healthcare movement in the UK placed artists, including writers, in healthcare settings 'in order to humanise the whole delivery of clinical care' (Sampson 1999: 9). *Survivors' Poetry* was founded in 1991 to promote and publish the poetry of 'survivors of the UK mental health system'. Speaking for the survivor movement, in the 1990s Ron Bassman commented that 'as people whose feelings, thoughts, and experiences have been described, judged, and interpreted by others, survivors insist on speaking for themselves and defining their own experience' (Bassman 1997: 239). Policy changes also produced openings for arts practices by shifting the emphasis in patient and doctor roles. Increasing concern with transparency, for example, is reflected in the Data Protection Act of 1998 that gave patients in the UK statutory rights to have access to their medical notes.

Arenas for the patient's voice also opened up during the late-twentieth century in published literature, online forums and the popular media's coverage of health matters. ERW may be seen as another manifestation of this trend. Grassroots social and political action from the 1960s paved the way for patients to articulate first-hand views of conditions lacking compassionate collective narratives. This movement produced a few literary gems, such as Christopher Nolan's fictional autobiography *Under the Eye of the Clock* (1987) about his cerebral palsy. However, in the late-twentieth century publishing houses were sometimes cautious in championing the patient's point of view. Following the surge of HIV/AIDS in the 1980s, authors such as Adam Mars-Jones and Edmund White in *Darker Proof: Stories from a Crisis*, Alan Hollinghurst (2005) and Michael Cunningham (2003) included AIDS as part of the central narrative of their novels. However, Thom Gunn is the only well-known British-born poet of the period to have tackled the subject directly, in *The Man with Night Sweats* (1992), and he had moved to the US long before. At this time, political activism and the development of effective medicines had more visible effects on the stigma surrounding HIV/AIDS than literary writing.

It was not until the twenty-first century that significant numbers of patient voices were heard in pathologies, film adaptations and online health forums. Will Self (2011), on being diagnosed with *polycythaemia vera*, a blood condition, recounts how he arrives to see his GP having self-diagnosed using information on the internet and proceeds to demonstrate mastery of clinical terms. Poet June Hall provides another example of a writer-turned-patient crafting language to critique and partially master her emotions, or at least to reflect on them differently. In 'Snakes' (2004) the neurologist's matter-of-fact prognosis for Parkinson's disease segues into the recipient's emotional response and the effect on her sense of hope. I use these examples not as illustrations of ERW but of the emergence of patients' narratives in published literature that corresponds to the interest in patients' voices in therapeutic work.

Gwyneth Lewis' long poem 'A Hospital Odyssey' illustrates the increasing confidence of writers in seeking to articulate personal perspectives on, and thus make their own meanings out of, health crises that affect them. The character of 'Maris' attends hospital with her husband, who is having treatment for cancer. Lewis' poetic gaze takes the reader inside the body like a powerful microscope and then looks at the hospital's interiors with human eyes, before looking far beyond to the sea and the stars like a telescope. The poem's language incorporates medical terms and the latest stem cell science. A screen shows magnified images of 'white and red corpuscles – erythrocytes/and leukocytes, each one a world/like a planet'. Her husband's bone marrow 'looked like a coastline on its glass slide/an aerial reconnaissance photo/of channels scoured by hostile tides'. Maris says:

...poetry excels at close-up and slow-motion,
it alters how we see space and time,
makes us their masters by changing their signs
for a while. This is why art is medicine

of kinds, although I'd take the chemo
as well as iambic tetrameter,
if I were ill enough and had to.

(Lewis 2010: 109)

Lewis suggests how poetry affects writer and reader by altering pace, shifting perspective and allowing control of perceptions. Further, this process suggests that 'art is medicine', though with the caveat that medicine's remedies are also desperately needed. Such published texts provide eloquent testimony of the patient's changing position with regard to narratives of illness.

Techniques

The section that follows provides a description of some of the techniques that I use in ERW sessions. The examples are snapshots of the process by which writing approaches and exercises are chosen, which bear in mind the need to structure activities according to pace and the participant. The first example discusses a general process, while the second two are specific case studies of work with patients.

1. Reading a text

A poem or other text is chosen that provides thematic or emotive resonance for the participant as well as an example of poetic form. In such sessions the choice of text is important and must take into account accessibility, subject matter, tone, relevance in relation to participants' interests, identity and aspects of health and well-being (Field 2006: 97–99). A poem read with one participant is Wendell Berry's 'The Peace of Wild Things' (Berry 1998). Berry's evocation of a peaceful place by water where he experiences relief from despair, fear and grief is a meditation that connects landscapes of mind, nature and 'wild things'. The participant's own recollections of a similar peaceful place can provide a context to explore their thoughts and feelings without becoming overwhelmed. Jane Speedy notes that narratological interest in such evocative texts can leave 'gaps or "liminal" spaces for possibilities' (Speedy 2004: 27). In Berry's poem, the poet describes an actual liminal space between sleep and waking, between earth, water and sky, in which consciousness shifts towards a sense of peacefulness and connection with natural and animal worlds.

2. Exploring images and discovering metaphors

In another session, ERW was used with a participant who mentioned feeling anger about the effects of her medical treatment. She was invited to explore these emotions by writing the words 'anger is' in a list repeatedly and adding different associations using verbs, nouns and adjectives. Given the option not to share the writing, she found that repetition brought more unusual ideas to mind and some vivid images. These images functioned metaphorically by gathering different elements of experience: a recollected real landscape, the emotions associated with it and her connection with other people and times. In such facilitated writing metaphor operates not merely as a poetic device, but rather is 'a way of linking up the disparate elements of ourselves and our world; a way of enabling the voices of these elements – normally clamouring silently – to speak and be heard' (Bolton and Lathan 2004: 117). It can connect the writer to 'sub-symbolic emotion and experience' and activate 'images which then form the basis of emotional schemas' (Robinson 2000: 5). Images conveyed in written words form a compact, discrete and intense 'vessel of meaning' linking inner and outer worlds, and can crystallize semi-symbolic images so that multiple aspects of experience can be conveyed to oneself and the facilitator. In the example discussed here, the participant discovered that her anger was many things, including a majestic mountain and a spiky holly bush, a bomb, dancing 'dervishly' and a silent stare; it was both mobile and still, empowered and aggressive. She remarked that noticing these aspects surprised her and that discussing them made her feel differently about her anger.

3. Improvization and flexible perspectives

In another case, we used ERW to develop themes through staged writing and reflection. The participant's concrete imagining of an abstract phenomenon, emotion or state gave options for looking from different points of view. The participant imagined his grief in bereavement as an old coat and proceeded in guided stages to write from the point of view of himself wearing the coat and then as the coat itself. He embellished the description of the coat so that it gained features such as grey-beige colours and ragged sleeves, one of which is impossible to put on. From the point of view of the coat, he wrote that the coat wanted to be worn, but did not like its colours or ragged sleeve and realized that the wearer was made uncomfortable by having his arm twisted to put it on. The participant was interested by the idea of grief being an 'arm-twister' and the notion that the coat had compassionate intentions in wanting to make the wearer warm, and he began to see it in a different way.

Literary language, medical language

Creative writing differs from spoken versions of the patient's story in medical consultations. ERW offers a performative element when a piece of writing is read out, and words become embodied through the use of voice, breath and sound. The alternation of talk, writing and reflection creates a rhythm that is different from that of a typical clinical consultation, and could be said to connect participants with 'the activities that mark us as human ... (that) pulse, fade out, and pulse again in human tissue, human nerves, and in the elemental humus of memory, dreams, and art ... ' (Rich 2001: 1). Mediation by a writer-facilitator is also different from that of the doctor. These factors influence how and what the patient articulates.

Below are examples of poetry by people who are both writers and patients: Roy Bayfield, whose first collection of poems arose from writing during recovery from heart surgery; and participant Claudia Haslam who wrote in sessions in hospital and who has given her permission to publish two haiku here. While such examples offer insights into how imaginative and poetic language works, it is important to emphasize that ERW is primarily about process and that written outcomes can be much less formed, coherent or finished than these examples. Facilitated writing activities can be carried out by people with varying degrees of confidence with literacy: scribing and oral telling are options too. Encouragement is given to anyone interested in participating, as accessibility is a main aim. Participants regularly comment that experiences in school convinced them they were 'not creative' or 'not good at this kind of thing' and that sessions help to overcome that conviction.

In 'Cardiac Cowboy Saloon', Bayfield draws upon the figure of a cowboy from his recollections of Western films to express woundedness and changed identity:

> We are feeble desperadoes
> grizzled from the frontier
> of bodies and time, caught
> stumbling from the goldrush,
> backshot, bad-luck cards dropping
> to a sterile tavern
> floor
>
> (Bayfield 2010: 10)

In this poem the men on the ward are heroic in their battles with physical challenge and suffering, yet in their vulnerability they are very unlike macho cowboys:

minor lavatorial triumphs
are cause for common celebration.
Plastic tubes dangle brightly,
like borrowed tribal jewellery.
Our scars prove us to be hard
men

(Bayfield 2010: 10)

Bayfield reflects on the writing process in the *Lapidus Journal*: '[i]llness had reduced my independence, and treatment involved profound surrender to the healthcare process. By contrast, writing gave me a vast and wild freedom, with the autonomy to interpret experiences as I wished' (Bayfield 2011: 4). He assumes a more potent position in relation to his illness by drawing on a figure of male heroism existing in a 'free' and 'independent' exterior location to explore the experience of being a patient weakened and confined to a ward. His poem evokes comic and tragic aspects of the experience and allows a typically male figure of heroism to be questioned as well as associated with coping with illness, perhaps implicitly also questioning 'masculinized' models of medical practice that frequently employ military metaphors – the 'magic bullet', 'fighting disease', 'killer cells' being 'zapped'.

Haslam used the Japanese haiku form to reflect on and communicate the frightening and painful experience of losing her hair because of chemotherapy:

A winter's night grips
My fragile bones, my face rasped
Raw by frozen tears.

Like Voldemort, me,
Hairless chemo patient, though
Less snaky, with specs.

(Haslam 2012)

The haiku form has three lines with five, then seven, then five syllables. Such use of few lines and syllables involves distilling experience and rendering it succinctly, yet leaving space for the emotional tone to be felt. The evil character Voldemort from J. K. Rowling's *Harry Potter* novels is used to allow the juxtaposition of suffering and deft self-deprecating humour. Commenting on the writing process, she remarked: 'it helped me to put into words what I was experiencing and feeling' and 'it is so helpful to be with others who can validate experience' (Haslam 2012).

While clinical discourses often emphasize 'terms of scientific certainty' and 'maintenance of the physician's authority' (Crawford 1993: 131), poetic writing can express lived experience that is 'extraordinarily muddled and chaotic, certainly not made up of clear beginnings, middles and ends' (Bolton 2000: 20). Narratologist Jerome Bruner suggests that accomplished writing 'creates not only a story, but also a sense of its contingent and uncertain variants' (Bruner 1986: 174). Diagnosis of a life-threatening illness such as cancer can provoke shock, fear, sadness and a sense of life narrative being interrupted or even calling its meaning into question. Other conditions such as depression and post-viral syndrome, or the negative emotional effects of a physical illness such as a stroke or injury, likewise tend to provoke questioning:

> [M]ost people would probably agree that they spend as much time reflecting privately on events, as they do articulating their thoughts and feelings to others. This has had obvious adaptive value in helping people take stock of changing conditions, make plans to overcome what is changeable, and adjust to what is not... [but this] can nonetheless lead to problems when these mental scenarios become intrusive on our thinking.
>
> (Brennan 2004: 37)

The goal of this reflection is not merely being able to conceive of problems, but finding ways to express them, to move them from 'within' to 'outside' in ways that include some sense of coherence.

Writer-facilitators tend to have heightened awareness of the multiple possible meanings in narratives and time to listen to these when working with patients. Introducing writing into the clinical environment opens possibilities for varied styles and paces of discourse and this can have profound influence on patients' experience of illness and treatment. As Jane Speedy argues, '[c]onversations that explicitly contain the possibility of poetic writings seem qualitatively different to other kinds of therapeutic conversations. The notes taken, questions asked, and spaces entered all appear to be shaped to some extent, by these possibilities' (Speedy 2005: 283).

Patients as experts

ERW techniques, which encourage a reflexive stance towards existing narratives, frequently employ published texts with patients and doctors to open up a critical and discursive space. Literature as artefact combines with writing as process to produce narratives not only of an individual's illness, but of the relationship between patient and clinician that may be reconfigured in ways that are potentially therapeutic in that they invite the story of illness – and of medicine – to be jointly authored. Through struggle, experimentation and uncertainty, a multi-faceted, more satisfying story may emerge. The goal is not merely to acclimatize the patient to illness, but to challenge powerful interpretations of illness that may restrict options for health.

Alan Bleakley's chapter in this volume argues that the medical humanities can provide a critical counterweight to reductive biomedical science and that arts interventions, especially drawing on the avant-garde, have the power to unsettle yet offer meaning to illness. ERW too can illuminate 'complicated truths' (Frank 2010: 5): it is no mere salve. The 'well-being' it endorses is not limited to making individuals 'feel better' but extends to adjusting the ethos and systems of care. For medical students, reflective writing and reading may draw attention to how value judgements as well as factual evidence influence identification and categorization of disorders (Spitzer 1981) or how cultural factors such as stigma influence the naming of disease, as with neurasthenia in Asian cultures (Schwartz 2002). Doctor-writers provide valuable insights from both angles. For example, studying William Carlos Williams' (1984) descriptions of the lives of patients, Dannie Abse's (2003) evocation of the experience of a patient on an operating table, or oncologist Siddhartha Mukherjee's (2011) 'biography of cancer' encourage a critical reappraisal of both doctors' and patients' experiences. Roter and Hall (2006) offer a meta-analysis of research into communication in medicine, confirming that patients value being listened to and that doctors talk too much, interrupt too much and close down consultations too early. How then is it possible to hear the patient's point of view in busy, target-driven medical practice? Perhaps the answer lies in accepting that any view is partial and provisional and in allowing multiple viewpoints.

The need for developments of this kind is supported by my own research. I conducted a thematic analysis of written feedback comments provided by 40 participants of ERW sessions between 2007 and 2011, which were held either in groups at Bristol's Brooklea Health Centre or in one-to-one sessions and groups at the Bristol Haematology and Oncology Centre (Hamilton 2013). The limitations of this methodology must be acknowledged, such as a small sample size and the possibility of participants' responses being shaped by deference to the facilitator. However, the study provides useful starting points for further analysis. Participants mentioned the following as being valuable to them, in order of frequency:

1. The opportunity to reflect on or revise (often painful) personal narratives

'It's like having another sense awakened – you get a different way of thinking about things'.

2. The opportunity and new ways to express feelings and thoughts

'When I started I realized it wasn't like being taught to write, but about expressing things in my own way; I felt I was able to articulate my feelings, explore further and then share with those who had been through similar things'.

'Almost always I came away from a session with an enormous sense of release and therefore much calmer'.

3. A positive change in emotions and confidence

'[I]t gave me confidence; [writing] gave me back some control'.

'[T]he sessions have had an effect on my feelings and how to share them'.

4. Artistic pleasure, distraction

'I would literally just be messing about...on the brink of tears, and find that I'd made a poem, or some crazy little collage. I was so pleased with one that I got a photocopy'.

'[The sessions] gave me something pleasurable to think about at a time when I was going through treatment'.

5. Being listened to / sharing with others

'I felt I was able to articulate my feelings, explore further and then share with those who had been through similar things'.

'This sense that your feelings are valuable; valid; worth expressing – this is what is helpful to me'.

6. Developing resources for self-care

'I think the tools I have gained will help directly/indirectly about the feelings about myself'.

Further indications that participants valued the writing sessions were regular attendance, positive feedback during and at the end of sessions and requests that sessions continue for others. Participants also explicitly associated the effects of ERW with increased self-perceived 'well-being'. Interestingly, very few mentioned improvements in physical health in reporting well-being, even where this was the reason for seeking medical help in the first place. Their interpretation of achieving 'wellness' involved medical care but was not solely confined to it, a consideration that aligns both with attention to 'whole person care' being provided in some medical education faculties and with my argument for an expansion of concepts of health and by extension of what is health-promoting.

The principles of narrative therapy developed by Michael White and David Epston (1990) could also provide a useful platform from which to develop ERW and articulate its therapeutic strengths. In narrative therapy, people are viewed as experts in their own worlds, even if they are not yet aware of this 'expertise'. The therapist then attempts to foster collaborative modes in which the person is encouraged to review life narratives and identify his or her own resourcefulness. Both practices involve 'the identification or generation of alternative stories that enable them to perform new meanings, bringing with them desired possibilities – new meanings that persons will experience as more helpful, satisfying, and open-ended' (White and Epston 1990: 15).

Is writing therapeutic?

The findings from my own small sample above can be helpfully situated against a number of meta-studies on the impact of therapeutic writing. I cite a selection here to indicate the problems associated with trying to find 'one size fits all' answers about the relationship between arts and health using empirical and large-scale studies. I do not claim that these examples provide full coverage of the extensive and complex literature on links between arts and health. The work of Rosalia Staricoff (2004) provides the closest that we have to such a 'full' literature review. She cites nearly 400 papers showing a positive impact of arts interventions on health outcomes, and states that:

> The use of literature, creative writing and poetry in mental health services produces significant benefits for both the patient and the care provider. It enables patients to regain control over their own inner world, increasing their mental well-being. It helps the nursing and medical staff to understand the cultural, social, ethnic and economic factors influencing the behaviour of patients.
>
> (Staricoff 2004: 20)

However, patients should not be treated as homogeneous. GPs Mugerwa and Holden (2012: 662) list studies in which therapeutic writing was beneficial to people with conditions such as high blood pressure and rheumatoid arthritis, and in which no beneficial effect was noted, for example in people with migraine and lung disease. Researchers acknowledge the influence on outcomes of unexplored variants in these studies with regard to disease types and writing protocols, which future studies will need to address in more detail. Mugerwa and Holden also refer to a meta-analysis (Frattaroli 2006) drawing on 146 randomized control studies where most outcome types (psychological health, physiological functioning, reported health, subjective impact of the intervention and general functioning) showed positive and significant effect sizes; health behaviours showed positive but non-significant benefit. Undesirable outcomes such as increase in negative mood immediately after writing about traumatic events (Bell-Pringle *et al.* 2004: 341) is one indicator that supportive facilitation can be a crucial determinant of outcomes as well as an ethical consideration.

Studies collated by Stephen J. Lepore and Joshua M. Smyth analyzing 'the writing cure' also provide a range of findings, many suggesting writing's beneficial effects. However, the editors note that '[a]lthough health measures are a convincing outcome measure, researchers and policy makers must also appreciate their crudeness' (Lepore and Smyth 2002: 288). Early studies of the therapeutic effects of writing by psychologists James Pennebaker and Sandra Beall (1986) used short- and long-term physiological, health and self-report measures of health. Subsequent studies have assessed the benefits of emotional disclosure (Petrie *et al.* 2004), of not suppressing negative emotions and of 'buffering' negative thoughts (Lepore and Smyth 2002). However, mechanisms for writing's benefits remain unclear.

A sample of different studies points to some of the difficulties of achieving consistency and reliability of research outcomes regarding writing's effects. For example, Schoutrop *et al.* (2002) examine the impact of writing on the processing of stressful events, Klapow *et al.* (2001) show a reduced use of outpatient services and Gidron *et al.* (2002) show a reduced number of clinic visits. In the Schoutrop study, closer analysis of the impact of writing on effects of the trauma was not followed up. The Klapow study's conclusions were critiqued by Wood (2007) on the basis of interpretation of somatic and distress scores and within-group variability. The Gidron study, like many others, used a small sample (41). Since writing interventions are at the interface of therapeutic/medical and literary paradigms, designing and delivering studies is inevitably complex. Variables include the number and duration of sessions, writing instructions, follow-up, profile of participants, aims and facilitation or lack of it. Wright and Cheung Chung (2001) highlight the difficulty in bringing both literary and scientifically oriented practitioners' knowledge and skills to bear.

The difficulties associated with such empirical studies indicate that existing health measures themselves require scrutiny. A robust philosophy of healthcare that allows for debate may be more open to new frameworks of 'therapy' alongside the use of consistent research protocols. In this way an evidence base for ERW might be developed that challenges as well as complements the growth of biomedicine.

Outlook

Increasing an evidence base for writing interventions requires funding and resources. Auto-ethnographic studies such as those employed by Kim Etherington (2003) align well with narrative practices and could be cost-effective to design and implement, but for these to be more acceptable to an evidence-based clinical practice, more work is required in engaging with epistemological bases of practice in more philosophical debate. Allowing the patient's own words to be central in this is important. Medical humanities offer a promising forum for devising research studies that could further build bridges between medicine and writing. As psychoneurobiology brings new understandings of mind and body interactions and as mental health becomes an increased priority for services treating ageing populations, writing practices may attract even greater interest as a sustainable resource for patients. They do not deny, avoid or diminish illness as clinically defined or treated, but allow it to exist within the context of other types of experience. For both doctor and patient, the heart of the matter at the intersection of medicine and literary arts could be not so much to do with the flesh – 'what is matter?' – or even the problem – 'what's the matter?' – but instead about meaning – 'what matters?' Answering that question requires all the resources at our disposal, including openness and imagination.

References

Abse, D. (2003) 'In the Theatre' in D. Abse, *New and Collected Poems*, London: Hutchinson.

Adams, K. (1990) *Journal to the Self*, New York: Warner Books.

Bassman, R. (1997) 'The Mental Health System: Experiences from Both Sides of the Locked Doors', *Professional Psychology: Research and Practice*, 28: 238–42.

Bayfield, R. (2010) 'Cardiac Cowboy Saloon' in R. Bayfield, *Bypass Pilgrim*, trans_genre_books.

Bayfield, R. (2011) 'Eight Times to the Green Heart: Walking, Writing and Rehab', *Lapidus Journal*, 6. Online. Available: http://lapidusjournal.org (accessed 2 July 2012).

Becker G. (1978) *The Mad Genius Controversy*, London: Sage.

Bell-Pringle, V., Jurkovic, G. and Pate, J. (2004) 'Writing about Upsetting Family Events: A Therapy Analog Study', *Journal of Contemporary Psychotherapy*, 34: 341–9.

Berry, W. (1998) 'The Peace of Wild Things' in W. Berry, *The Selected Poems of Wendell Berry*, Berkeley: Counterpoint.

Bolton, G. (2000) *The Therapeutic Potential of Creative Writing*, London: Jessica Kingsley Publishers.

Bolton, G. and Lathan, J. (2004) ' "Every Poem Breaks a Silence that had to be Overcome": The Therapeutic Role of Poetry Writing' in G. Bolton, S. Howlett, C. Lago and J. K. Wright (eds) *Writing Cures*, London: Brunner-Routledge.

Brashers, D. E. (2001) 'Communication and Uncertainty Management', *Journal of Communication*, 51: 477–97.

Brennan, J. (2004) *Cancer in Context*, Oxford: Oxford University Press.

Bruner, J. (1986) *Actual Minds, Possible Worlds*, Cambridge, MA: Harvard University Press.

Carlos Williams, W. (1984) *The Doctor Stories*, New York: New Directions Publishing.

Crawford, T. H. (1993) *Modernism, Medicine, & William Carlos Williams*, Norman: University of Oklahoma Press.

Cunningham, M. (2003) *The Hours*, London: Fourth Estate.

Etherington, K. (2003) *Trauma, the Body and Transformation*, London: Jessica Kingsley Publishers.

Field, V. (2006) 'Writing from Published Poems' in G. Bolton, V. Field and K. Thompson (eds) *Writing Works*, London: Jessica Kingsley Publishers.

Flint, R., Hamilton F. and Williamson C. (2004) 'Core Competencies for Working with the Literary Arts for Personal Development, Health and Well-Being'. Online. Available: www.lapidus.org.uk/resources/index.php (accessed 2 July 2012).

Foucault, M. (1975 [1963]) *The Birth of the Clinic: An Archaeology of Medical Perception*, trans. A. M. Sheridan Smith, New York: Vintage Books.

Frank, A. W. (2010) *Letting Stories Breathe*, Chicago: University of Chicago Press.

Frattaroli, J. (2006) 'Experimental Disclosure and its Moderators: A Meta -Analysis', *Psychological Bulletin*, 132: 823–65.

Gidron, Y., Duncan, E., Lazar, A., *et al.*, (2002) 'Effects of Guided Written Disclosure of Stressful Experiences on Clinic Visits and Symptoms in Frequent Clinic Attenders', *Family Practice*, 19: 161–6.

Greifer, E. (1963) *Principles of Poetry Therapy*, New York: Poetry Therapy Center.

Guglani, S. (2011) 'Medicine Unboxed', *Lapidus Journal*, 5:3. Online. Available: http://lapidusjournal.org (accessed 9 November 2012).

Gunn, T. (1992) *The Man with Night Sweats*, London: Faber and Faber.

Hall, J. (2004) 'Snakes' in *The Now Of Snow*, Bath: Belgrave Press.

Hamilton, F. (2012) 'Language, Story and Health', *Journal of Holistic Healthcare* 9: 17–21.

Hamilton, F. (2013) 'A Thematic Analysis of Participants' Feedback in Writing Sessions in a Primary and a Secondary Care Setting in the NHS'. Online. Available: www.lapidus.org.uk/index.php/resources/evaluation/ (accessed 2 January 2013).

Haslam, C. (2012) 'Instant Anthology', unpublished poetry anthology.

Hollinghurst, A. (2005) *The Line of Beauty*, London: Picador.

Journal of Poetry Therapy (1987–), Philadelphia: Taylor & Francis.

Klapow, J. C., Schmidt, S. M., Taylor, L. A., *et al.*, (2001) 'Symptom Management in Older Primary Care Patients. Feasibility of an Experimental, Written Self-Disclosure Protocol', *Annals of Internal Medicine*, 134: 905–11.

Lepore, S. J. and Smyth, J. M. (2002) *The Writing Cure: How Expressive Writing Promotes Health and Emotional Well-Being*, Washington DC: American Psychological Association.

Lewis, G. (2010) *A Hospital Odyssey*, Northumberland: Bloodaxe Books.

Mars-Jones, A. and White, E. (1988) *The Darker Proof: Stories from a Crisis*, London: Faber and Faber.

Mugerwa, S. and Holden, J. D. (2012) 'Writing Therapy: A New Tool for General Practice?', *British Journal of General Practice*, 62: 661–3.

Mukherjee, S. (2011) *The Emperor of All Maladies*, London: Fourth Estate.

Mulley, A., Trimble, C. and Elwyn, G. (2012) 'Stop the Silent Misdiagnosis: Patients' Preferences Matter', *British Medical Journal*, 345: e6572.

Nolan, C. (1987) *Under the Eye of the Clock*, London: Pan Books.

O'Donohue, J. (1999) *Anam Cara: Spiritual Wisdom from the Celtic World*, London: Transworld Publishers.

Pennebaker, J. W. and Beall, S. K. (1986) 'Confronting a Traumatic Event: Toward an Understanding of Inhibition and Disease', *Journal of Abnormal Psychology*, 95: 274–81.

Petrie K. J., Fontanilla I., Thomas M. G., Booth R. J. and Pennebaker J. W. (2004) 'Effect of Written Emotional Expression on Immune Function in Patients with Human Immunodeficiency Virus Infection: A Randomized Trial', *Psychosomatic Medicine*, 66: 272–5.

Poetry Society (1996) 'Report on Health, Healing and Personal Development', unpublished report.

Progoff, I. (1992) *At a Journal Workshop*, 2nd edn, New York: Jeremy Tarcher.

Rich, A. (11 March 2001) 'Credo of a Passionate Skeptic', *Los Angeles Times*. Online. Available: www.english.illinois.edu/maps/poets/m_r/rich/onlineessays.htm (accessed 3 March 2013).

Robinson, M. (2000) 'Writing Well: Health and the Power to Make Images', *Journal of Medical Ethics: Medical Humanities*, 26: 79–84.

Roter, D. and Hall, J. (2006) *Doctors Talking with Patients/Patients Talking with Doctors: Improving Communication in Medical Visits*, Connecticut: Praeger.

Sampson, F. (1999) *The Healing Word*, London: Poetry Society.

Schoutrop, M. J. A., Lange, A., Hanewald, G., *et al.* (2002) 'Structured Writing and Processing Major Stressful Events: A Controlled Trial', *Psychotherapy and Psychosomatics*, 71: 151–7.

Schwartz, P. Y. (2002) 'Why is Neurasthenia Important in Asian Cultures?', *Western Journal of Medicine*, 176: 257–8.

Self, W. (21 October 2011) 'Will Self: The Trouble with My Blood', *The Guardian*. Online. Available: www.guardian.co.uk/books/2011/oct/21/will-self-blood-disease (accessed 2 July 2012).

Speedy, J. (2005) 'Using Poetic Documents: An Exploration of Poststructuralist Ideas and Poetic Practices in Narrative Therapy', *British Journal of Guidance & Counselling*, 33: 283–98.

Speedy, J. (2004) 'The Contribution of Narrative Ideas and Writing Practices in Therapy' in G. Bolton, S. Howlett, C. Lago and J. K. Wright (eds) *Writing Cures*, London: Brunner-Routledge.

Spitzer, R. (1981) 'The Diagnostic Status of Homosexuality in DSM-III: A Reformulation of the Issues', *The American Journal of Psychiatry*, 138: 210–15.

Staricoff, R. L. (2004) *Arts in Health: A Review of the Medical Literature*, London: Arts Council.

Thompson, K. (2010) *Therapeutic Journal Writing*, London: Jessica Kingsley Publishers.

White, M. and Epston, D. (1990) *Narrative Means to Therapeutic Ends*, Adelaide: Dulwich Centre.

Williams, W. C. (1984) *The Doctor Stories*, New York: New Directions Publishing.

Wood, G. (2007) *Written Emotional Disclosure for Lay Caregivers of Older Adults*, Ann Arbor, MI: ProQuest Information and Learning Company.

Wright, J. and Chung, M. C. (2001) 'Mastery or Mystery? Therapeutic Writing: A Review of the Literature', *British Journal of Guidance and Counselling*, 29: 277–91.

Section Four

Performance

10 Performance anxiety

The relationship between social and aesthetic drama in medicine and health

Overview

Emma Brodzinski

Contemporary dramatic practice has problematized the relationship between art and everyday life and highlighted reciprocity between different spheres of experience. This chapter focuses on reciprocity between performance and medicine, seeking to provide a conceptual framework and contextual background for the case study chapters that follow. The chapter takes a broad view of performance – from stage performance, through television (TV) drama, to the performance of everyday life – in order to consider the different facets and manifestations of the relationship between what I identify as 'social' drama and 'aesthetic' drama.

Performance and medicine: Models of reciprocity

French performance artist Orlan tells the story of how, in 1978, she became very ill while attending a conference where she was due to speak. Orlan was taken to hospital but requested that a camera crew accompany her and document the resulting emergency surgical procedure for an ectopic pregnancy. She insisted on having only local anaesthesia in order to remain able to observe and comment upon her own body being opened up. The documentation of this surgical encounter was then, at Orlan's request, screened in the slot allocated to her within the symposium. From 1990 until 1993 Orlan engaged in a series of surgeries entitled 'The Reincarnation of Saint Orlan'. She took the notion of an operating *theatre* literally and staged a series of cosmetic procedures intended to reconstruct her face in the likeness of representations of the feminine taken from celebrated works of art. Orlan viewed her project as engaging with the status of the body in a technologized culture, questioning biological limits in the context of cutting edge technology that can re-shape the body.

Orlan stated that the operating theatre became her artist's studio. The artist took up the central role of the patient yet sought to make an artistic intervention within medical discourse. Throughout her surgeries, she remained a conscious and active participant, often reading from philosophical texts as the surgery progressed. Orlan states that the impression that she hoped to give the audience was that of 'an autopsied corpse that continues to speak, as if detached from its body' (Orlan 1996: 90). As well as positing the sentient patient as a threat to the unquestioned authority of the medical practitioner, Orlan's intentions can be read in terms of employing the thrills of the early modern anatomy theatre. The anatomy theatres of the Renaissance were seen as places of entertainment as well as education; many lay people paid the entrance fee to sit alongside medical practitioners and witness the display of the body framed by grand processions and musical accompaniment. Orlan's contemporary practice, and the public attention it has received, appears to echo this appeal and demonstrate an ongoing fascination with what literary scholar Jonathan Sawday terms the 'ill-defined things at the outer limits of life and death' (Sawday 1995: 43) that converge around the anatomized body, as well as an interest in the operating theatre as a performance space.

The operating theatre orientates the spectator towards a heightened awareness of the surroundings. It is a site where the body is opened and most vulnerable – literally a space of life and death. Medical sociologists such as Nicholas Fox have explored the performative structures that surround the contemporary operating theatre. Fox's *The Social Meaning of Surgery* (1992) carries out a detailed examination of the ritual practices of the operating theatre and considers elements such as special clothing and the organization of space. Fox's study draws on the seminal work of sociologist Erving Goffman, who explored everyday life as drama and had a particular interest in the dramaturgical elements of the hospital. Goffman's enquiry considers the norms and conventions of the hospital theatre. He observes that:

> [I]n the operating-room measures are taken to ensure the audience, whose members number only one, is soon oblivious to the weaknesses of the show, permitting the operating team to relax and devote itself to the technological requirements of actions as opposed to the dramaturgical ones.
>
> (Goffman 1976: 213)

It seems that Orlan engages with the drama of the hospital theatre and combines it with the demonstrative intentions of the anatomy theatre. In asserting herself as an active patient, Orlan can be seen to highlight the weakness of the 'show'. She describes her intervention as a process that is 'de-sacrilizing the surgical act' (Orlan 1996: 90). Not only does Orlan refuse the role of passive patient, she also works to highlight the theatricality of the hospital theatre through the use of ridiculous props – such as plastic lobsters – and elaborate costume by designers such as Paco Rabanne. Employing excessive paraphernalia can be seen to highlight the fact that objects and clothes with special significance are always employed within the operating theatre but their normality makes them invisible. The painting of the walls and costuming of medical staff also disrupt the usual scripting of roles as, in this context, the patient can be seen to be controlling the space.

Orlan's deconstruction of the operating theatre is also part of the impulse behind her public screening of events. In displaying actions that are usually hidden from view, or carefully edited within television documentaries, Orlan seeks to destabilize the mystique of surgery. In her seventh surgery, her subversive activity extended to inviting her audiences to interact with the processes of the operating theatre via satellite, fax and telephone, opening the room to those outside and disrupting its status as 'one of the most inaccessible 'back-spaces' of the modern hospital' (Fox 1992: 14).

Orlan uses her artistic practice to enact a feminist critique of surgery and open up wider discussion concerning identity. She states: 'My body has become a site of public debate that poses crucial questions for our time' (Orlan 1996: 88). The permanent changes to Orlan's own body and her personal investment in the work give it a particular quality. Live Art practice, which challenges the boundaries of art and life, can be traced back through the experimentation of the Modernist avant-garde but, more particularly, to developments in the neo avant-garde, which took hold in 1970s. Orlan asserts:

> My work emerged during the seventies…when art was engaged with the social, the political, the ideological; a period when artists were very invested intellectually, conceptually and sometimes physically in their work.
>
> (Orlan 1996: 85)

During the 1970s a range of practitioners embraced the use of the artist's own body as material. These artists sought to explore emergent radical political agendas – particularly anti-establishment and feminist principles – through corporeal expression. Orlan began working within the Fluxus movement, which resonated with her interest in socially engaged practice. She staged a number of performance events including her 'MesuRAGE' series, where she used her body to measure national monuments with the intention of highlighting patriarchal values embodied within cultural institutions. This type of experimental performance can be understood within the wider counter-cultural movement that sought to critique social grand narratives and promote the personal as political. There was an emphasis on direct experience, and aesthetic events were perceived as potential visible socio-political actions that could serve to instruct consciousness and feedback in to the drama of everyday life.

Orlan posits that '[c]osmetic surgery is one of the sites in which man's power over the body of woman can inscribe itself most strongly' (Orlan

1996: 91). What is significant within her practice is the framing of the work as an aesthetic action and the foregrounding of cosmetic surgery as a medium of exploration rather than as a means to a desired outcome. For example, for forty-one days after the seventh operation-performance *Omnipresence* (until her face was completely healed) an installation was mounted in the Centre Georges Pompidou, Paris. Each day a photograph of Orlan in her post-operative state was mounted in the gallery above one of Orlan's computer-generated images of idealized beauty. Unlike pictures published by cosmetic surgeons showing an imperfect 'before' shot and a well-crafted 'after', the images of Orlan's bruised face and bleeding wounds following surgery highlighted the violence done to the body in the pursuit of idealized beauty. In foregrounding the reciprocity of art and life, Orlan's work posits surgical practice as another kind of performance.

The case study of Orlan provides a useful starting point for enquiry for this overview chapter on medicine and performance. Her work raises many of the matters that I intend to explore in more depth. I have touched upon the notion of medicine as performance and the hospital as a theatrical space. I have opened up productive encounters between performance and medicine and the role of the artist's critique. I have also indicated how reciprocity can be understood at a deeper level, in terms of a blurring of boundaries between art and life. In order to explore this last element in more detail I will be drawing on a theoretical model initiated by American performance-maker and scholar Richard Schechner and developed by British anthropologist Victor Turner.

Developments in counter-cultural art practice and non-matrixed performance work, which was not mimetic or involving acting in the conventional sense but rather focused on participants' real responses, demanded a new kind of conceptual framework in order to read the subtlety of the relationship between art and life. Research carried out in the social sciences during the 1960s and 1970s played a major role in shaping contemporary performance studies and its understanding of emerging performance practices. Schechner was a pioneer of the integration of developments in social science, especially anthropology and sociology, and performance analysis. The melding of theoretical strategies not only opened up new areas of interest to performance scholars, but also facilitated a more complex examination of what it is to play a role and how that playing may enact social critique. In theorizing the new form of performance work, Schechner studied staged performances and their reflection of everyday life, as well as considering everyday life 'as if' it were a performance. Significantly for this study, Schechner looked at the inter-relationship between the two and attempted to codify the relationship between everyday life – termed 'social drama' – and 'crafted' events – termed 'aesthetic drama'. Schechner identified what he called an 'infinity loop' (Schechner 1988 [1977]: 190) which connects social and aesthetic drama in a self-perpetuating circuit. When considering medicine and performance within this model, investigation may focus on the way in which aesthetic representations of clinical practice may impact upon its practice within the social realm.

Turner criticizes Schechner's commingling of the aesthetic and the social. He acknowledges mutual influence but sees it in a more segmented and linear fashion – theatre shapes life, which then shapes theatre, which then shapes life. While I prefer to speak in Schechner's terms of aesthetic drama – which has further ramifications than a stage and allows for a blurring of boundaries between 'real' life and staged life – I think that Turner's term 'latent' is very useful. He states that the manifest social drama feeds into the latent realm of the stage drama phraseology that, as well as providing an impression of a particular culture at a particular time, allows for a future that bears traces of that moment. Turner suggests that the reflection of society provided by stage drama (as he calls it) 'is a metacommentary...on the major social dramas of its context' (Turner 1985: 300-1). The suggestion here is that the stage drama may be able to provide deconstructive readings through foregrounding the techniques that make up social dramas. Turner's identification of the 'implicit rhetorical structure' is useful in allowing for a notion of speech acts that are embedded within a culture and enacted as part of overt social dramas and it is these rhetorical structures that I turn to next.

Performance as medicine

Scholarship in the medical humanities has been influenced by the work of theorist Michel Foucault, who explored medical practice as a rhetorical structure. In *The Birth of the Clinic* (1963) Foucault considers the medical drama of the teaching hospital and examines the frameworks that establish the defining power of doctors and facilitate the patient's entry into prescribed narratives. While he is attentive to the spatialization of pathology and the way in which disease is related to context, Foucault places an emphasis on the verbal articulation of the pathological and suggests that medicine works on speech-acts. While Turner states that those in the community who have authority carry out redressive acts (1982: 92), Foucault's work seeks to identify those with the power to enact the statements. He argues that, through articulation, the person in authority (the doctor) actualizes disease. So, a 'seeing' becomes a 'saying' and what is unseen is actualized through diagnosis.

Foucault's emphasis is on the exposure of the constructed nature of what is considered 'natural', to reveal normalizing mechanisms. While there are connections with the work of Orlan, Foucault's focus is on how power is productive of identities and practices and on how it is enacted through systems and institutions. As sociologist Nikolas Rose suggests, his examination of the truth claims of medicine works through an exploration of the performative character of clinical discernment (Rose 1994: 62). For

Foucault, clinical thought relies on subjective perception within an aesthetic framework that makes the physician nearer to an artist than a scientist. Foucault quotes physiologist Pierre-Jean-Georges Cabanis: 'Everything, or nearly everything, in medicine is dependent on a glance or happy instinct, certainties are to be found in the sensations of the artist himself rather than the principles of the art' (quoted in Foucault 1997 [1963]: 120). Foucault highlights how subjectivity functions in the division of the sick from the well and focuses on the notion of the physician's gaze as the authenticating vehicle of medicine. He argues that it is the gaze that is the basis of medical knowledge and investigates the training of the aesthetic eye in the lecture theatres and on the wards of the teaching hospital.

Foucault's work is not without critique. Bleakley *et al.* note that, due to recent changes in medical education, Foucault's model of the gaze – derived from early modern practice – is outdated (Bleakley *et al.* 2011: 86). They go on to suggest that contemporary diagnosis is usually a collaborative process and promote a broader understanding of medical education and practice. Bleakley *et al.* assert that the 'gaze' is no longer the province of a single doctor, but is distributed across a range of artefacts such as imaging equipment and across the collaborative input of multiprofessional clinical teams and their patients.

Returning to the work of Goffman might serve to unpack the dynamics of identity construction that Bleakley *et al.* foreground. Goffman's work is centred in the realm of social drama. Goffman, like Foucault, is interested in the performative in a phenomenological sense and considers social construction and the construction of reality as shaped by social forces; however, Goffman works the other way around, employing drama as an analogy that enables him to explore role playing in social encounters. Goffman worked alongside Schechner and Turner on the New York University (NYU) Performance Theory course and his work foregrounds the importance of role-play in social life and opens up the everyday as a site for performance. While Turner identifies acting as an ambiguous word, Goffman is careful to maintain the distinctions between drama and everyday life. He says of *The Presentation of Self in Everyday Life*: 'This report is not concerned with aspects of theatre that creep into everyday life. It is concerned with the structure of social encounters' (Goffman 1976: 246).

The medical profession is one of Goffman's main case studies in his examination of the presentation of self before others. He examines the training and professional conduct of practitioners and observes the way in which events are framed within the social drama of clinical practice. He differentiates between the back region where performances may be rehearsed, such as the coffee room or lecture theatre, and the front region where performances are delivered to an audience of other social actors. As an interactionalist, Goffman focuses on external relations and is sensitive to the improvisatory elements within a human encounter. Goffman clarifies the difference between behaviour and performance – raised in the work of Schechner – and places an emphasis on audience. Goffman's work also importantly raises matters of 'idealization' and the tendency of performers to offer their observers an impression that is idealized in several different ways and provides models of performance and response.

The shifts in thinking following on from studies such as Goffman's and *Boys in White* by Howard Becker *et al.* (1977), which focuses on the cultur- alization of male medical students in an American medical school in the 1970s, can be related to changes in medical education. As many authors within this volume have noted, the publication of *Tomorrow's Doctors* by the General Medical Council in 1993 (revised in 2003 and 2009) recom- mended that UK medical schools move away from a model of imparting knowledge to delivering an educational experience that encourages critical analysis and the development of clinical skills. Medical schools responded with innovations in the undergraduate curriculum that included an under- standing and practice of communication skills as an essential aspect of medical education, promoting the ability to work well as part of a team and establish effective relationships with patients. Medical schools now commonly have courses in communication skills although there is consid- erable variation in the way that communication studies are taught. In the context of medical education, Bleakley *et al.* note that '[l]iterature (includ- ing drama) is the discipline approach par excellence for drawing out character, delineating role and articulating issues of identity' (Bleakley *et al.* 2011: 116). There is an understanding of the value of aesthetic drama and its relationship to social drama through activity such as rehearsing scenes, for example the breaking of bad news, and of employing fictional frameworks for exploring empathic response.

Sociologist Simon Sinclair employs Goffman's classic study to explore contemporary medical training. His book *Making Doctors: An Institutional Apprenticeship* (1997) is an account of medical training undertaken at University College London Medical School in the late 1990s. In charting this moment in the development of medical training, Sinclair examines the stages on which the medical students perform. The lecture theatre and the operating theatre are the most obvious of the dramatic settings and, in the later stages of their training, the students are involved in the theatrical spectacles of ward rounds, whose elaborate stage management is noted in Atkinson (quoted in Sinclair 1997: 32). Sinclair moves from Goffman's analysis to an examination of performance in a more overtly theatrical manner, in that he pays attention to productions such as the medics' panto, where the grotesque and parody can be understood as excessive modes of rehearsal for the performances the students are required to give in every- day life.

This work posits an interesting perspective on the hospital as a perform- ance venue. Diagrams in Sinclair's book clearly chart the development of clinical performance practice. The pre-clinical students are concerned with marking themselves off from the lay-world while, for the clinical students, the most important definition is between their official and unofficial role(s). Once individuals take on the role of 'Houseman' – a gendered term now abandoned, as junior doctors in the UK are called 'Foundation' doctors – the unofficial backstage has shrunk and official stages expanded. Sinclair highlights the ward rounds as occasions where students play roles as both actors and audience. The consultations take place with curtains drawn round the bed and students present the constructed history of their patient according to conventions such as standing to the left of the head of the patient's bed. Sinclair's study documents a student who deliberately exaggerated his presentation and was congratulated on his style by his superiors (Sinclair 1997: 217). He also describes a film shown just before clinical finals that gave advice about verbal and physical presentation alongside clinical topics (Sinclair 1997: 242).

Presentation is seen as an important matter for clinical practice. As Sinclair points out, consultants often make an assessment of a houseman through her/his performance on ward rounds. The students appear to be aware of the pressure to perform in an overt way. Those who spoke to Sinclair complained: 'It's all so theatrical! Be slick at this! Be slick at that! We need acting lessons!' (Sinclair 1997: 241). Indeed, the students approached their presentations in the manner of drama students, rehearsing together, offering directorial notes on each other's performances and sharing advice on stage fright. Interestingly, the medical students were quite cynical about the new courses on offer in doctor–patient communication and communication skills. Such modules were seen to be apart from the clinical training as they were taught by psychiatry away from the wards.

While there is value in reading Sinclair's work as a historical text in relation to the British context, his model still holds good elsewhere. Lorelei Lingard, a leading Canadian medical educator with a PhD in practices of rhetoric, suggests that 'old-style' communication models may be perpetuated in practice even within the context of new teaching methods. In particular, a study by Lingard *et al.* (2002) of communication within the operating room (OR) focuses on the role of novices within the OR and the way in which they are enculturated. Lingard suggests that the novice adopts one of two strategies in response to difficult situations: either to withdraw from communication or to mimic their teacher. This mimicry may be ridiculed by other team members, but Lingard *et al.* suggest that established patterns of communication and professional stereotypes may be transmitted as an 'embedded curriculum' and that 'those who talk the talk are assumed to be clinically competent' (Lingard *et al.* 2002: 237, 233). We might use Goffman's notion of idealization, as an impression that is idealized from clinical superiors, in order to understand how rhetorical strategies may serve to shape social exchanges.

In their OR study, Lingard *et al.* discuss the way in which the real dynamics of the clinical team may differ from the caricature represented in TV dramas such as *ER* or *Chicago Hope*. They argue, unsurprisingly, that communication is much more nuanced within real-life social drama, but it is interesting that they make overt comparison between the two. Sinclair's study suggests that, in order to deliver the performance demands they encounter, medical students may use the TV medical drama as a model for practice. Such dramas are certainly points of identification for students as would-be professionals, yet Sinclair proposes a more complex inter-weaving of the aesthetic and social drama. He argues that, especially for pre-clinical students who have no ward experience, the performative models given in media representations may be the only reference points they have to develop their own performance style. This assertion seems to be supported by research such as that by Matthew J. Czarny *et al.*, whose recent survey of 477 pre-clinical and clinical medical students at Johns Hopkins Medical School, found that 84 per cent of students watched TV medical dramas (Czarny *et al.* 2008: 3). Czarny *et al.*'s study raises concerns at this commitment to the consumption of television doctors, as it seemed that the pre-clinical students were more willing to take the televisual representation as accurate. The study notes: 'When compared to clinical medical students or nursing students pre-clinical students more frequently rated... depictions as adequate of artificial and transplanted organs... and confidentiality' (Czarny *et al.* 2008: 5). Czarny *et al.* acknowledge that medical educators may find the influence of such programmes on trainee health professionals concerning.

Medicine as performance

The notion of medicine as performance ties back more generally to Goffman's notion of the performative aspects of medicine, but the following section will consider the more formalized concern of performances depicting medicine and the inter-relationship between these (aesthetic) performances and the social drama of medicine. I will examine how medical dramas, both on television and on the stage, reflect and reinforce contemporary ideas and concerns. In this section I am going to focus on medical dramas in particular although, of course, in what media sociologist Lesley Henderson terms the 'medicalisation of the mass media' (Henderson 2010: 199) medical-related storylines are popular more generally in soap operas and documentaries. Henderson goes on to note that, alongside the police, doctors receive the lion's share of professional representation on television (Henderson 2010: 199). My focus in this section is on how the overt televisual performance feeds in to expectations and/or the delivery of clinical practice.

Doctors in TV medical dramas are portrayed in true-to-life situations and the makers of hospital dramas are often keen to stress the 'reality' of their programme and it is this that may be seen to appeal to the students of Czarny's study. Episodes of medical dramas will often deal with current medical issues. Programme-makers also commonly have medical advisers who work on the show. For example, *The Full Medical*, a BBC documentary detailing the making of *Casualty*, includes a scene being choreographed around a technical description of treatment. The actor looks on as the medical advisor demonstrates at which line a particular instrument should be applied. This scenario, where the imitation of a doctor's actions by an actor for presentation to an audience that may well include medics, clearly follows the arc of the feedback loop that Schechner proposes. The medical aesthetic can be seen to shape the product but is also subject to individual bias. In his account of his role as medical advisor on *Casualty*, accident and emergency (A&E) doctor Geoff Hughes describes dealing with letters of complaint from other clinicians who disagreed with his personal interpretation and felt that practice was not accurately represented (Hughes 1996: 300).

The TV drama is, fundamentally, presenting a fabrication. Bleakley *et al.* note that, in an age of collaborative practice, 'the staunchly individualist hero-doctor is no longer the ideal' (Bleakley *et al.* 2011: v). Yet medical dramas often present maverick medics as central characters. These figures are not only larger-than-life personalities, they also follow extremely unusual medical careers. A comparison between the work patterns represented on *ER* and career paths in everyday life by Alan Duncan and Harlan Gibbs foregrounds that, in order to preserve the continuity of characters necessary for a television drama, rotations in the emergency room (ER) are longer on the TV programme and people do not take any time to study for professional exams.

TV medical dramas appear to uphold the supremacy of clinical practice. In her seminal study on medics in the media, journalist Anne Karpf suggests that '[t]he visual grammar of medical programmes tends to reinforce the doctor's centrality and authority…the medical gaze prevails' (Karpf 1988: 12). This points to the fact that TV medical dramas privilege the medical practitioner rather than the patient and the cameras follow the movements of the medical staff. This is partly to do with their role as active agents within the drama and also connected to that fact that they are the points of continuity – the characters that are seen every week and that keep the attention of the audience, although this is not applied to the secretarial and portering staff who are seen as supporting roles. While Karpf's study may be seen by some as dated, Henderson's more recent work identifies the continuing importance of the 'committed physician who is always willing to break the rules and gain the best care for patient' (Henderson 2010: 206) in contemporary dramas such as *Scrubs* and *House*. She states 'these contemporary programmes have more in common with the early doctor shows than we might imagine' (Henderson 2010: 206–7). Indeed, Rebecca Chory-Assad and Ron Tamborini's content analysis study of clinicians on television in 2001, while acknowledging that the portrayal of doctors may be less complimentary than they were in earlier periods, nevertheless note that the representation of medical staff was positive overall (Chory-Assad and Tamborini 2001).

Karpf's study notes that the way in which the medics are framed by the camera reinforces medical discourse, observing that medics are commonly framed in mid-shot where close distance invites involvement. Institutional corridors and tracking shots of the efficient medical team or lone doctor running to a patient are popular images of the medical drama that promote the professionalism of their subject group. The notion of medicine as an objective science is also reinforced through the programme format itself in that the more you see, the more you understand, which Karpf notes supports the empirical fallacy of clinical practice. In the medical drama, diagnoses are made at high speed using the backdrop of medical technology that Goffman identified as an important element of staging within his observation of the social drama of clinical practice. Karpf identifies the climax of TV drama as the surgical operation, arguing that:

> Surgery occasions the icon of the medical drama, the operating theatre scene: with its close-ups of masked, gowned and concerned doctors...its cutaways to respirator and cardiograph...the mounting drama of the doctor's clipped instructions as bleeps of danger accelerate.
>
> (Karpf 1988: 184)

The drama of the operating theatre is something that the TV drama can do extremely well, using footage of real operations in order to maintain the 'realism' of the product. It seems to be that the 'hot' medicine of casualty is deemed more suitable for TV medical drama. Atkinson describes the characteristics of this type of clinical practice:

> [T]he 'hot' medicine taught in casualty...is entirely different from the 'cold' medicine of normal teaching on the wards...'hot' medicine is marked by its immediacy, when neither patient nor student has had the chance to rehearse the history and the whole business is less stage-managed, and medical action must often be taken there and then.
>
> (Quoted in Sinclair 1997: 32)

Sinclair's analysis fits with Goffman's notion of disguising procedure through improvisation. Goffman cites the medic as an 'obvious' example in that, when dealing with a patient, s/he must simulate a memory of and connection with them (Goffman 1976: 58). Hot medicine displays the medic at his/her best. However, the suitability of hot medicine for TV may not only be in its immediacy and drama, which also applies to surgical procedure. Rather than the slow decline of degenerate illness, acute disease is an episode of illness that leads to crisis – and crisis, as Turner has highlighted, is a crucial element in drama. Illnesses in medical dramas can be identified as liminoid phenomena in that they usually involve what psychiatrists call psycho-social transitions, in which 'old patterns of thought and activity must be given up and fresh ones developed' (Karpf 1988: 190). Hot medicine provides drama, tension and resolution that reinforce medical discourse. The acute incident also allows for an episodic structure – it is literally kill or cure – and a high turnover of storylines and guest artists.

The representation of medicine can be quite different within theatrical texts. Within live performance it is extremely difficult to stage the technical aspects of 'hot medicine'. Indeed, the degenerative illness is better suited to the stage and there is a great tradition of tragic heroes/heroines whose decline is tracked through epic drama.

In thinking through the relationship between social and aesthetic drama I wish now to turn my attention now to a stage drama which not only dialogues with the social drama of illness and cultural anxieties around its treatment, but also with media representations of that experience. *W;t* (also styled as *Wit*) by Margaret Edson is a contemporary text that that employs the techniques of tragic drama in its presentation of terminal illness. The play focuses on the fictional story of Vivian Bearing PhD, an eminent scholar of the Holy Sonnets of John Donne, who is diagnosed with metastatic ovarian cancer. The action follows the course of Vivian's treatment, including her enrolment on an experimental medical research project, and delivers a personal perspective on the process of dying which culminates in Vivian's death. Within the text, a primary concern appears to be the exploration of the medical management of terminal cancer and this is enacted through examining an individual's encounter with the institution of medicine. Edson clearly states that her work is informed by her experience of working in an AIDS-oncology unit and that concerns raised by that experience led her to write a handbook for families on dying and mourning. The play *W;t* came out of the same period and was undertaken because she 'needed to see such a play and it hadn't been written' (quoted in McFerran 2000). In the play, Edson appears to be working to develop a character and a situation that reflect the realities of everyday life and, in so doing, provide a model for mourning that may be seen as a theatrical version of her handbook.

In her examination of the practice of medicine, Edson capitalizes on the metaphor of the anatomization of the body by medics in a manner that appears sympathetic with a Foucauldian analysis of medicine as an aesthetic endeavour and, by making her central character a literary scholar, Edson highlights this critique. The character of Vivian engages with clinical practice at a level that displays an awareness of the centrality of professional language within medicine. In assessing her situation, the character states: 'My only defence [against the onslaught of the physicians] is the acquisition of vocabulary' (Edson 2000: 28). The character of Vivian likens herself to a poem and, at one point in the London production, presented at the Vaudeville Theatre in March 2000, she was shown with the words of a Donne poem projected onto her. This mise-en-scene could be seen to be a visual representation of her understanding that she is a body onto which the doctors project the theoretical paradigms of their research project. Yet, within the play, the voice of the patient is seen to remain the true authority. This perspective provoked a protracted correspondence in *The New York Times*, at the time of the MCC Theater production in the City (1998). Abigail Zuger MD asserted:

> Sixty years ago Paul Muni as Louis Pasteur and Ronald Colman as the fictional Dr Arrowsmith thrilled and inspired their audiences. Now the pendulum has swung around: It is the patients who are the heroes, while the doctors have receded into sketchy caricatures.
>
> (Zuger 1998: 2)

Vivian certainly is the fullest drawn character within the piece and the figure with whom the audience are encouraged to identify. The play opens as follows:

> VIVIAN BEARING *walks on [sic] the empty stage pushing her IV pole. She is fifty, tall and very thin, barefoot, and completely bald. She wears two hospital gowns – one tied in the front and one tied in the back – a baseball cap, and a hospital ID bracelet. The house lights are at half strength.* VIVIAN *looks out at the audience, sizing them up.*
> VIVIAN *(in false familiarity, waving and nodding to the audience).* Hi. How are you feeling today? Great. That's just great.
>
> (Edson 2000: 1; original emphasis)

In the London production the lights were up in the house as well as on the stage for this section, which enabled the performer to make eye contact with the audience. This direct address from the stage is not only startling in its acknowledgement of the audience as witnesses to the event, but it also resists the convention of the passive patient as information is gathered both from and about Vivian. In placing Vivian as narrator of her own story, Edson structures her work in a different way from the conventional TV medical dramas, in which bodies of patients come and go and are seen from the medical perspective. Also, unlike TV drama in which the cliffhanger is often whether a life can be saved, in *W;t* the audience are told what the outcome will be. Vivian says in her opening speech: 'It is not my intention to give away the plot; but I think I die at the end' (Edson 2000: 2). This acknowledgement allows the audience to pay attention to the *process* of dying.

The temporality of the dying and mourning process is foreshortened by the structure of the play. As Aristotle noted in *The Poetics* (330 BCE), the craft of theatre-making relates to the selection and employment of materials ordered in terms of aesthetic time and, within *W;t*, illness and disease is shaped within a carefully structured narrative arc. This point is brought to the fore at the beginning of the text when Vivian states: 'They've given me less than two hours' (Edson 2000: 2). It is clear to the audience that the scope of the play's events happens within the limits of the time it takes the character to die. I would suggest that the temporal dimensions of the piece allow for sensitivity to the deprivations that the character is undergoing, yet it also serves to remind the audience of the theatricality and distance. As I have already mentioned, dying is carefully structured within the text. The character of Vivian asserts:

> In this dramatic structure you will see the most interesting aspects of my tenure as an in-patient receiving experimental chemotherapy for advanced metastatic ovarian cancer. But as I am a *scholar* before ... an impresario, I feel obliged to document what it is like here most of the time, between dramatic climaxes. Between the spectacles. In truth it is like this: *She ceremoniously lies back and stares at the ceiling...* If I were writing this scene, it would last a full fifteen minutes. I would lie here and you would sit there. *She looks at the audience, daring them.*
>
> (Edson 2000: 21–2)

This speech is interesting in that it highlights the relationship between the social and aesthetic drama and reminds the observers that they are witness to a theatrical presentation that is being staged for their benefit and in which the process of dying has been edited and made easily accessible, even entertaining. This self-reflexivity differs from the TV drama's approach that obfuscates in its editing.

The climax of the play is Vivian's death and she tells the audience that she is going to 'leave the action to the professionals' (Edson 2000: 47). Unlike other tragic dramas, Edson's text does not subscribe to what Macintosh describes as 'the big speech convention' (Macintosh 1994: 91). Instead of delivering summative comments, Edson leaves the audience to make sense of the final actions of the piece that opens up the space for their own readings and projections. In leaving the audience alone – that is without the narrator figure of Vivian who has been the guide through the rest of the play – Edson can be seen to deliver a sense of helplessness and lack of comprehension that may be true to the experience of mourning in everyday life. The violence of the action at the end of the play is certainly disturbing. Vivian, as an active protagonist, recedes leaving the focus of attention on Jason Posner MD, a clinical fellow who, throughout the play, has been shown to value his research objectives above his clinical obligations. The character of Posner comments that the courses devoted to cultivating communication skills are 'a colossal waste of time for researchers' (Edson 2000: 35).

While, during the course of her illness, the character of Vivian had reflected on her career as an unforgiving and aggressive academic and had come to value the importance of personal kindness, Jason's final moments within the play are shown in a less positive light. Finding Vivian without a pulse, he calls the code team. He deliberately ignores Vivian's request to be Do Not Resuscitate (DNR), with the justification that 'She's Research [sic]' (Edson 2000: 54). The brutal enactment of the cardiopulmonary resuscitation (CPR) procedure, in which the body is stripped and manually manipulated, is exacerbated by the fact that Susie (Vivian's primary nurse and supporter of her DNR decision) and Jason literally fight over the body. This is not a play that glamourizes or even appears to endorse the use of CPR. Indeed, this appears to be another site of Edson's criticism of current medical practice as the medical establishment can be seen to be inflicting trauma rather than allowing for a peaceful death.

While the suspicion of medical educators towards TV drama has been previously noted in this chapter, it is interesting to observe that productions such as *W;t* have been employed within clinical training. For example, University of California, Los Angeles (UCLA) implemented an end-of-life educational programme called the *Wit* Educational Initiative (WEI) that ran between February 2000 and January 2002. Live stagings of *W;t* in medical settings combined with follow-up discussion and a detailed guidebook that was produced particularly to foster 'humanism, empathy, and self-reflection in the care that medical trainees provide to dying persons' (Lorenz *et al.* 2004: 482).

Linda Deloney and C. James Graham's report on the project recorded that, in the evaluation of the programme, great emphasis was placed on the emotional impact of the dramatic performance and the potential of theatre for 'emotional learning' (Deloney and Graham 2003: 249). Students attending the programme reflected on the way in which their medical education may have served to suppress their impulses for compassion. This can be seen to support the findings in a study by Mohammadreza Hojat *et al.* (2004), which documents the decline in empathy in medical students in their first year of clinical experience. While empathy generally reduced, Hojat *et al.* noted the largest falls were in response to the statements: 'It is as important to ask patients about what is happening in their lives as it is to ask about their physical complaints' and '[t]he best way to take care of a patient is to think like the patient' (Hojat *et al.* 2004: 937). Hojat *et al.* recommend 'empathy training' as a remedy for empathy fatigue and texts such as *W;t* can be seen to offer the opportunity to think like a patient and understand the benefits of that encounter and/or the problems that arise due to lack of empathic engagement (Hojat *et al.* 2004: 938).

Performance anxiety: Responses to medical performance

Having considered different modes of representation, this section will examine their impact and explore how both the general public and more 'specialized' audiences such as trainee doctors respond to what they see on television and in the theatre. Critics have discussed the impact of the dramatic or aesthetic representation of doctors and it has been proposed that television programmes have an effect on the relationship between medics and patients due to what is termed the 'cultivation effect' (quoted in Quick 2009: 43). This can be helpful for medics, in that people have positive expectations of care, but there is also worry in the medical community that programmes create unrealistic expectations. Susan J. Diem, John D. Lantos and James A. Tulsky are three clinicians who voiced their concerns about the historical over-representations of successful CPRs on television. They argue that TV programmes over-represent cardiac events requiring resuscitations in children and young people and under-represent cardiac arrests in the elderly which, in real life, is the primary type of cardiac failure. They also highlighted the way in which a successful outcome for CPR is over-represented. This, they felt, was significant as they suggested that 70 to 90 per cent of the US public gain their knowledge about CPR from TV and overestimate their own chances of survival after resuscitation (Diem *et al.* 1996). The difference between the representation of CPR in the mainstream TV drama and the self-reflexive staging of the stage drama *W;t*, where the emphasis is on an individual's story rather than the work of the medical team, may suggest a role for the performing arts in the arena of managing expectation.

There has also been concern in the medical community about the effect of TV drama on the expectations of the level of care that the patient receives in ER/A&E. Neal Baer MD, the producer of *ER*, states that a 'real-life' representation of an ER would be 'boring' and that, in order to create interest 'we take some license with reality' (Baer 1996: 1605). Thus, procedures are performed more quickly than in a real ER. In this context, where the reality and fiction are blurred, over-representation of medical miracles becomes problematic because it raises patients' real-life expectations and, for American medics, threatens litigation. Donald E. Larsen and Irving Rootman's study shows that a patient visiting a doctor comes with an image of the physician's role and how it should be performed. The authors posit that '[t]he more a physician's role performance meets a patient's expectations, the more satisfied the patient will be with the physician's services' (Larsen and Rootman 1976: 30). These expectations, however, may not all be positive. Michael Pfau *et al.* offer analysis on mediated representation of medics and employ Goffman's concept of the frontstage and backstage as a model for investigation. They note that:

> In terms of front regions, network television depictions of physicians have changed very little over the years...what has changed is that contemporary prime-time television depictions of physicians feature both front and back regions. Today's programs often probe deeply into the physicians back regions, revealing occasional uncertainties in diagnoses and mistakes in treatments, and exposing unflattering personal traits...These images can undermine established institutions.
>
> (Pfau *et al.* 1995: 444)

Pfau *et al.* open up a consideration as to how public access to backstage behaviours may undermine trust in professionals. Here viewers are witness to the human processes that make up the practice of medicine that is usually kept out of sight of the patient – in Goffman's terms, the processes that maintain the 'front'.

Baer's analysis picks up the theme of the doctor's attempt to control the flow of information. He suggests that the real problem is not the dramatization of medicine, but the fact that if the majority of patients are learning about CPR from TV it is because their physicians are not discussing it with them. He observes that '[i]n a 1984 study, Bedell and Delbanco found that physicians were unlikely to discuss CPR with their patients even if they believed that their patients should participate in decision making on this issue' (Baer 1996: 1605). Baer suggests that this topic needs to be discussed more openly with the processes of medicine becoming more transparent. There have indeed been moves within more recent medical practice to empower patients and involve them in making choices about their care. This has bought into focus the notion of the 'art' of medicine and the development of appropriate education, as clinicians have to facilitate the clinical encounter in ways that meet not only patients' expectations, but also expectations of other clinical colleagues in team settings.

The reflexive practitioner can be seen as central to contemporary clinical practice. The recent shift towards evidence-based medicine within the UK, as noted in many chapters of this volume, has placed a renewed emphasis on individual clinical expertise and the tacit knowledge acquired by physicians. There has been considerable discussion about evidence-based medicine in the *British Medical Journal*. In correspondence in the letters pages Chambers, a clinician, highlights the importance of the quality of the relationship between doctor and patient, noting that this might be therapeutic in its own right. He also emphasizes the significance of the individuality of each encounter and the importance of the physician responding in the moment to the particularity of the case history and allowing for diagnostic uncertainty (Chambers 2004). Thus, evidence-based medicine opens up the matter of subjectivity and even draws into possibility the admittance of failure. Huw Davies and Joseph Lampel, in their interrogation of performance indicators, promote the adoption of the 'learning organisation' model within the health sector as one that may succeed in 'performing'. They highlight the importance of the team and communication but, interestingly, they also highlight learning from failure:

> [L]earning organisations are the antithesis of bureaucracies: they are decentralised, team based, and encouraging of open communication; collaboration replaces hierarchy, and the predominant values are those of openness and trust... [L]earning organisations fight the natural

tendency to bury failures. They recognise that there is much to be learned from a detailed examination of failing.

(Davies and Lampel 1998: 161)

Boldly stated, there is, and in many ways rightly so, an emphasis on success within health settings and a culture of risk aversion. There has also been a belief in the power of medical science to provide positive outcomes. With an opening up of understanding and willingness to view, engage with and reflect upon performance there may be the opportunity for the aesthetic drama to explore failure or at least the strenuous effort to achieve.

In her study of the poetics of contemporary performance theatre, performance scholar Sara Jane Bailes (2010) posits failure as a significant artistic trope. Bailes discusses how highlighting the shortcomings of the performance event invite critical reflection in the audience and an awareness of the slippage between the real and the fake. Experimental theatre companies such as Sheffield-based Forced Entertainment work with the uncertainty of the live event and the constant threat of accident or mistake and use it to invite a conversation about the effort it takes to maintain the performance. So, for example, their production *First Night* (2001) explores the dynamic of the theatrical event itself and what happens when it all goes wrong. Initially, a line-up of eight performers in spangly costumes with rictus grins greets the audience. These figures address the audience directly and initially make promises of a great show and engage in a series of incompetent vaudeville-style acts until one of the performers calls to the audience:

> You look at us and see glamour and inspiring people, but inside there's a lot of self-doubt...No, but seriously – it's quite a stressful job. We come out here and we give our all – and sometimes it just about takes its toll.

(Forced Entertainment 2001: 74)

This works as part of the interrogation of the dynamics of performance but also connects with an ongoing theme of an investigation into the idea of the 'professional'; the work that a performer has to do and how their success might be measured. Rather than seeking ways to fix the world they inhabit, the performers present their endeavours to live with difficulty. This may prove to be instructive within the medical arena – as Kenneth Ludmerer (1999) asserts, one of the real flaws in medical education has been 'the failure to train learners properly for clinical uncertainty' (quoted in Bleakley *et al.* 2011: 25). The realm of health and care is, rightly, risk averse but there is no doubt that accidents do happen. This acknowledgement of difficulty and suffering within the aesthetic drama may be useful to the social drama of medicine in the discursive space that it opens up. Within the work of companies such as Forced Entertainment there is an understanding of dialogue and the importance of the human encounter as well as the fragility and fractures in communication. Bleakley *et al.* quote research that suggests 70 per cent of medical errors can be seen to be the result of miscommunication in team settings and that 50 per cent of such errors can be addressed through better education in communication and teamwork (Bleakley *et al.* 2011: 263). Rather than more conventional communication skills courses, perhaps the anti-aesthetic drama might provide models for practice?

Conclusion

In *Perform or Else* (2001), performance scholar Jon McKenzie reflects on recent developments in performance studies, and examines the way in which the concept of 'performance' has been taken up within contemporary society in the developed world. McKenzie also notes how different aspects of the performing culture may relate to one another, as well as impact upon the individuals who function within it. Healthcare is required to perform and deliver results, and the effects of interventions are measured. NHS 'performance indicators' have historically been predominately technical, such as the percentage of patients able to see a GP within 24 hours. Recently, however, there has been more emphasis on outcomes and room within the feedback for patient response. For example, the UK Department of Health GP Patient Survey (run most recently from January to September 2012) reflects upon the quality of care a patient feels they have received in terms of accessing services and consultation. This is perhaps where a more conventional understanding of performance might come into play as the human encounter is evaluated and it may be interesting to reflect upon what benchmarks the patient is assessing the doctor's performance against and where those models may originate from.

This chapter has explored factors relating to reciprocity between performance and medicine in order to provide a conceptual framework and contextual background for the case study chapters by Jessica Beck and Phil Jones that follow in this section. Beck and Jones do not explicitly discuss performance in terms of the drama of everyday life, as in this overview. However, their work broadly connects to this chapter's emphasis on the value of understanding performance as a part of life, which can be extended to considering the performance of emotions and the perceived external signs of improved well-being. Performance studies allow for the analysis of the relationship between aesthetic representation and social drama, and seek understanding of performance as medicine and medicine as performance, as well as highlighting cultural anxieties such as the treatment of uncertainty in medical practice and the way in which this may be seen as a poetics of failure. With developments in medical education in which, for example, students are learning to 'act' with compassion in simulated settings and through reference to medical drama, the reciprocal loop between the aesthetic and social drama appears to be both robust and complex.

References

Aristotle (1992 [330 BCE]) *The Poetics*, trans. T. Buckley, New York: Prometheus Books.

Baer, N. (1996) 'Cardiopulmonary Resuscitation on Television: Exaggerations and Accusations', *The New England Journal of Medicine*, 334: 1604–5.

Bailes, S. (2010) *Performance Theatre and the Poetics of Failure*, London: Routledge.

Becker, H., Geer, B., Hughes, E. and Strauss, A. (1977) *Boys in White: Student Culture in Medical School*, Chicago: University of Chicago Press.

Bleakley, A., Bligh, J. and Browne, J. (2011) *Medical Education for the Future: Identity, Power and Location*, London: Springer.

Chambers, J. (2004) 'The Rich and Fertile Tapestry of Evidence', *British Medical Journal*, 312: 71.

Chory-Assad, R. and Tamborini, R. (2001) 'Television Doctors: An Analysis of Physicians in Fictional and Non-Fictional Television Programs', *Journal of Broadcasting and Electronic Media*, 45: 499–521.

Czarny, M., Faden, R., Nolan, M., Bodensiek, E. and Sugarman, J. (2008) 'Medical and Nursing Students' Television Viewing Habits: Potential Implications for Bioethics', *The American Journal of Bioethics*, 8: 1–8.

Davies, H. T. O. and Lampel, J. (1998) 'Trust in Performance Indicators?', *Quality in Health Care*, 7: 159–62.

Deloney, L. and Graham, C. (2003) '*Wit*: Using Drama to Teach First-Year Medical Students about Empathy and Compassion', *Teaching and Learning in Medicine*, 15: 247–51.

Diem, S., Lantos, J. and Tulsky, J. (1996) 'Cardiopulmonary Resuscitation on Television – Miracle and Misinformation', *The New England Journal of Medicine*, 334; 1578–82.

Edson, M. (2000) *W;t*, London: Nick Hern Books.

Forced Entertainment (2001) *First Night*, Sheffield: Forced Entertainment.

Foucault, M. (1997 [1963]) *The Birth of the Clinic*, trans. A. Sheridan, London: Routledge.

Fox, N. (1992) *The Social Meaning of Surgery*, Buckingham: Open University Press.

General Medical Council (2003) *Tomorrow's Doctors*, London: General Medical Council.

Goffman, E. (1976) *The Presentation of Self in Everyday Life*, Harmondsworth: Penguin.

Henderson, L. (2010) 'TV Medical Dramas: Health Care as Soap Opera', *The Socialist Register*, 46: 198–215.

Hojat, M., Mangione, S., Nasca, T., Rattner, S, Erdmann, J., Gonnella, J. and Magee, M. (2004) 'An Empirical Study of Decline in Empathy in Medical School', *Medical Education*, 38: 934–41.

Hughes, G. (1996) 'Casualty: The BBC Series – The Role of the Medical Adviser', *Journal of Accident and Emergency Medicine*, 13: 299–301.

Karpf, A. (1988) *Doctoring the Media: The Reporting of Health and Medicine*, London: Routledge.

Larsen, D. E. and Rootman, I. (1976) 'Physician Role Performance and Patient Satisfaction', *Social Science and Medicine*, 10: 29–32.

Lingard, L., Reznick, R., Espin, S., Regehr, G. and DeVito, I. (2002) 'Team Communications in the Operating Room: Talk Patterns, Sites of Tension, and Implications for Novices', *Academic Medicine*, 77: 232–7.

Lorenz, K., Steckart, J. and Rosenfield, K. (2004) 'End of Life Education Using the Dramatic Arts: The *Wit* Educational Initiative', *Academic Medicine*, 79: 481–6.

Macintosh, F. (1994) *Dying Acts: Death in Ancient Greek and Modern Irish Tragic Drama*, Cork: Cork University Press.

McFerran, A. (23 April 2000) 'Putting Cancer Centre Stage', *The Sunday Times*. Online. Available: www.sunday-times.co.uk (accessed 17 August 2012).

McKenzie, J. (2001) *Perform or Else: From Discipline to Performance*, London: Routledge.

Orlan (1996) 'Conference', in D. McCorquodale (ed.) *Orlan: This Is My Body... This is My Software*, London: Black Dog Publishing.

Pfau, M., Mullen, L. and Garrow, K. (1995) 'The Influence of Television Viewing on Public Perceptions of Physicians', *Journal of Broadcasting and Electronic Media*, 39: 441–58.

Quick, B. (2009) 'The Effects of Viewing Grey's Anatomy on Perceptions of Doctors and Patient Satisfaction', *Journal of Broadcasting and Electronic Media*, 53: 38–55.

Rose, N. (1994) 'Medicine, History and the Present', in C. Jones and R. Porter (eds) *Reassessing Foucault: Power, Medicine and the Body*, London: Routledge.

Sawday, J. (1995) *The Body Emblazoned: Dissection and the Human Body in Renaissance Culture*, London: Routledge.

Schechner, R. (1988 [1977]) *Performance Theory*, 2nd edn, London: Methuen.

Sinclair, S. (1997) *Making Doctors: An Institutional Apprenticeship*, Oxford: Berg.

Turner, V. (1985) *On the Edge of the Bush: Anthropology as Experience*, Tucson, AZ: University of Arizona Press.

Turner, V. (1982) *From Ritual to Theatre: The Human Seriousness of Play*, New York: Performing Arts Journal Publications.

Zuger, A. (15 December 1998) 'When the Patient, Not the Doctor, Becomes the Hero.' *The New York Times*. Online. Available: www.nytimes.com/1998/12/15/science/essay-when-the-patient-not-the-doctor-becomes-the-hero.html (accessed 2 March 2013).

11 Theatre, performance and 'the century of the brain'

Influences of cognitive neuroscience on professional theatre practice

Case study

Jessica M. Beck

The relationship between neuroscience and professional theatre has developed exponentially over the last ten years. Indeed, this burgeoning relationship is evident from a sudden shift in the literature, visible not only in academic journals and publications, but even apparent in a casual trip to the National Theatre bookshop. Among the acting books, alongside Stanislavsky's *An Actor Prepares,* new titles using the words 'cognitive' and 'neuroscience' have appeared on the shelves. Examples of recent publications include: *Embodied Acting: What Neuroscience tells us about Performance* (Kemp 2012); *Toward a General Theory of Acting: Cognitive Science and Performance* (Lutterbie 2011); *The Actor, Image, and Action: Acting and Cognitive Neuroscience* (Blair 2008); and *Engaging Audiences: A Cognitive Approach to Spectating in the Theatre* (McConachie 2008) (see also Paavolainen 2012; Rokotnitz 2011; Soto-Morettini 2010). Theatre practitioners Brian Astbury (2011), Mick Gordon (2010) and Katie Mitchell (2009) have begun citing the work of neuroscientists such as Antonio Damasio, Michael Gazzaniga, or Joseph LeDoux. There are even books using cognitive science to re-explore Shakespeare (Cook 2010; Tribble 2011).

Theatre makers are interested in the neuro- and cognitive sciences for a variety of reasons: to explain what we already intuitively know – or what performers and audiences are already doing; to give us better insight into working with actors; and also because most (good) theatre makers have an insatiable curiosity. Theatre director Peter Brook believes that through discoveries in neuroscience, such as research into mirror neurons, science has 'finally started to understand what has long been common knowledge in the theatre' (Rizzolatti and Sinigaglia 2008: ix). Acting teacher and scholar Rhonda Blair is interested in 'how science might help us better understand what actors do when they act' (Blair 2009: 93). Director Mick Gordon maintains that 'we can best serve the theatre by integrating our new knowledge of the workings of the mind to help us make better work' (Gordon 2010: 71). Perhaps even more interesting is the direct collaboration between scientists and artists on theatrical performances. Recent plays created from neuroscientific/theatrical collaboration include *On Ego* and *On Emotion* (Gordon and Broks 2005/2008) and *2401 Objects* (Barker *et al.* 2011).

To those outside the theatre, our recent fascination with neuroscience may seem odd. However, as Joseph Roach explores in his book *The Player's Passion: Studies in the Science of Acting* (1993), a relationship has long existed between the sciences – biological, psychological, neurological – and the performing arts. Roach's survey follows the close correlation between acting theory and the scientific understanding of the body throughout history:

> Conceptions of the human body drawn from physiology and psychology have dominated theories of acting from antiquity to the present. The nature of the body, its structure, its outer dynamics, and its relationship to the larger world that it inhabits have been the subject of diverse speculation and debate. At the center of this ongoing controversy stands the question of emotion.
>
> (Roach 1993: 11)

Roach's 'question of emotion' is a recurring theme throughout the relationship between science and the performing arts. As a theatre director myself, my own quest to better understand emotion in performance took me as far as Cachagua, Chile, to work with a neuroscientist who studied the physiological changes that occur during an emotion (Beck 2010). In London, the Wellcome Trust – a charity dedicated to improving health – has been instrumental in introducing scientists to theatre makers and partially funding their collaborations. Recent examples include Analogue Theatre – which will be discussed in more detail – and The Articulate Hand, the partnership of theatre maker Andrew Dawson and neuroscientist Jonathan Cole.

The collaboration of scientists and theatre makers also coincides with the general emergence of the medical humanities over the last thirty years. Anton Chekhov (1860–1904), perhaps one of the most influential playwrights of the twentieth century, was also a doctor. In a letter to a fellow writer, Chekhov considers the similarities between art and science from his unique vantage point:

> [T]he sensitivity of the artist may equal the knowledge of the scientist. Both have the same object, nature, and perhaps in time it will be possible for them to link together in a great and marvelous force which at present is hard to imagine.
>
> (Quoted in Coope 1997: 49)

The 'object' to which Chekhov refers is us – human beings. In theatrical practice human beings are the main subjects of our storytelling, plays or narratives, while the performers – human beings themselves – are the instruments to tell those stories. The shared 'nature' between art and science is one of curiosity and investigation. Theatre makers are continually asking questions about human behaviour, society, and how we function. This curiosity is evident in how performers 'work' on themselves to better their craft, as well as in the stories that we tell through performance. And one could also argue, at least when comparing theatre and medicine, that both disciplines also have the potential to heal.

The aim of this chapter is to survey and investigate the role of cognitive sciences in professional theatre practice. The first section will cover the history and context of this subject throughout the twentieth century and up to the present day, highlighting the shift from psychology to the neurosciences, as well as the move towards collaboration with scientists. The second section will cover some recent examples of theatre makers in Britain engaging with neuroscience in their professional work. Finally, I will consider what the cognitive sciences offer theatre makers, and how we can further develop the interplay between the medical sciences and theatre makers.

The twentieth century: Body and mind

At the turn of the twentieth century Konstantin Stanislavsky (1863–1938), an actor and director of the Moscow Art Theatre (MAT), began developing a system for actor training and pioneered the rehearsal process. Stanislavsky staged most of Chekhov's work, and Bella Merlin even suggests that Chekhov's writing, in particular *The Seagull*, 'was the catalyst which provoked Stanislavsky into applying new laws to the *acting process* in order that it too might be structured' (Merlin 1999: 224; original emphasis). Stanislavsky was the ultimate magpie, drawing upon science, art and non-western systems, such as yoga, to inform his theatrical practice. Scientists and psychologists such as Charles Darwin (1809–1882), Ivan Petrovitch Pavlov (1849–1936), William James (1842–1910) and Theodule Ribot (1839–1916) influenced Stanislavsky's work. Today, Stanislavsky's system is considered 'the most influential actor-training system in the western world' (Whyman 2008: x), and most theories of acting developed during the twentieth century – whether consciously or not – have roots in his work.

The American William James and the Frenchman Theodule Ribot can be seen as the most significant psychologists influencing Stanislavsky's work. James introduced the view of emotions as perception of bodily changes in what became later known as the James–Lange theory of emotion.[1] In his essay 'What is an Emotion?' (1884), James maintains: '*the bodily changes follow directly the* PERCEPTION *of the exciting fact, and that our feeling of the same changes as they occur* IS *the emotion*' (James in Lange *et al.* 1922: 13; original emphasis). Stanislavsky scholar Rose Whyman points out that 'in reference to acting, [the James–Lange theory] was purported to indicate that adopting the appropriate action would result in experiencing the appropriate emotion' (Whyman 2008: 60). James' view of emotion made an important contribution to Stanislavsky's development of his technique 'method of physical actions' and Vsevolod Meyerhold's 'biomechanics'.

James' theory is sometimes reduced to a linear cause and effect sequence, but acting theorist Richard Hornby is certain that James did not intend 'to shift the seat of emotions from inside to the outside, but to reject the duality all together' (Hornby 1992: 126–27). This rejection of duality is central to Ribot's view of emotions and his use of the term 'psychophysio-logical', which Stanislavsky would later apply to the actor's process – as 'psychophysical'. In his 1897 publication *The Psychology of the Emotions*, Ribot maintains '[n]o state of consciousness can be dissociated from its physical conditions: they constitute a natural whole, which must be studied as such' (Ribot 1911 [1897]: 112). In acting terms, Stanislavsky wanted his perform-ers to 'work' on themselves and develop a 'psychophysical' relationship between body and mind, asserting that 'in every action there is something psychological, and in the psychological, something physical' (quoted in Carnicke 1998: 139). Acting trainer and director Phillip Zarrilli notes that in this case 'psycho': [D]oes not mark the recent Western invention of psychologices of the self/individual as in the compount "psychological," but rather refers to another meaning of the Greek *psyche*: the vital princi-ple – namely, the *élan vital* or the enlivening quality of the (actor's) breath/energy' (Zarrilli 2007: 636). Remnants of these ideas can be found in the work of Michael Chekhov's 'psychological gesture'.

While psychology was an important influence on acting theory at this time, Hornby emphasizes that the contribution was typically 'from behav-ioralists and experimentalists like Ribot, James, Lange and Pavlov rather than from psychoanalysts like Freud or Lacan' (Hornby 1992: 187). There is no evidence to suggest that Stanislavsky was familiar with the work of Sigmund Freud (1856–1939), and Whyman insists it was 'through the influ-ence in Russia of German philosopher Edouard von Hartmann [that] Stanislavsky inherited and appropriated pre-Freudian concepts of the *unconscious*' (Whyman 2008: 4). However, acting scholar Robert Gordon points out that the vocabulary used in Stanislavsky's system (which includes terms such as unconscious, motivation and subtext) 'has become the actor's equivalent of the pseudo-Freudian jargon of popular psychology' (Gordon 2006: 56). It is only in the public's view that acting is more closely associated with popular psychology.

Stanislavsky's system did not become prominent in Britain until the 1960s, perhaps because the MAT never performed in London (Gordon 2006: 71). In Britain, actor training only became a 'legitimate' form of education in the early 1900s with the formation of two drama schools: Elsie Fogerty's Central School (now the Royal Central School of Speech and Drama or RCSSD) and Sir Herbert Tree's Academy of Dramatic Art (now the Royal Academy of Dramatic Art or RADA). In the 1930s, theatre companies began to form their own schools, and in 1934 Michael

Saint-Denis and George Devine (both of whom would later open The Old Vic School in 1947) opened The London Theatre Studio. Saint-Denis was the nephew of Jacque Copeau (1879–1949). Copeau believed in training actors in a similar manner to Stanislavsky, but did not directly draw from medicine or science. Like Stanislavsky, Copeau was interested in mending the mind/body division that was a challenge for actors to overcome. Saint-Denis brought Copeau's ideas to Britain, and is responsible for the inclusion of the Alexander Technique – a body–mind technique used to improve alignment and posture – in British actor training programmes. As Robert Gordon notes, 'Saint-Denis was thereby provided with a pseudo-medical principle in support of his notions of integrated corporeal expression' (Gordon 2006: 154). In addition to Stanislavsky's legacy, theatre makers in the twentieth century also made explorations into non-western paradigms – such as Kathikali dance drama and martial arts such as Tai Chi and Aikido – and bodywork based on human skeletal structure using practices such as the Feldenkrais Method and, again, the Alexander Technique.

The case study of Stanislavsky indicates some important shifts over the course of the twentieth century, highlighting the way in which scientific theories about links between body and mind appealed to some key individuals in theatre practice and education (although not universally and not with immediate success in Britain). It also indicates how the nature of those perceived links and the sciences to explain them have changed over time. Furthermore, the period also saw a marked change in the nature of collaborations between theatre and science.

For the majority of the twentieth century, the predominant interaction between scientists and theatre practitioners was one-way, with the theatre makers taking the ideas that appealed to them. In the 1970s a shift occurred, and scientists began to collaborate with actors. RADA hired psychologist Brian Bates to teach their actors about psychology. Originally planning to offer seminars, Bates quickly realized that the actors were more interested in 'getting up on their feet':

> Discussions about the psychology of madness were punctuated by demands to be allowed to 'get up and try it, act it, see how it feels'. [...] All of this was very far from the original intention: that I should offer psychology to the actors. For I soon realised that actors are intuitive, creative psychologists.
>
> (Bates 1986: 9)

It was also in the 1970s that Susan Bloch, a professor of neurophysiology at the University of Chile, was invited by the university's theatre school to teach psychology to their students. Rather than teach a theoretical course on psychology, Bloch made a proposition 'to create a practical workshop for the study of emotions, with an interdisciplinary collaboration between scientists and theatre experts' (Bloch 2006: 25). Bloch teamed up with colleague Guy Santibáñez-H. and a leading theatre director, Pedro Orthous. The researchers set out to examine the physiological changes that occur during the expression of human emotion by monitoring respiratory movements, heart rate, arterial pressure and changes in muscular tonus in subjects (a combination of patients, drama students and psychology students) who under hypnosis were reliving emotional experiences from their lives (Bloch *et al.* 1987). The research suggested 'the existence of a *unique* association between particular bodily changes and a corresponding subjective experience' (Bloch and Lemignan 1992: 32; original emphasis), which led Bloch to identify six effector patterns that she considers to be 'basic emotions' – anger, tenderness, fear, eroticism (also referred to as sexual love), sadness and joy.

Each emotion evidenced a distinct pattern of physiological changes. Bloch and her colleagues noted that while many of the changes that occurred were controlled by involuntary mechanisms, others were not. Those responses that could be controlled voluntarily included breath, facial musculature and postural attitude. The research revealed that if one can learn to activate the voluntary aspects of the pattern together at the same time – breath, facial expression and postural attitude – one can phys-iologically activate that emotion. This ability to activate a particular emotional effector pattern was called the BOS Method (named for Bloch, Orthous and Santibáñez-H.). General Pinochet's takeover of Chile put an abrupt end to their working relationship, and Bloch moved on to the Institute of Neuroscience of the University Pierre et Marie Curie in Paris. Bloch was determined to continue this study of emotion and resumed her research with fellow Chilean expat Horacio Muñoz, a theatre director work-ing in Denmark with Teater Klanen. From this experience the BOS Method evolved into 'Alba Emoting'[2], a psychophysical technique intended to serve as a tool for actors to effectively induce the physiological changes that occur with an emotion. For actors, the connection between breathing and emotion is nothing new, with roots tracing back to the ancient Indian text the Natyashastra (Nair 2007). However, Bloch and her research team were among the first to explore this relationship in the context of Western science, articulating phenomena that many performers have been intu-itively embodying for centuries.

In the 1980s, psychologist Paul Ekman, who is renowned for his work with facial expression recognition, conducted a study working with actors from the American Conservatory Theater in San Francisco. Ekman and his team studied six 'target' emotions, considered to be universal – surprise, disgust, sadness, anger, fear and happiness. Each subject was given precise instruc-tions to move the muscles of their face, rather than told to adopt an emotional expression. While holding the expression for ten seconds, data on certain physiological changes were collected, including changes in heart rate, temperature of the left hand and right hand, skin-resistance and

forearm flex or muscle tension (Ekman *et al.* 1983: 1208). Similar information was also collected when the actors were asked to 'relive' an emotional
experience, what Lee Strasberg calls 'emotional memory'. Ekman's research
discovered that:

> [P]roducing the emotion-prototypic patterns of facial muscles in
> action resulted in autonomic changes of large magnitude that were
> more clear-cut than those produced by reliving emotions.
>
> (Ekman *et al.* 1983: 1210)

Performance scholar Richard Schechner comments on the results of the
study, maintaining that:

> [Ekman's] work was a flagrant demonstration of "mechanical acting" –
> the kind despised by most American performers, but exactly what is
> learned by Indian young boys beginning their studies as performers in
> kathakali dance-theater.
>
> (Schechner 1988: 264)

As with Bloch's work, Ekman's research 'validated' through Western
science ideas that performers have been embodying for thousands of years.
Bloch and Ekman are familiar with each other's research. Ekman has some
disagreements 'in regard to [Bloch's] choice of emotions and the specifi-
cation of the particular facial expressions that characterize each emotion'
(Ekman in Bloch *et al.* 1988: 202). While there is evidence of shared
emotions, scientists do not agree on a definitive list. However, Ekman does
agree in general with Bloch's findings and his own unpublished research
found that 'when subjects make facial expressions respiration falls into
place' (Ekman in Bloch *et al.* 1988: 202).

In terms of a medical paradigm, the ideas of James and Ribot on the
physiology and psychology of emotions respectively (via Stanislavsky) have
held the most sway in twentieth-century acting theory. However, at the
beginning of the twenty-first century, there has been a definite shift into
the realm of cognitive science, and specifically cognitive neuroscience,
shaping up to be what acting teacher and scholar Rhonda Blair describes
as 'the Century of the Brain' (Blair 2009). The shift is evident in theatre
scholarship, actor training and plays produced in the last decade.

In *Performance and Cognition: Theatre Studies and the Cognitive Turn*, editors
Bruce McConachie and F. Elizabeth Hart identify a 'cognitive turn' among
theatre scholars that potentially challenges 'several of our current
approaches to the study of theatre and performance' (McConachie and Hart
2006: 1). The sudden rise in the use of the 'C-word' is largely university-
driven in both United Kingdom and the United States. In Britain, The
University of Kent recently founded a Centre for Cognition, Kinesthetics and
Performance and in September 2012 held a symposium on Affective Science

and Performance. In June 2012, the Wellcome Trust, in collaboration in with RCSSD, held a conference for puppeteers and neuroscientists entitled *Objects of Emotion: How our Minds Bring Things to Life*. In addition to universities, organizations such as the Wellcome Trust and the National Endowment for Science, Technology and the Arts (NESTA) have played an important role in facilitating and funding many of these collaborations between neuroscience and performance. However, available funding and university research are only partial contributing factors.

Some of Stanislavsky's ideas have seamlessly resonated with discoveries in the cognitive sciences, for instance, the idea of the 'psychophysical' links with the concept of 'embodied mind'. Cognitive linguist George Lakoff and philosopher Mark Johnson maintain:

> The embodied mind is part of the living body and is dependent on the body for its existence. The properties of the mind are not purely mental: They are shaped in crucial ways by the body and brain and how the body can function in everyday life.
>
> (Lakoff and Johnson 1999: 565)

This view challenges the dominance in Western culture of Cartesian duality, which considers the mind and body as separate systems. For Rhonda Blair, cognitive science recognizing the embodied mind is crucial:

> One of the key implications of this is that actors do not need to 'make up' or construct a way of mending the splits in themselves; they need to develop a more accurate picture of themselves as being already necessarily integrated.
>
> (Blair 2008: 17)

Working with actors from the basis of the integrated whole is important to overcoming our Cartesian inheritance. And while the idea of the actor's psychophysical connection between body and mind is not a new concept, 'cognitive science provides an empirically derived theoretical basis for the description of psychophysiological activities involved in acting' (Kemp 2012: 18).

For example, theatre practitioner Brian Astbury uses language from the cognitive sciences to enhance his work with actors in the rehearsal room. Astbury's theory is that an actor's natural defences can interfere with good acting. In order to overcome these barriers, Astbury developed physical exercises where the primary objective is for the actor to engage with the 'cognitive unconscious' (Kilhstrom 1987; Reber 1996), the aspect of the mind that is just out of awareness, also called a 'tacit knowing' or knowing more than we are explicitly aware of. Related to the idea of the embodied mind, the body is a type of 'cognitive unconscious to which we have direct access; and metaphorical thought of which we are largely unaware' (Lakoff and Johnson 1999: 7). Astbury refers to most of his exercises as 'Left-Brain Disabling Devices', which attempt to overcome left-brain analytical dominance with right-brain 'creativity'. There is a claim by neurobiologists that so-called 'uncreative' people 'have marked hemispheric dominance, with the left hemisphere suppressing creative states and processes. By contrast, creative people are said to have less hemispheric dominance' (York 2004: 6). Phillip Zarrilli also discusses left- and right-brain differences in his actor training system (Zarrilli 2009). Such ideas are cited here as theories that are particularly useful in establishing bridges between performance and medicine, but are not universally accepted and should be approached with caution.

Theatre scholar John Lutterbie's *Toward a General Theory of Acting*, explores using Dynamic System Theory (DST) as a possible approach to understanding acting. Lutterbie maintains that DST 'effectively refutes Descartes's claim that the mind and the body are distinct, insisting instead on the intricate, inextricable interweaving of mind, body, and world' (Lutterbie 2011: 79). Bruce McConachie considers what research in cognitive science reveals about the behaviour of audiences. McConachie (2008) explores spectatorship through ideas such as conceptual blending and mirror neurons, using these notions to debunk theories such as suspension of disbelief and semiotics. However, while it is tempting to look to neuroscience for 'explanations' about how actors – or audiences – work, we must remember to view this phenomenon as a moment in time. As Roach's history of acting theory suggests, theatre practitioners have always and will continue to follow and be informed by advances in medicine and science.

Neuroscientists and theatre makers in the twenty-first century: 'A great and marvelous force'

In 2003, high-profile theatre and opera director Katie Mitchell embarked on a fellowship researching the later work of Stanislavsky, funded by NESTA. Mitchell discovered that Stanislavsky had been influenced by the theories of William James on the physical origins of emotions. Interested in determining whether James' view still 'held water', Mitchell found that James had a champion in neuroscientist Antonio Damasio. His 'somatic-marker' hypothesis is a further developed version of James' work. Damasio explains:

> The process does not stop with the bodily changes that define an emotion, however. The cycle continues, certainly in humans, and its next step is the *feeling of the emotion* in connection to the object that excited it, the realization of the nexus between object and emotional body state.
>
> (Damasio 1994: 132)

During the workshop, Mitchell and her actors read Damasio's *Descartes' Error* (1994) and *The Feeling of What Happens* (1999). In a recent interview, Mitchell described the process explaining that she 'would literally work through the book in a rehearsal room with performers and go "okay, so anyone understand this? Can we translate this into anything practical or useful in our working practice?" ' (Mitchell 17 September 2012). Damasio mentions six 'primary' emotions (the same as Ekman's) – happiness, sadness, fear, anger, surprise and disgust – and the company began by re-enacting moments from their lives when these emotions were very clear. They found Damasio's view of a 'gap' between the physical expression and conscious recognition of emotion useful, and then began building characters from 'physical frames', experiencing the physiological changes of the emotion first, resulting in 'bigger' movements. The company realized that 'theatre tends to do a more discreet version of life' (Mitchell 17 September 2012). It was becoming clear to Mitchell that 'in order for the audience to know what the emotion is, [the actors] need to do the physical frames that happen as the body responds before it hits consciousness' (Mitchell 17 September 2012). Now Mitchell needed to test these ideas in front of an audience.

Iphigenia at Aulis by Euripides was Mitchell's first production to incorporate this research, staged at the National Theatre in 2004. The actors began by building their characters with their newly acquired knowledge about emotion. In Mitchell's words, the company 'cut through the jungle that is psychology and found something which seemed simpler and more concrete and more graspable, called biology' (Mitchell 17 September 2012). Mitchell also employed Damasio's theory of background emotions, choosing for all the characters to engage in 'fear'. According to Damasio, background emotions are detected by 'subtle details of body posture, speed and contour of movements, minimal changes in the amount and speed of eye movements, and in the degree of contraction of facial muscles' (Damasio 1999: 52). To achieve this background emotion of unease 'no one was ever allowed to sit still, everyone always had to move all the time' (Mitchell 17 September 2012). The impact of Mitchell's work on the biology of emotions on the production is noted in reviews and articles. Kim Solga recalls her experience watching Iphigenia and Clytemnestra, played by Hattie Morahan and Kate Duchêne, after Iphigenia pleads in vain with her father Agamemnon for her life. Solga describes the scene:

> Morahan and Duchêne are overwhelmed by their emotions in a manner that is rarely seen in British (or North American) stage realism. They seem unable to get up [...] they duly force a cheerful, journeying tune, through convulsive tears and loud gasps that punctuate the song, awkwardly, with upset that seems somehow too real, too much, for a play. They grab at each other's faces, desperate for last touches of comfort.
> (Solga 2008: 147)

Solga's account suggests that Mitchell's use of Damasio's research was noticeable and effective. The entire experiment was pivotal for Mitchell:

> As a result of these discoveries my relationship to the audience radically changed. It was no longer essential for the actors to feel the emotions; now what mattered was that the audience felt them. What was essential was that the actors replicated them precisely with their bodies.
>
> (Mitchell 2009: 232)

Mitchell was able to find this precise physical vocabulary with her actors using Damasio's research.

In a similar manner to Mitchell, I was able to employ the research of Susana Bloch to develop a physical vocabulary in the rehearsal process and to enhance the staging of a production. In 2011, I directed Samuel Beckett's *Play* at the University of Exeter as part of my doctoral research. This Beckett piece features three actors encased in urns up to their necks, speaking text at rapid speed when prompted by a swivelling light controlled by a fourth actor or 'inquisitor'. Beckett's later plays usually contain strict instructions for the actors that involve intense physical demands or restrictions. In *Play*, Beckett's notes to the actors consist of 'faces impassive throughout' (Beckett 2006: 307) with the further instruction that their voices should be 'toneless except where an expression is indicated' (Beckett 2006: 307).

There are only three places in the script where Beckett actually does indicate expression, where he specifies 'vehement', 'hopefully' and 'wild laughter'. In order to help the actors fulfil Beckett's wishes, I turned to the work of Bloch.[3]

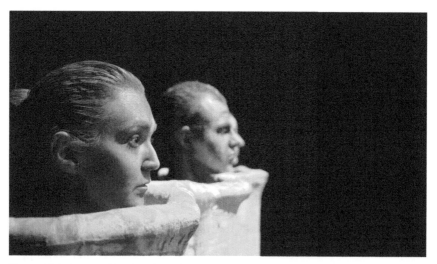

Figure 11.1 Lauren Shepherd, Callum Elliott-Archer and Symmonie Preston in *Play*.

Source: Photograph by Benjamin J. Borley. Reproduced with permission of Benjamin J. Borley

The rehearsals for *Play* began with an intensive week of Alba Emoting training. By increasing their awareness of facial-postural-respiratory effector patterns, the actors were able to use Alba Emoting to eliminate any *unwanted* physiological patterns. For the rehearsal process of *Play*, Alba Emoting became a kind of *via negativa* or a 'technique of elimination', which rids 'the organism of its resistance to the psychophysical process of playing a role' (Slowiak and Cuesta 2007: 20). In this case, Alba Emoting was used to rid the organism of the unwanted physiological traces – rather than resistance – of the emotional effector patterns. With new awareness, the actors could avoid being swayed by the emotion implicit in the lines of text.

Other theatre directors have directly collaborated with neuroscientists, rather than drawing on their theories as in the examples above. Mick Gordon, artistic director of On Theatre, has co-written two plays with neuropsychologist Paul Broks – *On Ego* (2005) and *On Emotion* (2008) – both of which played at the Soho Theatre, London.

The purpose of Gordon's company On Theatre is to explore different facets of humanity and modern life by creating 'theatre essays' on a variety of subjects. When I asked Gordon about the importance of cognitive science in his work, he admitted a particular fascination with neuropsychology, which, in Gordon's opinion, is 'at the frontier of the most interesting work that is being attempted to understand why we are, what

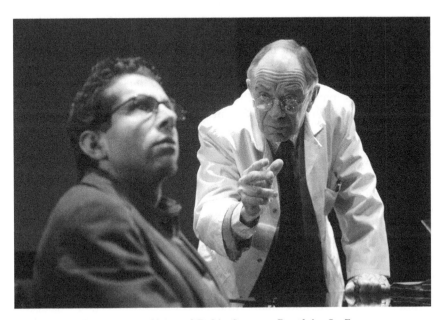

Figure 11.2 Elliot Levey as Alex and Robin Soans as Derek in *On Ego*

Source: Photograph by Manuel Harlen. Reproduced with permission of the Soho Theatre

and who we are' (Gordon 25 September 2012). Prior to his work with Broks, Gordon spent five years working with a variety of psychologists from different backgrounds experimenting with ways to use their case studies or therapeutic techniques in a theatrical context at the National Theatre Studios and the Royal Festival Hall in the UK, as well as the Oscar Korsunovas Theatre in Lithuania. Reflecting on those workshops, Gordon found the realm of psychology in this context a bit 'woolly', and struggled to find 'a dramatic purchase on psychology as theatrical material' (Gordon 25 September 2012). Then Gordon read Broks' book *Into the Silent Land* (2003), a collection of short stories/meditations on life drawn from Broks' years of experience as a neuropsychologist. Gordon became especially interested, as neurologists 'are actually dealing with certain factual things that they know about the brain because of brain damage' (Gordon 25 September 2012). Gordon suggested to Broks that they collaborate. *On Ego* questions our perception of identity, self and ego (and the fragility of that perception), while *On Emotion* explores whether or not humans are merely the puppets of our own emotion.

Other theatre directors have sought to represent the process of brain science, rather than to draw upon concepts or to collaborate with scientists. In 2011, the theatre company Analogue won *The Scotsman's* prestigious Fringe First Award at the Edinburgh Festival for its production of *2401 Objects*. The focus of the play was the infamous amnesiac Patient HM, or Henry Molaison. Plagued with highly disruptive seizures, Molaison – at the age of 27 – underwent an experimental procedure in 1953 to remove the hippocampus, a part of the brain concerned with consolidating short-term into long-term memory. The seizures stopped, but unfortunately the procedure left Molaison unable to form new memories (Miller 2009). Henry spent the rest of his life in care, as Patient HM, an important research specimen. *2401 Objects* focused on Henry's life, but also the beginning of his life after death as part of The Brain Observatory's archive. In 2009, neuroanatomist Jacopo Annese began Project HM – the dissection and documentation of the brain of Henry Molaison – 'the most studied human being in the history of psychology' (Miller 2009: 1634).

Over a two-day period in December, Annese carefully dissected and photographed Molaison's brain to create what he hopes to become a 'Google map of the brain' (Barker and Jarvis 14 July 2012). The dissection was streamed live on the internet, which is how Hannah Barker and Liam Jarvis, the founders of Analogue Theatre, first discovered Molaison's story. (Such a 'performance' connects to Emma Brodzinski's discussion of Orlan's surgery as performance art, in the overview chapter of this section.) Viewers could watch the entire procedure, hear the music playing in the laboratory and post comments. This 'performance' in itself was not without controversy, and many viewers communicated their distaste.[4] Katherine Sweaney insists that 'many who raised objections were disturbed by what they perceived as the exhibitionist nature of exposing someone's

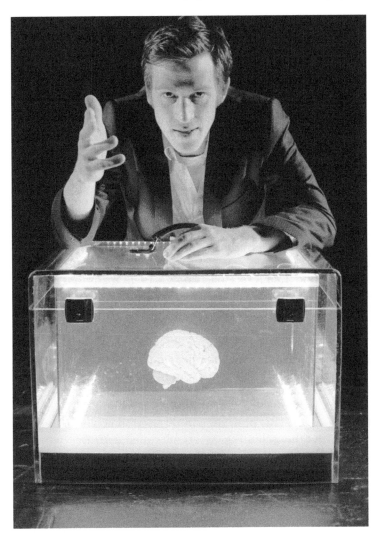

Figure 11.3 Paul Hassall representing Dr Jacopo Annese in Analogue's *2401 Objects*
Source: Photograph by Paul Blakemore. Reproduced with permission of Analogue Theatre
© Analogue

body online' (Sweaney 2012: 192). The founders of Analogue Theatre decided to contact Annese. In a recent interview that I conducted, Barker and Jarvis (14 July 2012) revealed they had no idea when the project first began that Annese would become such as integral part of the production.

The title – *2401 Objects* – refers to the number of pieces into which Molaison's brain was separated. The play opened with the recorded voice of Annese welcoming the audience to the performance:

Ladies and Gentlemen. Hello, this is Dr Annese from San Diego. I have been asked to say what do I do for a job and it is not an easy answer at the moment because I thought I was an anatomist, and I think I became more of a storyteller, and I tell stories about patients who have something wrong with their brains.

(Barker *et al.* 2011)

Gradually, the recorded voice of the real Annese gives way to an actor, and eventually to the story of Henry. While *2401 Objects* is primarily about the life of Molaison, Project HM and the collaboration with Annese – from the dramaturgy to the design – informed the construction of the play. The steel-framed set with moving parts that they cleverly coined as a 'Macrotome' was:

[I]nspired by the cryomicrotome which was used to dissect Henry Molaison's brain; the blade cuts once across the brain to remove a micro thin slice, and then resets to its original point ready to repeat the same process.

(Barker *et al.* 2011)

Even the music to score the scene changes was inspired by the music Annese was listening to in the wet laboratory during the live dissection. Annese himself became an artistic component of the play.

Analogue Theatre's collaboration with cognitive scientists was not limited to Annese. Analogue had been building a relationship with the Wellcome Trust from previous projects, and received some research funding and contacts with other scientists. As a result, when *2401 Objects* toured around the UK and in Germany in 2011 and 2012, in most locations the company was able to team up with local neuroscientists to offer post-show discussions and events. Some of the scientists included Professor Richard Morris of Edinburgh Neuroscience, who works at the University of Edinburgh at the Centre for Cognitive Neural Systems; Professor Thomas Back who specializes in human behavioral neuroscience; Ian Varndall, head of British Neuroscience Association; and Hanna Pickard of the Centre for Neuroethics at Oxford. Audiences in Germany were also able to take the 'star test'[5] – which Patient HM was subject to take repeatedly throughout his lifetime, and even dissect mouse brains with a mini cryomicrotome. The production and the additional events were intended to engage audiences in a discussion about identity, ethics, and – perhaps serve as a memorial to Henry Molaison – rehumanizing the life behind Patient HM. What Jarvis or Barker had not anticipated was the effect that this exchange between science and art would have on the scientists:

Richard Morris commented that the play had made him really think about the relationship that he has with his patients, made him really think about the kind of scientist he is, the kind of way he wants to work with his patients in the future – which is a wonderful thing to say. When we were sort of thinking about the impact that we can have as theatre-makers and what the work can do, that's one of the really significant things that we can do [...] not just engaging with the public, but also engaging with scientists and try to get them engaged with the emotional life of the patients.

(Barker and Jarvis 14 July 2012)

In this instance, the theatre had something to learn from the neuroscientist, and the neuroscientist from the theatre.

Conclusion

As we have seen, cognitive neuroscience can change the way theatre makers think about theatre, the way in which we work with actors, and how we engage with audiences. While there may be contributing factors – such as specific funding streams – theatre makers are simply following the current science and understanding of human biology as they always have done. As medicine, science, and the arts are all engaged in a process of human exploration, it is no wonder that there will be overlapping interests and curiosities.

Is there a danger in theatre makers commandeering the research of scientists? Perhaps. Blair warns that 'popular writings about science can easily be adopted or appropriated by those of us who aren't scientists in reductive and misrepresentative ways' (Blair 2009: 93). In the interview with Analogue, Jarvis confessed that 'the exciting thing – and the problematic thing – about interdisciplinary work is that you don't know what you don't know' (Barker and Jarvis 14 July 2012). So even when research *is* appropriated accurately, how do theatre makers know that the research is solid? The research of Damasio, for example, is the most frequently cited among theatre scholars and practitioners, and his books are hugely popular and accessible to a 'civilian' audience. However, within the field of cognitive neuroscience, Damasio's work is not without criticism. Max Bennett and Peter Hacker, in their book *The History of Cognitive Neuroscience*, dedicate the latter part of a chapter to making a long list of objections to Damasio's research – including his 'somatic marker hypothesis'. Bennett and Hacker maintain:

Damasio's theory of the emotions is a modification of [William] James's. But James's theory is sorely defective from a conceptual point of view, and cannot serve as the conceptual framework for the experimental and neurological investigation of the emotions.

(Bennett and Hacker 2008: 194)

Jarvis is apprehensive about the application of cognitive science to theatre and performance scholarship:

I think applying medical language to theatre processes is sort of unquestioning to that language. I feel as though in certain modes of theatre scholarship that language is used to authenticate the work that theatremakers are doing, and I think that's the very least that cognitive neuroscience can do [...] I don't look to cognitive science to affirm what I'm doing.

(Barker and Jarvis 14 July 2012)

I agree with Jarvis on this point. As a theatre director, I do not need cognitive science to affirm the work I make. However, it is fascinating to discover more about the human organism, especially when this knowledge translates into concrete and practical tools to use in the rehearsal room, as was true for the use of Alba Emoting in *Play*, or Damasio's work in *Iphigenia at Aulis*. When I asked whether Mitchell thought more directors should be looking to neuroscientists, Mitchell reflected:

The only sadness I have is that I couldn't get [Damasio's work] to spread further in my field. [...] Because I just think it would really enhance a theatre culture, which is into vague expressions of emotion and speaking language with posh voices. This could really help create much more architectural definition to our theatre making and a real sharpness of understanding for the audience.

(Mitchell 17 September 2012)

Mainstream theatre practices have yet to embrace cognitive science with the enthusiasm of the academics. Astbury feels similarly about actor training at drama schools:

Unfortunately, far too many training systems tend to encourage the use of the conscious left brain and ignore the wonders of the right. The result: dull, restricted, out-of-the-moment acting, able to deliver only one thought process at a time, not the multi-leveled complexity of the most ordinary of us human beings.

(Astbury 2011: 85)

Nonetheless, it appears as though performers are on the precipice of a paradigm shift. And whatever 'dangers' there may be when trying to 'validate' art with science, theatre makers should not be deterred from *engaging* with science. In this chapter, we have seen cognitive neuroscience provide a concrete vocabulary for the rehearsal room (Mitchell 2009; Beck 2010), help audiences contemplate what it is to be human (Gordon and Broks 2005, 2008) and rehumanize what has been reduced to medical experimentation (Barker *et al.* 2011). The most exciting possibilities concerning collaborations between scientists and artists have yet to be realized. With the production of *2401 Objects*, a neuroscientist was challenged to rethink the way he treats his patients. In summary, it is the *mutual learning and development* between artists and scientists that will create Chekhov's idea of a 'great and marvelous force'.

Notes

1 Carl Lange, a Dutch psychologist, independently posed the same theory (Whyman 2008: 59).
2 Named partly for a production of Lorca's *The House of Bernarda Alba* performed by Teater Klanen.
3 I had been studying Alba Emoting since 2007, worked with Bloch in 2008 and am now a certified instructor of the technique (CL5).
4 For an in-depth discussion of Project HM as a performance, see Sweaney 2012.
5 A psychological test in which Henry would have to draw a star with his fingers while looking at a mirror. Henry's improvement showed that he did have some ability to learn certain motor skills.

References

Astbury, B. (2011) *Trusting the Actor*, United States: CreateSpace Independent Publishing Platform.

Barker, H., Hetherington, L. and Jarvis, L. (2011) *2401 Objects*, London: Oberon Books Ltd.

Bates, B. (1986) *The Way of the Actor*, London: Century Hutchinson Ltd.

Beck, J. M. (2010) 'Alba Emoting and Emotional Melody: Surfing the Emotional Wave in Cachagua, Chile', *Theatre, Dance and Performance Training*, 1: 141–56.

Beckett, S. (2006) *The Complete Dramatic Works*, London: Faber and Faber.

Bennett, M. R. and Hacker, P. M. (2008) *The History of Cognitive Neuroscience*, London: Blackwell Publishing.

Blair, R. (2009) 'Cognitive Neuroscience and Acting: Imagination, Conceptual Blending and Empathy', *TDR: The Drama Review*, 53: 92–103.

Blair, R. (2008) *The Actor, Image, and Action: Acting and Cognitive Neuroscience*, London: Routledge.

Bloch, S. (2006) *The Alba of Emotions: Managing Emotions through Breathing*, Santiago: Ediciones Ultramarinos PSE.

Bloch, S. and Lemignan, M. (1992) 'Precise Respiratory-Postoro-Facial Patterns are Related to Specific Basic Emotions', *Bewegen & Hulpverlening*, 1: 31–40.

Bloch, S., Orthous, P. and Santibáñez-H., G. (1988) 'Commentaries on "Effector Patterns of Basic Emotions"', *Journal of Social and Biological Structures*, 11: 201–11.

Bloch, S., Orthous, P. and Santibáñez-H., G. (1987) 'Effector Patterns of Basic Emotions: A Psycophysical Method for Training Actors', *Journal of Social and Biological Structures*, 10: 1–19.

Broks, P. (2003) *Into the Silent Land: Travels in Neuropsychology*, London: Atlantic Books.

Carnicke, S. M. (1998) *Stanislavsky in Focus*, Los Angeles: Harwood Academic Publishers.

Cook, A. (2010) *Shakespearean Neuroplay: Reinvigorating the Study of Dramatic Texts and Performance through Cognitive Science*, Baskingstoke: Palgrave MacMillan.

Coope, J. (1997) *Doctor Chekhov: A Study in Literature and Medicine*, Isle of Wight: Cross Publishing.

Damasio, A. R. (1994) *Descartes' Error: Emotion, Reason, and the Human Brain*, New York: Putnam.

Damasio, A. R. (1999) *The Feeling of What Happens: Body and Emotion in the Making of Consciousness*, New York: Harcourt Brace.

Ekman, P., Levenson, R. and Friesen, W. (1983) 'Autonomic Nervous System Activity', *Science*, 221: 1208–10,

Gordon, M. (2010) *Theatre and the Mind*, London: Oberon Books.

Gordon, M. and Broks, P. (2005) *On Ego*, London: Oberon Books.

Gordon, M. and Broks, P. (2008) *On Emotion*, London: Oberon Books.

Gordon, R. (2006) *The Purpose of Playing: Modern Acting Theories in Perspective*, Ann Arbor: University of Michigan Press.

Hornby, R. (1992) *The End of Acting: A Radical View*, New York: Applause Theatre Books.

Kemp, R. (2012) *Embodied Acting: What Neuroscience tells us about Performance*, London: Routledge.

Kilhstrom, J. F. (1987) 'The Cognitive Unconscious', *Science*, 238, 1445–52.

Lakoff, G. and Johnson, M. (1999) *Philosophy in the Flesh: The Embodied Mind and its Challenge to Western Thought*, New York: Basic Books.

Lange, C. G. and James, W. (1922) *The Emotions*, Baltimore: Williams & Wilkins Co.

Lutterbie, J. (2011) *Toward a General Theory of Acting: Cognitive Science and Performance*, London: Routledge.

McConachie, B. (2008) *Engaging Audiences: A Cognitive Approach to Spectating in the Theatre*, Basingstoke: Palgrave Macmillan.

McConachie, B. and Hart, F. E. (eds) (2006) *Performance and Cognition: Theatre Studies and the Cognitive Turn*, London: Routledge.

Merlin, B. (1999) 'Which Came First: The System or "The Seagull"?', *New Theatre Quarterly*, 15: 218–27.

Miller, G. (2009) 'The Brain Collector', *Science*, 324: 1632–36.

Mitchell, K. (2009) *The Director's Craft: A Handbook for the Theatre*, London: Routledge.

Nair, S. (2007) *Restoration of Breath: Consciousness and Performance*, New York: Rodopi.

Paavolainen, T. (2012) *Theatre/Ecology/Cognition: Theorizing Performer-Object Interaction in Grotowski, Kantor, and Meyerhold*, Basingstoke: Palgrave MacMillan.

Reber, A. S. (1996) *Implicit Learning and Tacit Knowledge: An Essay on the Cognitive Unconscious*, Oxford: Oxford University Press.

Ribot, T. A. (1911 [1897]) *Psychology of the Emotions*, London: The Walter Scott Publishing Co., Ltd.

Rizzolatti, G. and Sinigaglia, C. (2008) *Mirrors in the Brain: How Our Minds Share Actions and Emotions*, trans. F. Anderson, Oxford: Oxford University Press.

Roach, J. (1993) *The Player's Passion: Studies in the Science of Acting*, Ann Arbor: University of Michigan Press.

Rokotnitz, N. (2011) *Trusting Performance: A Cognitive Approach to Embodiment in Drama*, Basingstoke: Palgrave Macmillan.

Schechner, R. (1988) *Performance Theory*, London: Methuen.

Slowiak, J. and Cuesta, J. (2007) *Jerzy Grotowski*, London: Routledge.

Soto-Morettini, D. (2010) *The Philosophical Actor: A Practical Meditation for Practicing Theatre Artists*, Bristol: Intellect.

Solga, K. (2008) 'Body Doubles, Babel's Voices: Katie Mitchell's Iphigenia at Aulis and the Theatre of Sacrifice', *Contemporary Theatre Review*, 18: 146–60.

Sweaney, K. W. (2012) ' "The Most Famous Brain in the World": Performance and Pedagogy on an Amnesiac's Brain', *The Review of Education, Pedagogy, and Cultural Studies*, 34: 182–96.

Tribble, E. B. (2011) *Cognition in the Globe: Attention and Memory in Shakespeare's Theatre*, Basingstoke: Palgrave MacMillan.

Whyman, R. (2008) *The Stanislavsky System of Acting: Legacy and Influence in Modern Performance*, Cambridge: Cambridge University Press.

York, G. K. (2004) 'The Cerebral Localization of Creativity', in F. C. Rose (ed.) *Neurology of the Arts: Painting, Music, Literature*, London: Imperial College Press.

Zarrilli, P. B. (2009) *Psychophysical Acting: An Intercultural Approach after Stanislavski*, London: Routledge.

Zarrilli, P. B. (2007) 'An Enactive Approach to Understanding Acting', *Theatre Journal*, 59, 635–47.

12 Medical humanities, drama, therapy, schools and evidence

Discourses and practices

Case study

Phil Jones

This chapter concerns the relationship between the medical humanities, dramatherapy and therapeutic work with children. It will demonstrate the ways in which the relationship between the arts therapies and medical humanities can be both newly understood and offer particular and innovative value to the arts therapies. The chapter will illustrate how this new position can enable specific insights into contemporary dilemmas concerning dramatherapy for children in schools.

The chapter will firstly consider the historical relationship between the arts therapies and the medical humanities. It will examine the absence of mutual attention, and argue for the value of dialogue, between the two fields. This chapter breaks new ground in redressing this absence and in its proposal of how the relationships between the arts therapies and the medical humanities can be understood and positioned.

An illustrative example of research will be used to examine the potential of dialogue between the medical humanities and dramatherapy with children in educational settings. This is followed by material contrasting the ways in which the findings would be understood by the usual discourses in dramatherapy with the way in which the findings can be treated differently by including the arts therapies within the concerns and discourses of the medical humanities. This is linked to areas such as an understanding of tensions between clinical practice in schools, power and narratives of evidence or impact. The example is then drawn on to argue for the value of dialogue between dramatherapy and the medical humanities.

Dramatherapy

In his 'Handbook' of 1917, *Principles of Drama-Therapy*, Stephen Austin gives one of the first definitions of dramatherapy: 'the art or science of healing by means, or through the instrumentality, of the drama/or, by means, or through the instrumentality, of dramatic presentation' (Austin 1917: x). One way of reading this early articulation is to see it as representing an assertion of drama's relationship to health, which, during the twentieth century, would go on to be reflected in the development of a profession with a body of theory, practices and research (Jones 2007; Casson 1997). Following on from such first published forms of the term, the emergence of dramatherapy as a profession has taken place since the 1930s in a number of countries (Jones 2007: 45). My review of these developments notes a common route: of 'training programmes, the creation of professions governed by national associations along with state recognition and registration in some countries' (Jones 2007: 57). The Netherlands, United States (US), United Kingdom (UK), Ireland and Canada established the first postgraduate programmes, alongside levels of state registration, with more recent developments in Greece, India, Israel, Norway and South Africa (2007: 57). Such registration has seen dramatherapy become primarily defined and positioned within health service frameworks, rather than as a part of arts provision in every country it has developed (Jones 2005; 2007). One example of this defining and positioning is dramatherapy's state recognition in the UK by the Health and Care Professions Council (HCPC), alongside other 'health and care professionals' such as occupational therapists and practitioner psychologists (HCPC 2012). The HCPC *Standards of Proficiency – Arts Therapists* document describes dramatherapy as 'a unique form of psychotherapy in which creativity, play, movement, voice, storytelling, dramatisation, and the performance arts have a central position within the therapeutic relationship' (HCPC 2003: 9–10). This independent regulatory body 'protects' the title of 'dramatherapist': anyone using the title without training and registration can be subject to prosecution and a fine. It also 'assures high quality of training and high standards of service provision for most health professionals in the country' (HCPC 2012).

Another way of looking at Austin's early definition is to see it as reflecting tension in its use of the term 'or' within the phrase 'art or science' (Austin 1917: x). This chapter will examine the question of the relation of drama as therapy to its identity as art *or* science, which can be seen as a theme within the field's current development in response to contemporary debates about dramatherapy, efficacy and evidence (Andersen-Warren 2012; Leigh *et al.* 2012). The tendency in dramatherapy's approach to measuring its efficacy has been to locate its approach to gathering evidence using qualitative rather than quantitative methods. In schools this includes: children's use of story-making structures, drama-based evaluations in which clients use role playing and create improvisations as reflections on change, and strengths and difficulties self-report questionnaires (Winn 2009; Andersen-Warren 2012). Such positioning has been connected to traditions within theatre-based research that draw upon qualitative methodologies as the most appropriate to examine the drama or theatre space where, as Hughes *et al.* argue, mess, creativity and improvisation mean that researchers, and those being researched, need to be able to meet and capture 'experiences that confound expectations of an orderly, rule bound...universe' (Hughes *et al.* 2011: 188). They, for example, argue that the researcher needs to be able to improvise, to be flexible and open to events that unfold, and that too much 'predetermined design' (Hughes *et al.* 2011: 188) of research tools hinders the richness and efficacy of enquiry into drama. Because dramatherapy is rooted in drama its methods of understanding its processes have similarly, in the past, mainly reached to the qualitative (Jennings 1990; Landy 2001). Recent literature has, however, indicated a shift and a challenge to the field, as contexts such as schools are demanding evidence from a quantitative perspective (Jones 2012; Leigh *et al.* 2012). This chapter will argue for the value of dialogue between dramatherapy and the medical humanities in helping to understand and respond to this shift.

The medical humanities and the arts therapies: Mutuality, unease and absence of attention

In this volume Alan Bleakley defines the medical humanities as plural and as consisting of 'contested and fragmented fields', naming four of them: the humanities studying medicine, arts and humanities intersecting with medicine in medical education, arts for health and arts therapies. Medical humanities literature makes reference to the arts therapies and has made gestures towards them in relation to its theoretical framework (Evans and Greaves 2003; Downie and Macnaughton 2007). However, to date, this relationship is one of unease. A decade ago, Martyn Evans and David Greaves articulated the nature, scope and identity of the medical humanities – then in their 'first flush of youth' – as 'emergent' and as reflected by particular domains and relationships that had been given attention in research and in literature (Evans and Greaves 2003: 57). Evans and Greaves contrast these areas with others that were relevant but not yet investigated, and that formed questions concerning the boundaries *and* mission of the medical humanities. They note that, '[o]ne of these questions concerns its relationship to the "arts in health" movement, and thus to the therapeutic roles for creative and expressive arts in the clinical situation. This relationship is far from clear, and on examination it is a complicated and intriguing one' (Evans and Greaves 2003: 57). The literature since then has been typified by inattention and lack of ease in relation to the arts as therapy. Authors such as Robin Downie and Jane Macnaughton (2007) or Evans (2008), in defining the nature and extent of the medical humanities illustrate this unease:

> The term "medical humanities" tends to be used in three senses. These senses refer to three movements which may overlap, but are distinct in their aims, methodologies and participants. First there is what we may term "the arts as therapy". This is perhaps the oldest strand...we shall

not in this book be discussing the movement, which has its own extensive literature and distinctive philosophy.

(Downie and Macnaughton 2007: 8)

Evans examines the question 'What is "the medical humanities"?' and 'why
might its importance – if any – be shown' (Evans 2008: 56). Within his definition he considers 'the therapeutic use of particular arts practices and
"products" in the clinical or public health settings' (Evans 2008: 56), positioning them in a way that reveals the same dynamic as Downie and
Macnaughton, where these 'may be the subject of medical humanities
enquiry, and they may even be conditioned by medical humanities influences upon thinking in health care, but they are not my concern here'
(Evans 2008: 56).

Both sources contain a theoretical and philosophical acknowledgement of
the arts therapies accompanied by an exclusion in attention. In Downie and
Macnaughton, the gesture contains both a positioning of the arts therapies as
a 'strand' while locating their attention elsewhere, and noting that they have
their own 'distinct' identity – as if this means they need not be given attention
from the medical humanities. The implication here is that the arts therapies
are both 'of' the domain of the medical humanities but also 'apart', and that
the field's literature, as it stands, deems it as not needing attention within the
gaze of the medical humanities. Evans (2008) frames them in a different, but
related, manner. The therapeutic uses of the arts are 'distinct' from the
medical humanities, yet may be the subject of its attention in terms of
'enquiry'. The parallel with Downie and Macnaughton (2007) is that a
gesture is made that acknowledges connections and inclusions while turning
away from direct 'concern'. The unease can be defined as an uncertainty in
how to engage with the arts therapies. This combination of gesture of inclusion or relatedness accompanied by a turn away is reflected through much of
the literature in the medical humanities. The journal *Medical Humanities*, for
example, over the past decade has included numerous articles on the arts and
health (including Rothenberg 2006; Macneill 2011), but, while occasionally
mentioning the arts therapies, does not contain one article addressing the
relationship between the arts therapies and the medical humanities. Similarly,
the arts therapies in major journals such as *The Arts in Psychotherapy*, or in disci-
pline-specific journals such as *Dramatherapy*, have made no acknowledgement
of the potential relationship within the past decade.

What happens if we change this gesture of turning away *or* aside to one
that turns towards this area: what does it reveal? What might a direct gaze of
attention involve, and what might the implications of this revelation be? The
next section presents research into contemporary concerns in dramatherapy. This is followed by material contrasting the ways in which the findings
would be understood by the usual discourses in dramatherapy to the way in
which the findings can be treated differently by including the arts therapies
within the concerns and discourses of the medical humanities.

Illustrative research example

The research involved email interviews with 48 dramatherapists, identified by invitation to qualified therapists who were members of organizations such as the British Association of Dramatherapists, the Netherlands Creative Arts Therapy Association, and snowball sampling through less formal networks that cross international boundaries and included therapists in Canada, Taiwan, Malta, Belgium, Ireland, the USA and Australia. Despite the different national contexts in which these therapists worked, there were some significant similarities in their concerns about the future of dramatherapy in 'evidence-based' school cultures. While other chapters within this volume have considered evidence-based healthcare, it is thus important to remember that the healthcare environment is not the only place in which the arts, health and well-being intersect and in which arts therapies are under pressure to 'prove' their worth within this paradigm.

Half of those responding worked with children. Early accounts of the emergence of the arts therapies noted that schools were the sites of early pioneering work (Jennings 1990; Jones 2007). This contact has continued, though, as the research in the next section will show, it is perceived as being under threat. Vicky Karkou and Patricia Sanderson's UK survey (2006) of practitioners indicated that education was the second most frequently reported area for arts therapists to work in, with schools as a prominent site. A review of arts therapies practice in schools by Jenny Stacey contrasts the period 'following the second world war' with its 'wave of energy and curiosity' with recent changes in the 'educational and political agenda' (Stacey 2008: 219). Stacey characterizes the former, especially 'from the nineteen seventies', as a time when dramatherapy was becoming established in schools and that this reflected a 'mutuality' between therapy and schools (Stacey 2008: 219). Both were connected by 'education becoming more child-centred... and the social and emotional well-being of the child [as] a focus in which creativity and self-expression were important' (Stacey 2008: 219). This is contrasted with 'shifts' reflected by Standard Assessments Tests (SATS) introduced in the UK in 1991, league tables, initiated in 1992, and the 'culture change marked by OFSTED (Office of Standards in Education)' all of which 'focus attention' on 'monitoring and evaluation of schools' performance in terms of pupils' educational progress and whether schools provide value for money' (Stacey 2008: 219).

Other authors echo Stacey's position. Toby Quibell notes that, while schools are 'places rich with opportunity to make a positive contribution to the development of young people', this is becoming lost in the face of the 'pressures to raise standards year after year, school life often sidelines the emotional and social aspects of learning' (Quibell 2010: 114–15). Quibell also comments that 'references to systematically researched dramatherapy in schools are very hard to find' (Quibell 2010: 116). Karkou notes parallel patterns in a number of countries and that the field is encountering 'problems' in evaluation in relation to educational evidence and research. She notes that 'in recent years... evidence-based education has become an important characteristic' of the school environment (Karkou 2010: 14). The current situation thus constitutes a new challenge for arts therapists, who are required 'to develop ways of working that are tailored around the school culture' of monitoring of performance and academic outputs (Karkou 2010: 279). Katrina McFerran and Jennifer Stephenson note the 'spread' of 'evidence-based practice (EBP)... through... education', and distinguish 'interventions supported by "evidence" from "popular" practice, that is, interventions that are widely supported by schools but not founded on empirical research' (McFerran and Stephenson 2010: 259–60). Authors such as Deborah Shine note tensions between government-initiated demands emerging from OFSTED and arts therapy practice in schools, where 'the various professionals and agencies involved do not share a professional language or culture. Subsequently different emphasis is placed upon monitoring and achievement of outcomes' (Shine 2012: 59). Shine argues for a 'new approach' to areas such as researching the effect of dramatherapy in order to meet tensions arising in relation to the divide between 'the demands' of a therapeutic agenda to meet children's emotional and psychological needs and educational settings dominated by impact constructed within agendas of academic attainment (Shine 2012: 59). Karkou notes 'the fact that there is limited research work completed and reported from the context' of schools and identifies the need for further enquiry (Karkou 2010: 10).

Despite this growing literature on evidence-based education, no research has been undertaken to establish practitioners' perceptions and experiences of this perceived shift or to understand the nature of this tension. The aims of the research responded to this gap within arenas within which dramatherapists practice, such as work with children in schools. The research aimed to address this need by inviting respondents to answer concerns such as:

1. Does the organization(s) or workplace(s) you are employed by, or work in connection with, ask for evidence or material on the efficacy of dramatherapy?
2. Please comment on whether you consider there to be adequate research based evidence available to support the field?
3. Do you have any views on the need for qualitative and/or quantitative published research into dramatherapy in your area of work?

The data collected have been analyzed thematically using the MAXQDA qualitative data analysis software. Themes were identified inductively from the raw interview data, and were used to identify common patterns across responses, as well as acknowledging individual experiences (Boyatzis 1998). The research does not claim to be representative of the field as a whole, nor would the scale of responses validate this. Rather it seeks to present the experiences and perceptions of those who responded, and, through excerpts, to illustrate the variety and detail of common themes. All respondents were asked to complete an informed consent form with guarantees of anonymity for themselves and the contexts they worked within. The only identifying detail would be the country of practice.

Sample of findings

Analysis of the responses identified the following common themes: the increased presence of what was described as an 'evidence based agenda' (Dramatherapist T, Canada) in schools and a 'provider culture' with low tolerance of qualitative findings – valuing quantitative research, especially of the 'gold standard' of the randomized controlled trial (Dramatherapist N, UK); a lack of quantitative research in dramatherapy; and an urgent need for particular approaches to develop to meet 'management… scrutiny' of impact (Dramatherapist P, UK). The following offers brief illustrations from the interview data from those working in schools to examine these themes, and reveals the detail of both commonalities and diversity within responses to the research questions.

In relation to the invitation for the question concerning schools 'asking for evidence or material on the efficacy of dramatherapy', a changing landscape was mentioned by a number of therapists and this was experienced as having particular challenges. The following extracts exemplify common patterns of connection:

> I've worked there for 10 years and until this academic year the school's management have not asked for evidence of the 'efficacy of dramatherapy'… This spring term however, the head teacher… asked for 'tracking' information about attendance, educational attainment and behaviour in respect of the children in dramatherapy… I have experienced this request as seeking 'proof' of the effectiveness of dramatherapy, but being measured predominantly in educational terms… The changes from government over the past two years have been and continue to be brutal, in my working experience. Anything that can't be 'proven' with some delusion of 'absolute science' seems to be suffering. The culture of low tolerance is jeopardizing the quality of well-being for many clients who are classed as 'in need' or/and 'vulnerable'.
>
> (Dramatherapist G, UK)

A dramatherapist from the Netherlands noted parallel concerns about the nature of measurement:

> The funders of fields of youth… mental health care ask dramatherapists to work evidence based. A theoretical/hypothetical explanation is

not enough anymore...The dramatherapists in the field...need reviews of existing effect studies and adequate Random Control Trials and quasi-experimental studies.

(Dramatherapist H, the Netherlands)

So much of performance in education is judged against quantitative data – OFSTED is still outcomes driven – dramatherapy falls short where quantitative data/research is considered and so does not fit in neatly to the management framework for scrutiny.

(Dramatherapist P, UK)

Here are illustrated connections and relationships within the major themes of a changed culture linked to requests for evidence viewed in specific ways. The extracts above locate this change as being driven in specific ways. The demands are located as 'outside' – from the 'head teacher', 'the funders', 'government', 'management' or the UK's OFSTED. They are not located within the work of the therapy or the pupils themselves in terms of the reasons the children come to therapy. The respondents explicitly stated that the concepts and criteria for 'evidence' are driven by externally set educational outcomes with no reference to an individual child's therapeutic goals or well-being. One notes a tension with 'OFSTED driven' criteria, the other with effectiveness being 'measured predominantly in externally set educational terms'. This seems to be implicitly linked to, as one respondent suggested, ways of measuring educational services such as SATS that do not 'see children's emotional and psychological needs' (Dramatherapist J, UK). The responses enabled further insights into the ways this 'seeing' was perceived. They noted measurements linked to educational effects or outcomes that were to be 'viewed' by adults outside the therapy. This was common to all countries. The majority of these criteria were linked to educational frameworks with external measures connected to both behaviour and school discipline:

The funders of this project are increasingly interested in the effectiveness of our approach. [...] We are also asked to identify the number of disciplinary actions that involve the children that we work with before and after treatment along with the child's attendance record.

(Dramatherapist L, USA)

Some noted specific measures – these were qualitative and based on, or connected to, self-reporting and therapist-completed formats. This was a theme that was reflected in particular ways in response to questions two and three. An illustrative example of this noted a range of measures: 'With younger children I use self-reporting "Hopes and Wishes"...I also use feedback forms for carers, parents, teachers, key-workers and managers' (Dramatherapist N, UK). Such ways of working were typical of responses in that they are located in small-scale research, and used qualitative measures based on devices such as story or role-play activities or self-reporting quest-ionnaires and testimonials.

Narratives about 'impact' and 'evidence' were much used in the inter-views, and there were commonalities in the ways these were positioned in the therapist responses concerning validation and a need to engage with quantitative methods:

> The research in our field tends to be qualitative and not quantitative and therefore funders do not consider it seriously. Moreover, the samples are small as was the case for the non-profit organisation I work for. Quite frankly without the 'gold standard' experimental design – with control groups and random assignment many foundations are suspect of findings . . . Absolutely, there is a need in order to prove our value in the schools.
>
> (Dramatherapist T, UK)

A number identified a tension within their responses to qualitative and quantitative methods, locating them within discourses of fear and anxiety. One such example linked it to 'magic' reduced by the scientific gaze:

> Some dramatherapists will argue that attempting to quantify our work will only serve to reduce to it what can only be observed objectively and consequently lose the appreciation in the 'magic' from what transpires invisibly between and within participants. Moreover, the artistic process and experience is inherently subjective. And dramatherapists might simply be afraid that we actually cannot empirically validate our work (and what would happen next, we dare not imagine).
>
> (Dramatherapist S, USA)

'Tradition' was often cited as a cause for current tension, with emergent calls for evidence framed by quantitative evidence contrasted with dramatherapy's tradition of using qualitative methods:

> While strengths of dramatherapy can include a client-centred approach and flexibility, this seems to have created a vacuum separat-ing dramatherapy from systems considerations and consistencies in outcome . . . There is little or no consistency for measures which could help communicate that efficacy or even define data'.
>
> (Dramatherapist N, Canada)

The following echoes this respondent's concerns about a vacuum, but combines a critique of quantitative-based approaches to researching impact with a contrasting expression to engage with this framework:

I do not agree with the fixation on quantitative data in education – judging schools only on pupil progress graphs. It tends to lead to inaccuracies and deliberate fixing of data and is of course subjective. However, producing some quantitative date would give us more of a foot in the door of education from where we can perhaps show/demonstrate the value of qualitative research and data'.

(Dramatherapist L, Australia)

Another theme concerned the 'voice' of the child clients: 'At a time when there is an increasing emphasis on externally set criteria to evaluate change, I find it hard to keep the client in the picture and this threatens the core of my beliefs about being an arts therapist' (Dramatherapist V, Taiwan). Here, the therapist positions research and evidence as concerning power and belief: externally set criteria are seen as not easily engaging with empowerment and the child's voice. The therapist sees these as central to his or her identity, work and conception of the role of the therapist-researcher as a powerful advocate. Therapists involved in the research often highlighted factors that emphasized the potency of dramatherapy research to engage with client languages and perspectives: 'We need more research especially as regards what sense and meaning children construct around the intervention alongside which aspects of the intervention children find most useful' (Dramatherapist L, Malta).

The responses bear testimony to a changed context of provision being linked to a demanded research 'evidence base' connected to externally set frameworks. These are identified as being linked to quantitative criteria developed to match educational goals and agendas and not the therapeutic needs of children. The research reveals a field with urgent needs. Such voices reflect a shifting environment constructed of developments that foreground particular tensions in relation to research and practice.

Reframing analysis: dialogue between dramatherapy and the medical humanities

How can the inter-relational possibilities of the medical humanities and the arts therapies be demonstrated in a consideration of the matters raised in the research findings? What is the nature of the task of examination or responding to the research questions, findings and their implications? One way would be to position the arts therapies and dramatherapy as part of the medical humanities. If dramatherapy became this, what would this mean, how could it be justified and how could the effect of this positioning be useful in understanding the research and its findings?

The literature on dramatherapy and research in schools focuses upon methodology, dilemmas concerning approaches and techniques and reports on clinical material, such as case studies (Domikles 2012; Feldman *et al.* 2009; Roger 2012; Smythe 2010; Tytherleigh 2010). This can be considered as revealing an absence of attention and engagement within the field's discourse. No attention is given to deeper philosophical and cultural concerns in relation to research or the clinical dilemmas and challenges encountered by therapists in schools. This is reflected by the therapists' responses in the data presented in the previous section, in which the discourse of the therapists was typified by attention to skills or specific methods, management accountability, changed demands from funders and changes in requirements of providers.

What happens if the research is positioned in relation to the medical humanities and their concerns? I want to use the research findings to examine the ways in which the arts therapies can be brought into the kinds of discourses that the medical humanities concern themselves with. I will illustrate how this relationship is possible and valid, and reveal the ways this can be useful to the arts therapies. The analysis will reframe discourse away from the normal concerns with skills and method as indicated above and will engage with the data in dialogue with medical humanities perspectives.

If dramatherapy is 're-positioned' in this way, it can become connected to aspects of the medical humanities' philosophical and theoretical concerns and goals. What are these and why are they relevant? Evans (2008) has distinguished various functions of the medical humanities, including the analysis of the practice of medicine. Downie and Macnaughton suggest that the medical humanities offer a particular kind of critical function where, for example, they can examine the purpose of health-related concerns and thereby challenge areas where 'medical practice and research' is accepted 'as a given' (Downie and Macnaughton 2007: xi). They argue that 'the humanities can recommend broader perceptions of and attitudes to health and how it may be enhanced' (Downie and Macnaughton 2007: 165). Shapiro *et al.*'s definition of the role and nature of the medical humanities emphasizes specific aspects of this process. They first show how the field of medical humanities draws upon 'methods, concepts, and content' from other humanities disciplines in order to 'investigate illness...healing, therapeutic relationships, and other aspects of medicine and health care practice', to 'reconceptualise health care' by encouraging practitioners to 'query their own attitudes and behaviours', and to offer 'integrated' perspectives on healing (Shapiro *et al.* 2009: 192). Here, they are arguing that the role of the humanities should be to offer particular, contrasting perspectives on conceptions of health, intervention and their role in reframing these within medicine. Their second point concerns power and narrative in health services. They argue that the medical humanities enable us to engage with the way 'certain biomedical narratives are privileged', those that are 'mechanistic (the body is a machine), linear (find the cause, create an effect), and hierarchical (doctor as expert)' (Shapiro *et al.* 2009: 194). The role of the medical humanities is to understand and challenge these narratives that 'marginalize the humanities, which don't neatly conform to this cultural model', to promote an expanded vision of medicine and medical education beyond the instrumental (Shapiro *et al.* 2009: 194). This 'expansion' connects to Bleakley's assertion, in his introductory chapter within this volume, that a key aspect of the medical humanities should be democratization and 'scepticism towards utilitarian models of health and well-being, seeing meaning in illness; provides a core, reflexive point of resistance to dominant, reductive biomedical science'. The relevance of these aspects of the medical humanities to dramatherapy connects to Stephen Pattison's 'purposes and hopes' for the role of the medical humanities to remain a 'broad church', as also discussed in Victoria Bates and Sam Goodman's introductory chapter. Pattison sees the 'effects' of the medical humanities in particular ways concerning equity and the creation of new knowledge:

> Equal space and respect would be accorded to practitioners, performers, theorists, and analysts from the various relevant arts, humanities, and medical practices and disciplines. Attempts would be made to try to break down barriers between these different groups and perspectives; work would be undertaken to build effective channels of communication, dialogue, and debate.
>
> (Pattison 2002: 34)

If transferred to dramatherapy, what can these dynamics offer? These ways of positioning the medical humanities could be reframed in relation to understanding the research findings, as:

1. Can the presence of the arts in a health/medical domain, in the form of dramatherapy, be viewed from the perspective of offering challenges to 'givens' in health provision and to the ways 'certain biomedical narratives are privileged' (Shapiro *et al.* 2009: 194)?
2. Can the role of the medical humanities in influencing 'practitioners' to 'query their own attitudes and behaviours' (Shapiro *et al.* 2009: 192) be useful in giving status to the role of humanities' conceptions of health and of the understanding of the nature of dramatherapy in schools?
3. Can the medical humanities, in relation to its role in trying 'to break down barriers between these different groups and perspectives' and its 'work... to build effective channels of communication, dialogue, and debate' (Pattison 2002: 34) be of use in responding to the research?

I will argue that this is the case and that this perspective has value. The next section addresses each of these questions and will illustrate how the perspective offers innovative possibilities in creating ways of gaining insight into the research findings, in addition to opening up a deep rationale that can be taken forwards to form agendas for directions in dramatherapy research.

The reframed analysis

Challenges to 'givens'

The previous section noted that the 'problem' as reflected both by the literature and the research participants' responses, tends to 'see' only in terms of method and clinical application. I want to approach the findings in relation to the medical humanities' concerns with deepening our awareness of the cultural position and potentials of dramatherapy.

Critical literature argues that dramatherapy came into existence in part as a response to recognition of the need and potential within domains that, by the twentieth century, were often separated: the theatre, play, psychiatry, ritual and education (Jennings 1990; Landy 2001; Jones 2007). Its existence in the twentieth century came about because of unrealized possibilities between different disciplines – created within the potential space between them. Its emergence and potency as a therapy did not arise within a single discipline, but from the potential of interdisciplinary engagement between areas such as theatre, education and health. From a historical perspective, two of the main contexts for dramatherapy's emergence are the theatre and locations of health provision such as the hospital, domains that still remain separate in many societies. This way of looking at the field suggests that dramatherapy's vitality and relevance is powered by an interdisciplinary dynamic. However, when considering the experiences reflected by the respondents within the research a more problematic situation emerges. It reveals a tension rooted in difference experienced as opposition rather than of interdisciplinary energy as positive and mutual.

As mentioned earlier, research methods that are becoming increasingly valued in national health systems or by education providers differ from those used and valued in theatre and, traditionally, in dramatherapy (Dokter and Winn 2009; Snow and D'Amico 2009; Jones 2012). The research data indicates a position where health and education services are, increasingly, valuing, or only recognizing, quantitative approaches to change and impact. In this way, the experiences of the respondents can be understood to represent dynamics concerning the relationship between health-based frameworks and those of the humanities. The extracts from the research illustrate the lived experience of this tension concerning, as one of the above respondents frames it, 'recent changes' linked to impact or evidence being understood in particular ways. Here, for example, is an emphasis on effect as measured by changed behaviours outside of the dramatherapy room and measurements as 'standard' that are developed outside the discipline of dramatherapy or having 'long histories' with which dramatherapy is seen to 'compete', as another respondent commented (Participant K, the Netherlands).

One way of understanding this is to see it as a challenge to existing discourses in educational services. Respondents noted a shift in the primary or sole means of assessing the impact of dramatherapy towards quantitative measurement – either of behavioural change outside of the therapy room or of academic results. The respondents often viewed these factors as needing to be met by the field finding ways in which quantitative frameworks for understanding the nature of health and change could be created and adopted by dramatherapists. They identified this as the developmental challenge for the field's future. However, when examined from the medical humanities perspective of giving status to the role of the humanities in an understanding of the nature of interventions in health provision, this can be seen as a matter related to power. Pattison's analysis of dominant discourses and powerful narratives of 'mechanistic (the body is a machine), linear (find the cause, create an effect), and hierarchical (doctor as expert)' (Shapiro *et al.* 2009: 194) can be identified as fuelling the pressure and othering of humanities perspectives and linked to an understanding of the othering in schools of dramatherapy's qualitative frameworks for understanding impact. Within this way of reframing the processes and experiences communicated by participants, the issues they identify can be understood and responded to differently as the next section will address.

Medical humanities and conceptions of dramatherapy

The experiences reported in the data can be reframed to reflect dramatherapy's challenge to dominant discourses within the education system that see change as being measured by quantitative frameworks for behaviour in classrooms or of clients' academic results. Rather than submitting to the power of such dominant discourses, options for alternative responses can be linked to another aspect of the medical humanities' concerns and mission. This concerns Pattison's advocacy of the insights and work of the medical humanities involving the breaking down of 'barriers between these different groups and perspectives' and its 'work . . . to build effective channels of communication' (Pattison 2002: 34). A different understanding of the research responses can envision a way forward, which lies in dramatherapy researchers and practitioners breaking barriers between frameworks and methodologies. By understanding the situation as representative of philosophical and cultural tension and divide, insight can be gained which enables the examination of dialogue or exploring of interdisciplinary value. The response becomes less a matter of how dramatherapists can develop methods of quantitative evaluation through their clients' classroom performance, and more of how mutuality between different approaches to health and well-being can be understood and sought. Rather than to fear or be anxious about this, the role of both can be to explore the nature of potentials across the cultural divide. Are there ways of framing and understanding both arts- and medical-based traditions in research to permit mutuality and mutual awareness, for example, in relation to shortcomings or new potentials within research? This approach posits difference not as entrenched, but as dynamic and as heralding new possibilities.

Medical humanities and breaking down 'barriers'

When viewed from this perspective, one of the crucial next phases for dramatherapy is to develop theoretical and methodological dialogues and routes to enquiry that fully meet an understanding of dramatherapy's potential relationships with quantitative and qualitative methodologies. Innovations in this meeting of the qualitative and quantitative could also explore the ways the languages of dramatherapy can form the methods of the research. Research that uses dramatherapy processes such as role, play, story making or improvisation need to be explored in ways that create dialogue between quantitative and qualitative methodologies. Research that uses qualitative enquiry into clients' experiences of dramatherapy can be used to develop further enquiry that uses qualitative data to form enquiry using quantitative approaches, for example. The developmental challenge for dramatherapy's future becomes reframed. The arts therapies are culturally important in holding and valuing the presence of the arts within domains that, within the emerging discourses of efficacy and impact in schools, do not easily engage with their role and approaches to intervention and meaning making. Any enquiry into arts processes in therapeutic work in schools needs to be reconsidered in dialogue with discourses concerning the cultural position and potentials of dramatherapy. Such enquiry would address, for example, topics such as the status given to the role of 'messy' processes such as improvisation and play in relation to evaluating and understanding therapeutic change for children in schools. This reframing demands a shift in the field's attention away from a sole engagement with technique, method and the immediate clinical encounter towards a dialogue with these broader, deeper concerns.

Conclusion

This chapter has argued for the value and potential that is unlocked by critical analysis of the discourses that lie within and beneath dramatherapists' experiences in work with children in schools. The value of this approach is understood in terms of both intellectual capital and the development of ways to address dilemmas in the discipline. Its potential lies in fresh insight, illumination and opportunities for resolving barriers.

The chapter has not paid close attention to the nature of dramatherapy as a profession or practice, in part because these matters are dealt with thoroughly in relation to different forms of arts-based intervention within this volume. Instead, it has offered a critical review of the absence of dialogue between the arts therapies and the medical humanities. The chapter has illustrated the potentials of this interdisciplinary attention and offered an example of these potentials linked to a specific piece of research. The chapter has also drawn on new research analyzing the voices of dramatherapists working with children in schools, particularly concerning the future of the discipline and its research. The chapter's innovation involved drawing on research into therapists' experiences of lived contemporary dilemmas and ideas to create a dialogue with the medical humanities. The innovative re-framing of dramatherapy within medical humanities' concerns and frameworks has enabled new insights into the data and the situation they represent. The understanding enabled by the dialogue creates: a way of understanding the phenomenon beyond and within their immediate manifestation; insight into the wider perspectives of theory, cultural tension; and ways of reconsidering and gaining an insight into the nature of a response to the lived direct experiences of dramatherapists.

Interdisciplinarity has been seen to be of value in offering potential for innovation in philosophy, theory and praxis (Jacobs and Frickel 2009), including the creation of insight in specific fields but also in the emergence and development of new fields. The arts therapies are hybrid and their development has been described as recognizing gaps and potential arising from developments, interactions and unease in fields of health, medicine, psychotherapy, education and the arts. Downie and Macnaughton asked if the arts therapies are, by their nature, a 'movement' within the medical humanities (Downie and Macnaughton 2007). This chapter has illustrated a different kind of relationship – of dialogue – with the medical humanities offering new insights into arts therapies' theory, praxis and research.

References

Andersen-Warren, M. (2012) 'Research by the British Association of Dramatherapists and Literature Review', in L. Leigh, I. Gersch, A. Dix and D. Haythorne (eds) *Dramatherapy with Children and Young People in Schools: Enabling Creativity, Sociability, Communication and Learning*, London: Routledge.

Austin, S. F. (1917) *Principles of Drama-Therapy: A Handbook for Dramatists, Dealing with the Possibilities of Suggestion and the Mass Mind*, New York: Sopherim.

Boyatzis, R. E. (1998) *Transforming Qualitative Information: Thematic Analysis and Code Development*, London: Sage.

Casson, J. (1997) 'Dramatherapy History in Headlines: Who did What, When, Where?', *Dramatherapy*, 19: 10–13.

Dokter, D. and Winn, L. (2009) 'Evaluating Dramatherapy. EPB and PBE: A Research Project', *Dramatherapy*, 31: 3–9.

Domikles D. (2012) 'Violence and Laughter: How Dramatherapy Can Go Beyond Behaviour Management for Boys at Risk of Exclusion', in L. Leigh, I. Gersch, A. Dix and D. Haythorne (eds) *Dramatherapy with Children, Young People and Schools: Enabling Creativity, Sociability, Communication and Learning*, London: Routledge.

Downie, R. S. and Macnaughton, J. (2007) *Bioethics and the Humanities: Attitudes and Perceptions*, Abingdon and New York: Routledge-Cavendish.

Evans, H. M. (2008) 'Affirming the Existential within Medicine: Medical Humanities, Governance, and Imaginative Understanding', *Journal of Medical Humanities*, 29: 55–9.

Evans, H. M. and Greaves, D. (2003) 'Coming of Age?', *Journal of Medical Ethics: Medical Humanities*, 29: 57–8.

Feldman, D., Jones, F. and Ward, E. (2009) 'The Enact Method of Employing Drama Therapy in Schools', in D. Read Johnson and R. Emunah (eds) *Current Approaches in Dramatherapy*, Illinois: Charles C. Thomas.

Health and Care Professions Council (HCPC) (2003) 'Standards of Proficiency – Arts Therapists'. Online. Available: www.hpc-uk.org/assets/documents/100004FBStandards_of_Proficiency_Arts_Therapists.pdf (accessed 21 November 2012).

Health and Care Professions Council (HCPC) (2012) 'Home Page'. Online. Available: www.hpc-uk.org (accessed 21 November 2012).

Hughes, J., Kidd, J. and McNamara, C. (2011) 'The Usefulness of Mess: Artistry, Improvisation and Decomposition in the Practice of Research in Applied Theatre', in B. Kershaw and H. Nicholson (eds) *Research Methods in Theatre and Performance*, Edinburgh: Edinburgh University Press.

Jacobs, A. J. and Frickel, S. (2009) 'Interdisciplinararity: A Critical Assessment', *Annual Review of Sociology*, 35: 43–65.

Jennings, S. (1990) *Dramatherapy with Individuals and Groups*, London: Jessica Kingsley Publishers.

Jones, P. (2005) *The Arts Therapies*, London: Routledge.

Jones, P. (2007) *Drama as Therapy*, London: Routledge.

Jones, P. (2012) 'Approaches to the Futures of Research', *Dramatherapy*, 34: 63–82.

Karkou, V. (ed.) (2010) *Arts Therapies in Schools*, London: Jessica Kingsley Publishers.

Landy, R. J. (2001) *New Essays in Drama Therapy: Unfinished Business*, Springfield, IL: Charles C. Thomas.

Karkou, V. and Sanderson, P. (2006) *Arts Therapies: A Research-based Map of the Field*, Edinburgh: Elsevier.

Leigh, L., Gersch, I., Dix, A. and Haythorne, D. (eds) (2012) *Dramatherapy with Children and Young People in Schools: Enabling Creativity, Sociability, Communication and Learning*, London: Routledge.

Macneill, P. U. (2011) 'The Arts and Medicine: A Challenging Relationship', *Medical Humanities*, 37: 85–90.

McFerran, K. and Stephenson, J. (2010) 'Facing the Challenge: A Music Therapy Investigation in the Evidence-Based Framework', in V. Karkou (ed.) *Arts Therapies in School*, London: Jessica Kingsley Publishers.

Pattison, S. (2002) 'Medical Humanities: A Vision and Some Cautionary Notes', *Medical Humanities*, 29: 33–6.

Quibell, T. (2010) 'The Searching Drama of Disaffection: Dramatherapy Groups in a Whole-School Context', in V. Karkou (ed.) *Arts Therapies in Schools*, London: Jessica Kingsley Publishers.

Roger, J. (2012) 'Learning Disabilities and Finding, Keeping and Protecting the Therapeutic Space', in L. Leigh, I. Gersch, A. Dix and D. Haythorne (eds) *Dramatherapy with Children, Young People and Schools: Enabling Creativity, Sociability, Communication and Learning*, London: Routledge.

Rothenberg, A. (2006) 'Creativity, Self Creation, and the Treatment of Mental Illness', *Medical Humanities*, 32: 14–19.

Shapiro, J., Coulehan, J., Wear, D. and Montello, M. (2009) 'Medical Humanities and Their Discontents: Definitions, Critiques, and Implications', *Academic Medicine*, 84: 192–8.

Shine, D. E. (2012) 'Fear, Maths, Brief Dramatherapy and Neuroscience', in L.

Leigh, I. Gersch, A. Dix and D. Haythorne (eds) *Dramatherapy with Children, Young People and Schools: Enabling Creativity, Sociability, Communication and Learning*, London: Routledge.

Smythe, G. (2010) 'Solution-Focused Brief Dramatherapy Group Work: Working with Children in Mainstream Education in Sri-Lanka', in V. Karkou (ed.) *Arts Therapies in Schools*, London: Jessica Kingsley Publishers.

Snow, S. and D'Amico, M. (2009) *Assessment in the Creative Arts Therapies: Designing and Adapting Assessment Tools for Adults with Developmental Disabilities*, Springfield, IL: Charles C. Thomas.

Stacey, J. (2008) 'The Therapeutic Relationship in Creative Arts Psychotherapy', in S. Haugh and S. Paul (eds) *The Therapeutic Relationship: Perspectives and Themes*, Ross-On-Wye: PCCS Books.

Tytherleigh, L. (2010) 'Dramatherapy, Autism and Relationship Building', in V. Karkou (ed.) *Arts Therapies in Schools*, London: Jessica Kingsley Publishers.

Winn, L. (2009) *The Use of Outcome Measures in Dramatherapy*. Online. Available: www.BADth.org.uk (accessed 21 November 2012).

Section Five

Music

13 Music, therapy and technology

An opinion piece

Overview

Paul Robertson

In this opinion piece, I write as an experienced musician who has played at the highest level of performance. I also write as someone who has employed music as therapy and who has studied both neuro-biological and cultural aspects of the impact of music upon the body, mind and spirit. After years grappling with the intangible and ineffable aspects of music I am as cautious about reducing its impact to either measured outcomes or neural firings as I am of considering even the most subtle musical analysis an explication of the musical experience. While each of these approaches has an important role and must be considered seriously, as a musician I am keenly aware of the difficulty, even the impossibility, of quantifying aesthetic human experience. Yet, as a devotee of the scientific method, I recognize the need for rigorous, replicable and meaningful analysis of music used therapeutically. So why do we feel the need to justify or explain beauty in order to be able to experience or value it? Accepting the notion that both the rational and subjective aspects of musical experience are necessary to its fuller appreciation, this chapter seeks to explore this tension between quantitative measures and qualitative experience in evaluating the impact of music on health, taking the interplay between the objective and subjective as an important way to talk about the medical humanities in general.

While accepting the importance of the many academic developments in the complex and diverse field of music therapies, the following chapter is neither intended as a literature review nor an analysis of the many studies that have taken place on the music/health relationship. Instead it is intended to be read as an opinion piece based on decades of working in the field of medical humanities (before it was so named), in which I have witnessed the rise of new technologies, evidence-based healthcare and the brain sciences, which have all shaped our contemporary understandings of the relationship between music, medicine and the mind. This chapter pays particular attention to music as therapy, complementing Helen Odell-Miller's case study on the professionalization of music therapy within this section.[1]

Despite its focus on music therapy, this is not merely an opinion piece on the 'impact of the arts on health'. I also seek to consider how developments in medicine and technology have shaped how we understand the reciprocal relationship between music and health. This aspect is also developed further in the case study by Zack Moir and Katie Overy within this section, which shows how new technologies since the Second World War have influenced musical experience. This current chapter presents a more personal perspective on the changes that have occurred in both fields in the last 70 years and the impact of such changes on the art/health relationship. I hope that this opinion piece is able to enrich the debate about the universal relevance of music as therapy and also stimulate questions about how we understand and measure the relationship between music, health and well-being.

Why medical humanities? Medical practitioners and music

Before moving on to discuss the relationship between medicine and music more closely, it is important to question why medical and healthcare practitioners are interested in music and musical interventions in the first place. I will concentrate on doctors. The answer may lie in fundamental overlaps between the natures of the professions. Although a broad generalization, as a string quartet player I was always aware that an unusually high proportion of our audiences seemed to be doctors. I would speculate that doctors and musicians share a high degree of empathy, together with a desire to 'place' or organize their feelings within a coherent rationale structure; they also create and explore therapeutic 'touch' within their respective disciplines. Another common trait between the two professions may be the desire to command and gain knowledge within areas of experience that are intrinsically unknowable (or at least defy everyday verbal expression) and challenging.

Despite much prevailing delusion regarding medical 'truths', the doctor's role is overwhelmingly, and indeed crucially, involved with the unknown and the unknowable – for example the patient's own experiences and beliefs, the real nature of healing (as opposed to treating) and the uncertainties of diagnosis. Medicine is as laced with uncertainty as is musical interpretation although, for obvious reasons, such uncertainty is perhaps more often welcomed within a musical context than in the medical arena. The tremendous value, actual and perceived, in naming illness can act as a limiter, placing a totemic structure upon treatment pathways. It is very clear that naming an illness can act as an effective shortcut with which to shape treatments and approaches. It can also help patients get a conceptual handle on their illness. However, we have become so culturally dependent on the naming of things that we have reached a point where often something is only considered real or recognized once it has been named. Patients often speak of a diagnosis being a validation – of their subjective experiences, and almost of themselves. The perceived value of naming may at times prove hazardous, both for medicine and for music. Within this system, the doctor–patient consultation, the narrative and the taking of medical histories loom very large. Synthesizing all this information into a single named and valid illness is a big responsibility, which draws upon the art of medicine alongside its science. Of course, the 'art' and 'science' of medicine are also not mutually exclusive categories.

It is possible to observe musical parallels here, particularly in relation to the interconnected factors of language, authority and expertise. Describing a particular musical journey as a 'symphony', for example, creates an often completely mistaken expectation as to its contents or intention. Renaming the same work a 'tone poem' or 'rhapsody' or 'invention' will alter the educated listener's reception of the music. By the same token, simply using any of these terms might alienate anybody who presumes the whole thing to be elitist. There seems to be a powerful authority exercised in both medicine and music once the 'expert' or 'interpreter' is able to define uncertainties and distill ambiguity into a single integrated whole. It is as rare for the musical performer as it is for the clinician to sustain clarity and dynamic authority while simultaneously acknowledging doubt and ambiguity. However, I must remark that this is exactly the quality that truly great players manifest. There is often a far greater depth of insight when a fine performer is discovering the musical truth in the moment of its performance rather than displaying predetermined certainties. Can the same be said of doctors? And if so, how does it manifest itself? I argue that much current medical education and practice will need reconstruction in order to embrace overt doubt and ambiguity. We should not view such doubt and inward reflection as a sign of either weakness or indecisiveness, but rather as an indicator of a higher competence in which the unknown and unknowable are acknowledged and even embraced. Many senior physicians would readily concede that part of their role involves carrying themselves confidently with certainty while functioning in an environment of constant ambiguity.

I have outlined what I believe to be some shared characteristics of music and medicine, and the importance of embracing uncertainty in both. This music–medicine relationship can be used productively, for example, with medical students. In recent years, I have led a Special Study Unit at the Peninsula Medical School in Truro based around music. Professor Anthony Pinching, an experienced clinician (now retired), joined me in these in-depth sessions with small numbers of fourth-year medical undergraduates. During this period a number of significant things gradually became clear. The strength and the weakness of musical experience is that the larger part of it remains implicit, and therefore often unrecognized, within our current cultural behaviours. Illustrating this, each year a number of bright young students would come along insisting that they knew nothing about music, and had no experience or knowledge of it. To begin with, this was quite off-putting – how to begin a conversation about a topic that was a complete mystery to one of the parties? In time, we discovered that in fact all these students actually had a very intimate relationship with all sorts of music, although often not within the narrow bandwidth of high-art classical repertoire. Simply exploring their current favourite listening would quickly uncover all sorts of powerful narratives, and some subtle defining marks of personal history and identity. From then on, some of their wider preoccupations as fledgling doctors would open up. All of these discussions reinforced in me the belief that, perhaps because of the largely unconscious process by which the brain learns to select what it consciously hears, we can be much affected by music while remaining overwhelmingly unaware of our own responses.

The ambiguities of music thus allowed students to produce their own meaning and reflect on their identities as doctors. Within the course, we also explored the potential therapeutic aspect of music for patients. What I would hope for from music, as an integral part of the medical humanities, is perhaps best illustrated by one student who insisted that she had no previous relationship with music. Her major motivation in choosing the music module was that she had observed great change in a deeply disturbed child, possibly autistic, during a session with a local music therapist. She was keen to understand what had been happening and why. As well as connecting much more personally with music in her own personal history, we were able to direct her towards literature that addressed these topics. She submitted a thoughtful essay discussing the role of music therapy and its possible inclusion within mainstream medicine, which finished with a single, simple challenge: 'What is the level of proof required before it would be negligent for a doctor *not* to prescribe music for a patient?'

This is a powerful validation for the place of the medical humanities in medical education, which to my mind – and in the light of the *Tomorrow's Doctors* guidelines from the General Medical Council in 1993 – needs little further proof. The role of the medical humanities in medical education has also been discussed extensively elsewhere in this volume. It is therefore not my purpose here to question the value of the relationship between music and medicine. Instead, I seek to address some of the more pertinent and challenging questions about proof that this student also raised.

Historical and cultural antecedents

Therapeutic musical interventions are probably as old as humanity. We might speculate that early practitioners were shamans, who considered themselves divinely inspired. Trances stimulated by music could apparently induce altered states while acting as a powerful cathartic force to expel alien or infectious possession. Within such a magical belief system, music is perceived to be an agency for such magical transference. Thus, the artist is conceived as a type of shaman and the musical inspiration taken to be proof of a special divine or even demonic possession. Shamans today, practicing in hunter-gatherer communities, such as the Inuit, use rhythmic music to go into trance and thereby enact healing of individuals or communities. The shaman's drum is thought of as an animal – indeed, is made from animal skin – on which the shaman rides to another world to gain the powers to conduct healing or receive insight. The rhythm of the drum is often combined with chanting, where shamans are inspired to make up songs or reproduce traditional forms. Enlightenment philosophers reacted towards the tradition of inspiration and trance, taking a more 'rational' approach to how music works. However, links between the artistic and the divine ritual continue even now. Humans still use music to celebrate in many formal rituals and celebrations. From a simplistic anthropological viewpoint, is there anything substantially different between our current musical rituals worldwide and what we would perhaps prefer to think of as having far more primitive origins?

Paying attention to history also highlights the long roots of links between medicine and madness, or at least mindlessness. Plato suggested that when artists are inspired they are – by definition – mindless or unable to use their rational intelligence. This anticipates the early use of music therapeutically for the possessed, epileptic and the cognitively and emotionally disturbed. An interesting strand is the periodic musical depiction of madness – as in the English Restoration fashion for 'mad songs'. Here again there was a, possibly somewhat prurient, fascination with an ability to depict altered states. Not only was music expected to work therapeutically, but also the representation of illness through songs has often been an important aspect of society throughout history. While this volume and this chapter focus on the period since 1945, such continuities in the societal importance of music must be remembered.

We should also pay some attention to the historical roots of the perceived relationship between madness and musical genius. In the Romantic musical period in particular, performers and managers, to enhance the appeal of artists, sometimes exploited such associations. Paganini established a supposed possession as the basis for his remarkable musical gifts. As a result of his tragic self-medication with both mercury and endless purgatives, he became increasingly spectral and bizarre in appearance, reinforcing the myths of divine possession. Many other composers entered this unfortunate class of mythic madmen, such as Berlioz (bi-polar and an opium addict); Mozart (chronic illness, plus much later 'romantic' myth-making); Beethoven (bi-polar and deaf); Schubert (syphilitic with mood disturbance); Scriabin (periodically delusional) among others. Pundits find much less to write about relatively well-adapted musical figures such as Saint-Saens (child prodigy, exceptionally gifted and successful and musically conservative) and Mendelssohn (exceptional child prodigy, highly successful career and conservative).

While this is necessarily a sweeping overview of some of complex history of the relationship between medicine and health, I have used it here to argue that one of the main truths of contemporary musical life in general

– and music therapies in particular – is that both are based in the most ancient, primitive and unconscious aspects of our humanity and cultures, and perhaps also of our biology. Therapeutic music can be both about entering altered states and treating altered states

Turning to more recent history, which is the focus of this current volume, we can see both continuity and change. While many of the same associations remain prevalent – such as music, madness and genius – there have also been specific technological and social developments that have influenced how we understand the relationship between music, medicine and health. Taking the United Kingdom as an example, the National Health Service (NHS) has promoted a rise in evidence-based healthcare in the last 70 years because of the importance of justifying the expenditure of public money. Music therapy has become interwoven with such debates, being evaluated in relation to its value for specific medical issues and particularly for mental health.[2] Such trends picked up after the 1940s because of the necessity of treating war veterans with psychological disorders.

In her contribution to this volume, Helen Odell-Miller also rightly highlights how the psychological disciplines have been particularly important for the promotion and recognition of music therapies within the NHS. I wish here to also pay some attention to the professionalization of music therapy and to its current nature. In music therapy currently, the therapeutic approaches developed by Paul Nordoff and Clive Robbins in the 1950s and 1960s are relatively in the ascendency, and increasingly receive a significant degree of clinical recognition. This includes becoming a recognized and regulated profession allied to medicine, largely due to the sustained efforts of the music therapy movement. Music therapy is now at least to some degree recognized and utilized as a valuable addition to other approaches in hospitals and other clinical settings. Yet it will be competing increasingly with a range of other therapies in any resource-limited health system, so it will have to make a persuasive case for its systematic application in defined clinical conditions. This of course brings us back to the pragmatic necessity of having an evidence base, not to mention a biological rationale, for using it in preference to some other approaches.

Largely based on extemporized musical dialogue and exchanges between the music therapist and client, this therapeutic approach is essentially aesthetic in character. My observation of such sessions reveals that they are largely based on two fundamental principles. Firstly, retrogenesis, which recognizes that human memory, identity and development tends to follow the principle of 'first in, last out' – the idea that our earliest experiences are our most tenacious ones. Since musical response is so precocious, established while *in utero*, most individuals have this as a kind of default system that can be accessed even when higher cognitive function is falling away, as in old age dementias. Secondly, the ability to lock in to the natural developmental stages that seem to be hardwired into our earliest development. Much of this normal development has a musical component, such as the increasingly subtle and complex prosodic exchanges between neonates and mother, leading to the universal language of 'motherese'. For those who do not undergo such development naturally, such as those individuals with Down's syndrome or autism, the possibility remains to replay such developmental windows later on in life with a gifted therapist as guide.

Another prime tenet of the music therapeutic process is now acknowledged to be the special musically mediated relationship between client and therapist. A 'therapist effect' is well recognized and studied in other clinical interventions. It is a moot point as to whether there is an additional element to this effect that is intrinsic to the use of music as the intervention and a musician as its mediator. These considerations speak strongly to the chamber musician in me – having a sacred regard for sensitivity of response and communication between performer and listener. It has also made conventional measured assessment extremely tricky, but not necessarily impossible, and has necessitated more nuanced qualitative and quantitative evaluations of the relationship between arts, communication and health. This relationship operates in terms of both clinical symptoms, particularly in relation to mental health, and a patient's experience or management of ill health, particularly in chronic conditions.

In addition to the rise in music therapy as a profession, there have been a number of practical developments within medicine and technology in the last 70 years, which have shaped how we measure the impact of music therapy. The arts/health relationship is a reciprocal one, as we have used new medical technologies to measure the impact of music on health. New technologies since the Second World War have influenced how we measure musical experience and have even influenced the nature of musical experience, as shown clearly by Zack Moir and Katie Overy's chapter on cochlear implants. More recently, within the so-called 'cognitive turn', we are able to observe and visualize the impact of listening to music on different parts of the brain. Although limited by the technical restrictions of the technologies involved, as well as the somewhat simplistic musical appreciation of some of the researchers, it shows how musical therapies have responded to the context of the late-twentieth century by finding new ways to quantify their worth. I will now consider these two interwoven matters in turn: the increasing need to measure musical experience and the impact of the rise of new technologies, including brain scanning.

Music therapy: Defining, capturing and measuring beauty

> Not everything that can be counted counts; and not everything that counts can be counted.
>
> Albert Einstein

Before I consider some of the questions around measuring the impact of music on health, I need to explain exactly what I mean by 'therapy'. I am focusing upon some significant approaches to music as a therapy since 1945, because I believe that they may well provide the framework for a new objective aesthetic both of music and its therapeutic applications. One of the dilemmas of our current materialistic view is confusion about the relationships between body, mind and spirit. In order to sit comfortably within our current scientific paradigm most doctors feel obliged to conform to a model in which higher human functions are conceived only as a by-product of our material existence. These functions include affect, cognition, moral conscience, consciousness and aesthetic feeling. Unfortunately such reductionist thinking leads to a coarsening of all finer experience. Joy becomes merely the healthy manifestation of 'well-being', which in turn must be an expression of physical health. While there is certainly a correlation between bodily health and the experience of spontaneous joy, it is not a self-defining one. If it were, how could we explain why so many people experience and spread joy while dying? By the same token, human happiness is not the sole preserve of the fit.

We must not be seduced, in my view, into a mere sentimental attachment of human existence for its own sake – longevity clearly does not equate to quality of life. However, we must surely seek to enhance and uplift the value of life in all circumstances. This must then include all those subtle experiences and relationships that serve to render life beautiful and meaningful. Surely this must embrace loving communication and the appreciation of the beautiful? In this sense much current clinical medical practice is simply inadequate. Reporting my own experience of a long hospital incarceration, while wholeheartedly applauding the exceptional surgical care I was fortunate to receive on the National Health Service, the lengthy recovery was much less positive partly because of the functionality of the experience. For me, the meaning and value of music therapy thus lies in its aesthetic nature rather than only its function.

I will now turn to consider three therapeutic applications of music: music in hospitals, music-thanatology and music environments. These three ways highlight the diverse forms that therapeutic music can take, which further problematizes the method of capturing and measuring them – a question that I will return to consider in due course.

Some might feel that arts performed in a hospital setting do not strictly constitute therapy, as there is no clear therapeutic relationship established in most hospital musical performances. While true, perhaps we should extend our model of therapy to embrace such altered dynamics, whether through a more general effect, or in a manner analogous to preventive medicine. Happily there has been some enthusiastic take-up of such alternative performance situations from within the music community, particularly supported by Yehudi Menuhin's delightful 'Live Music Now' programmes, which involve young players in performance situations outside the concert hall – such as prisons, hospitals and care homes. A veritable seachange of attitude has also taken place within music conservatories to favour such outreach activity.

As something of a pioneer in music in hospital, a few comments arise from my own experience. Musicians working in clinical settings need to consider their programming carefully. Along with many other novices, we began by naively assuming that we should choose light and happy music. Nothing could have been further from the truth. All the people in such settings are unsurprisingly far more mindful of their mortality. As a result, they seem more responsive to serious or poignant pieces and may be open to a far more profound musical understanding and repertoire than previously. This also questions the tendency to describe arts therapies as acting in the service of health and well-being (see Alan Bleakley's introductory chapter). Music for the soul can be challenging and engage a person with their deeper experience rather than merely providing light distraction or entertainment. The benefit of music therapy may then be for people to make greater meaning out of illness. They may find immense consolation that a composer has used his own suffering as a springboard for achieving something beautiful, truthful and uplifting. They may find solace in an emotionally engrossing event that can not only distract them from their present condition, but also allow them to engage – and equally importantly disengage – at will. Hospital and illness intrinsically involve, after all, a loss of the personal locus of control.

Music-thanatology is the playing of music for the dying, an enlightened and beautiful tradition now resurrected by Therese Schroeder-Sheker, who has established a movement largely focusing upon the end-of-life care for cancer sufferers in hospice and other care settings. Here the focus is almost entirely upon relief and refreshment rather than any attempt to cure. But all medicine is, or should be, about enhancing and, where possible, supporting health and well-being; only a rather small part of medicine can be realistically looking to cure. Because of the relative frailty and vulnerability of the typical hospice patient, music-thanatologists quite correctly seek to diminish their own role as performers, seeking rather to serve and reflect the patient's needs and changing state. It would be as inappropriate for such a bedside musician to indulge in technical pyrotechnics. This represents, for me, a noble practice that stands at another pole from the increasingly popular participatory programmes, which seek to involve patients and other vulnerable folk pro-actively in music making. Such programmes are many and various, but we can confidentially assume that a group of old folks getting together every week to sing in a choir or dance the popular favourites of their youth must be every bit as life-enhancing as fit young men electing to play team games, or mums meeting over tea, or believers participating in regular church events. Whether any of these activities can lead to better health outcomes will no doubt emerge. I personally have my doubts, although I can believe that socializing around musical activities may be effective simply because music taps in to ancient autonomic responses.

There is an interesting new movement in dementia care in which the built environment is used to reinforce normalcy and memory. I have had the pleasure of working closely with a leading practitioner of this approach, Dr John Zeisel. His working hypothesis is that people more easily know themselves when they inhabit familiar environments, and in many sense this is something we all experience. Radical, unexpected change disrupts our sense of identity and can easily lead to disorientation and depression. Hospitalization is such a circumstance, as is social disruption or sudden loss of home or health. Loss of a carer or a loved one will also challenge our identity and certainty. Importantly, such profound inner disturbance can also be induced by dementia or stroke, so that the familiar suddenly becomes alien and frightening. In due course, there may be drugs that can compensate in part for such internal loss of memory and coherence. However, in many ways a natural resource that is already fully functioning within all of us is our ability to recollect through early-established memories. Of these, because of its very early establishment within the auditory system, music is perhaps the most available and potent resource with which to reconnect with oneself. We would do well to pay much greater attention to the hidden potential that such 'hardwired' systems of response may be able to offer us. Designing healing environments must in the future incorporate aesthetic considerations as well as practical ones, since 'man does not live by bread alone'.

So, in the light of these varied forms of therapeutic musical interventions, how can we hope to measure them in the way that is increasingly expected in an evidence-driven healthcare system? Some elements of scientific culture seek to understand the influences of organized sound as a transaction between the player and the listener, mediating joy and beauty by way of the auditory system, and internally organized and processed within the brain by a complex network of sophisticated brain domains. While all of these processes are happening and are a necessary condition to experience sounds as music, they are sharply insufficient in explaining the joy or the beauty of music. It is generally and increasingly well accepted that music *can* have a role to play in enhancing well-being – even in a form that unsettles the listener – and thereby aiding healing. However, there is still a great deal of confusion as to the exact process by which music engages with our physiology to effect such positive change. In broad terms, we can say that the affective potency of music is differently framed in accordance with the cultural attitudes current to the social context. Musical experience and the influence of music on well-being vary across time and space. Improved medical understandings of the processes of listening can therefore be seen as providing little insight into musical experience, which is a subjective process. While the division between 'scientific' and 'artistic' methods of assessing music experience should not be overstated, there is evidently a divide between those who understand listening as a process and those who view it as an experience. These themes are also brought out in the Moir and Overy chapter within this section.

Many followers of Robbins and Nordoff have found themselves obliged to justify their efficacy through quasi-clinical studies and trials, which are deemed necessary only because of the prevailing cultural dependency upon the 'scientific' method. Science in this context is often narrowly defined, overlooking how scientific methods can include nuanced qualitative studies. The apparent division between qualitative and quantitative studies is more complex than it first appears. The very significant distinction of science is not in its originality of conception, but rather in the painstaking and objective manner with which it must seek to uncover the universality of its application. In the light of this definition of science, in a different context the rigorous refinement of a dedicated musical performer would also constitute a form of science. In time we may increase our appreciation of such creative repetition in order to create a new objective appreciation of much that is currently relegated to the vague, ill-defined or broadly aesthetic.

In the meantime, evidence-based healthcare demands a hypothesis (such as the therapeutic value of music) being tested by obtaining data that support or at least do not falsify it. For many therapeutic interventions, this can best be achieved through large-scale double-blind clinical trials. However, such an approach is often difficult to apply with the very personal and subjective experiences that typically mark out the transactions of a musically therapeutic relationship or process: firstly, the intervention is complex; secondly, the outcomes are multiple and complex and not readily reduced to measurable quantities. Systematizing them into something that can by analyzed on such a scale could potentially change the nature of the intervention. Yet there are some precedents, for example in complex physical or psychological therapies, where practitioners have freedom to conduct their individual therapies within a defined range and where measurable markers of effect are systematically monitored. Brain-scanning methods provide an ostensibly more objective approach to understanding the body–mind relationship and its connection to music but, as discussed below, to date they tend to leave the most profound questions of musical experience untouched. Music offers us a unique channel into ourselves, a precious role that cannot be deemed illegitimate just because we lack the means to objectify its inner workings.

As alluded to above, a general convergence between the expectations of medical scientific 'proof' and the assessments of music therapy have taken place, not least because of the various pressures of funding, qualification and attitudes within the dominant medical ethos. To a significant extent the schools of music therapy that currently enjoy the greatest general and clinical recognition are those that have sought to embrace the so-called scientific method, particularly Nordoff-Robbins, and the other broadly aligned schools who have situated themselves within the academic university system. These have also seemingly focused at least their public profile around fairly well-defined syndromes and areas or therapy, particularly autistic spectrum disorder, cerebral palsy and dementia. The work of Dr

Rosalia Staricoff also illustrates the value that changing the parameters of research can reveal. She conducted large-scale interviews and assessment of the effects of music upon patients, staff and visitors to the Chelsea and Westminster Hospital in the period 1999 to 2003.[3] While the nature of the research could only capture the subjective effect of having music present, such as reducing anxiety and pain, it would be a mistake to overlook the scientific basis of such large-scale qualitative studies.

New technologies: Quantifying and changing musical experience

Within this chapter I have argued that musical experience, culture and medicine are interwoven. The relationship between medicine and health is not a mere matter of the direct 'impact' of one on the other, nor is it easily measurable, but rather is both a personal and social aesthetic experience. In the late-twentieth century a number of important technological shifts also shaped musical experience and the ways in which it is measured and understood. I argue here that some of these developments have had an adverse effect on our understandings of the arts/health relationship, in terms of reducing it to a mechanistic process. However, in other ways they provide a means to quantify and measure musical experience for the purposes of gaining credibility in an increasingly evidence-based health-care system. I will consider three examples from the late-twentieth-century context: technology for measuring sound waves, auditory enhancement technology and the technology for studying unconscious responses to music (especially brain scanning and the 'cognitive turn').

Without seeking to homogenize the scientific community, as many have engaged extensively with qualitative research methods, there is a group of scientific thinkers who seek to capture the essential characteristics of music by way of purely mechanistic descriptions and analyses. One group has become convinced by the notion that musical affect can be captured and understood by means of studying the wave forms of musical sounds as they occur. A significant part of such music as wave-form work is the direct result of changes in technology. There has long been an appreciation of sound being a manifestation of wave form and for thousands of years philosophers have studied its laws. In more recent times much of the mechanism of sound as waves has been intensely explored both within and beyond the UK, for example, with the work of the nineteenth-century German scientist Hermann von Helmholz on sound and tone. Sound is clearly subject to the physical laws of molecular energy and flow. However, the assumptions we make in response to such an acknowledgment differ according to the evolving methods and limitations our technologies place upon our expectations. So what is specific about the technologies of the late-twentieth century?

In the nineteenth century molecular/wave energy was used to directly drive the vibrations of a needle upon soft wax, which created oscillations that could be reproduced. As with many forms of technology, the Second World War provided an impetus for – or at least an acceleration of – change. Magnetic tapes had been conceived of before the war but this technology became more sophisticated by the late 1940s and 1950s, spurred on by the capture of Germany's Magnetophon recorders. Sound waves were then directly captured and transformed into magnetic tape that could be manipulated, cleaned up and edited by cutting and splicing. This was the method of musical capture that typified my early recording experience in EMI's Abbey Road Studio One. The sound waves were captured in an analogue form and then transformed into physical form – the black vinyl record. There were even people who could actually read these disks by carefully looking at the contours of the wave shapes that could just be seen within the grooves of the long playing records. However, the current digitization of information including that of recording seemingly leaves no such trace. Partly for this reason many leading recording artists remain deeply uneasy with contemporary digital recording techniques, which they believe create a dehumanized and impersonal version of their music making. Such suspicion stems from the knowledge that unlike its analogue forbears, digitization involves the conversion of sound waves into numbers.

Manfred Clynes provides an important example of late-twentieth-century attempts to use new technologies of sound wave analysis to understand emotional responses to music. Having established himself as a highly successful concert pianist, Clynes migrated first to psychology and then to computer science. From the 1950s through to the turn of the century, his work combined neuro-science with new computer technologies for measuring sound waves. Indeed, his interest in the relationship between brain activity and music was such that in 1960 he invented the Computer of Average Transients (CAT) for measuring cerebral electricity; the relationship between music and medical technology was thus a productive one. His pioneering work in psychology included a remarkable approach to the measurement and capture of the 'fingerprints' of emotion. He recognised that in experiencing any emotion, a whole gamut of interconnected neuro-psychological changes sweep through the brain and body. His work thus largely pre-dated our understanding of how hormonal and neuro-chemical processes are integral in shaping affect.

Clynes also realized that such changes must simultaneously alter many other body systems, including the tone of muscles, and developed a device that could register subtle changes in muscle tone. He discovered that all humans share common traits of muscular/emotional response. For example, when 'primed' by way of verbal association, and irrespective of culture, all humans share an unconscious tendency to bear down and push away when experiencing anger, but will tend to lighten and draw towards themselves when feeling affection or love. In this way Clynes claimed to have captured 'hard' measures of subjective emotion. Having established his method of gestural emotion, which he called Centics, he used the resulting algorithms to seek out connections between these archetypal affective responses and the expressions of music. In effect, Clynes believed he had discovered a way of calibrating personal emotional gait with identity. Although many remain entirely sceptical of Clynes' claims because of the apparent immeasurability of emotional experience, I believe that his work was none the less seminal. At the very least it highlights the two-way relationship between musical technologies and the ways in which we have measured and understood musical experience temporally. His approach particularly impacted the development of new digital methods for correlating sound waves and brain activity in the late-twentieth century.

The belief that sound is waves of energy led to an apparently logical assumption that a full discovery of the laws of sound and the technology to capture it must also discover the fundamental processes of music. Since music is made up of combinations of sound waves, and since it is also so emotive and affective, one might assume that a direct algorithmic connection between these two could be established. The idea is therefore that this sound wave, or set of sound waves, can create that precise emotion. So, how much merit is there in such approaches? I believe that the idea that musical experience can be measured through sound waves is ultimately mistaken. Such claims are culturally specific and constantly in flux. Now there are many brain scientists who are convinced that the further development of brain science will reveal the nature of consciousness and musical experience. I argue that it will never be possible to comprehend the musical experience by continually parsing the sounds that make it up. The crucial piece that is missing from such an approach is precisely that which makes it valuable, namely our own personal experience. In this regard I would also point out that this opinion piece does not even begin to discuss whether good musical performance might enhance its effectiveness therapeutically. The reason for this is arguably self-evident: at present we have no idea how to 'objectively' measure musical excellence or musical experience.

Another piece of technology to be considered here relates to the development of auditory enhancement methods. These methods are distinct from the technologies discussed above for the measurement of sound waves, although their emergence and use were undoubtedly interconnected. Auditory enhancement methods provide an example of technology that links not to the *measurement* of musical experience but to its physical enhancement. As Moir and Overy show in their chapter on cochlear implants, the enhancement of music experience is a complex process. There have been many attempts – some more successful than others – to associate specific musical elements with precise and predictable physiological and neurological alterations, trying to establish a causal linkage. In the post-war period Alfred Tomatis, for example, was devoted to a rigorous study of the relationship between sound and the development of the auditory system. His technology of sonic manipulation, with which he sought bespoke auditory signals for the needs of the individual, was perhaps the leading method in the period following the Second World War. While his approach remains very interesting and much of his original research was ground-breaking in its time, history has dealt quite harshly with many of the specifics of his approach. However, this should not detract from the contemporary importance of his thinking and insights.

Tomatis developed an electronic system that could be calibrated to enhance and exercise the areas of weaker pitch response in the individual when listening to music or speech. This was based on the observation that if an individual could not hear a sound then the voice could not produce it. This can be viewed as a productive technology in terms of the arts, as it was not only designed for the listening of music but also to improve the tone of singers. In the long term, his method was overtaken by the computer manipulation of sound, which shows that rapid technological changes have both responded to and influenced musical experience. Even as some significant technological advances from the last generation are losing recognition, we see the emergence of a whole raft of potentially life-changing computer-based programs that could completely alter the listener's relationship to the world of music.

Finally, I wish to turn to the significance of studies of the brain and of unconscious responses to music for our understandings of the relationship between music, medicine, health and well-being. By a curious yet significant quirk of evolution, human beings seem designed not to recognize the potency of their musical responses. Since the auditory system develops very early in our development and because we are not designed to shut our ears, it is the brain itself that must filter out unwanted and unnecessary sounds. This can be easily illustrated if one sits for a while in a room with a ticking clock. Very soon we become completely unaware of the repetitious predictable ticking noise. The brain can even subsume, for example, continuous traffic sounds, so that it is only an unexpected disruption of the continuity of sound that will alert the conscious mind. Even more remarkable is the fact that we are also normally unaware of the vast inner world of sounds emanating from our internal physiological systems such as heartbeats, breathing and blood flow. Because we exclude internal and external sounds that we do not need to hear, much musical response also takes place unconsciously – one only has to think of the many music scores that so manipulatively direct our affective response in film, TV and advertising. However, such unconscious responses can now be measured and calibrated through brain technologies and brain-scanning techniques.

I am aware of one interactive technology that has successfully prototyped an intelligent system. This takes bodily information directly from the listener, using a discreet physiological monitoring device, and matches it the subject's level of physiological response. It then runs a search through any given track list for music that will match this level of response. This innovative system can then be programmed to entrain the listener towards a greater or lower level of arousal as they wish. The beauty of this system is that it does not attempt to make any aesthetic judgment. Geared as it is to the more primitive levels of response in our autonomic systems, it functions at this level of largely unconscious response and emotion. Fortunately such response is readily measurable, yet below the threshold of cognition. This puts the application of music at a similar level to drugs, such as beta-blockers, that lower autonomic response and control blood pressure. Interestingly, early tests seem to indicate broadly similar efficacy between such drugs and music.

The introduction of such highly informed interactive technologies will initially challenge the music therapy community, much as chess-playing computers at first seemed to compete with Grand Masters, or computerized diagnostic systems seemed to threaten the experienced physician. However, I am convinced that that they will not supersede the role of the music therapist – any more than they will make redundant the significant role of the interpreting musician. In time, they may allow for a raised aesthetic sense and emotional self-knowledge in people listening to music, which will actually facilitate a more-refined starting level for musical dialogue. Technology might be able to take over some of the complex yet basic tasks of the therapist, but will not, in our lifetimes, even get close to those flashes of inspirational intuition that make the therapist someone more than a mere practitioner, and someone more akin to an artist. However, a period of transition is likely to follow as roles and tasks adjust.

In the past decade, the focus of scientific research has travelled upstream from the peripheral auditory system to the brain, largely owing to dramatic advances in non-invasive brain-mapping technologies. We are beginning to discern aspects of what was once the implicit content of the artistic experience into some more specific observations. For example, important areas lie in the right cerebral hemisphere, which appear to represent musical syntax, intriguingly, in exact symmetry to equivalent left hemisphere areas known to represent linguistic syntax. One can envisage how such insights could influence future development and assessment of music therapy for patients with autism or learning disabilities. Moreover, in the medium to long term, brain mapping could become an 'objective' tool for justifying and even assessing the clinical application of music therapy. However, we should bear in mind that results gathered from, for example, positron emission tomography (PET) and functional magnetic resonance imaging (fMRI) can only be as insightful as the people applying them. Some forms of brain mapping are still relatively coarse and we should not fall into the trap of assuming they represent any form of uncontested 'truth'. The brain sciences are even now only barely scratching the surface of what constitutes our perception of the beauty or excellence, still less of how we construe the intrinsic value, of one piece of art from another.

In order not to overstate the notion of technology as a *purely* mechanistic and visual process, it is important to note here that the late-twentieth century has seen not only a 'cognitive turn' but a 'linguistic turn' in association with a postmodern age. While its impact has been more on the arts and humanities than the sciences, increasingly complex computer programmes for qualitative data analysis can be used to study the language of musical response; new technologies can thus be used to formulate sophisticated semantic ontologies of musical experience. I am again sympathetic with this notion but unfortunately, although for completely different reasons, I believe it to be as misguided as the other approaches that I have outlined in this section. The basic limitation of using language to precisely define mood was neatly summed up by Mendelssohn when he famously said that music is 'too precise for words'. While much of our perceived emotional response is culturally informed, *all* our valuations, assessments and verbal expressions about these different feelings are entirely socially formed. Emotive words will convey different meanings when translated not only between individuals, but also between different languages and cultures, even if we assume that there are cross-cultural emotional concepts.

This section has presented the problems associated with many new technologies for understanding musical experience, but I do not want to leave the reader with an impression that I believe that all attempts to capture musical experience are futile. While I believe that attempting to capture individual musical experience through brain scanning or linguistic analysis is inherently restrictive, each of these technologies helps us to understand a part of the impact of music on health, well-being and emotions. Music is a complex and multifarious event combining cultural, personal, biological and acoustic qualities. Because of this it is my contention that only a similarly multifaceted approach can even begin to capture its richness. In this it is perhaps a little like traditional medicines, which tend to be notoriously complex in their makeup. While it is certainly entirely reasonable to seek to capture and isolate the effective ingredients of such herbs and roots, one cannot then expect the end result to match the original in aesthetic interest.

I would expect certain approaches towards music as therapy to show efficacy even when practiced outside of a connected treatment. However, we shall only ever begin to realize the full potential of music therapy when it becomes an integral part of a wholly transformed aesthetic medicine. This may seem a long way off just now but I remain convinced, and history confirms, that such cultural shifts can take place very quickly. For these reasons I am wary of making judgements too glibly about the respective approaches described in this opinion piece. However, I am also fundamentally convinced that any approach – technological, methodological or analytic – that seeks to proselytize the idea that it somehow alone holds the secret to music as therapy should be viewed with extreme caution. Extreme dangers should also surround any approach that is completely seduced by the notion that everything it does can be captured, measured and assessed. As I have suggested throughout, any musical method that can be totally described in such a way is, of necessity falling far short of the musical experience itself. There is every honour in attempting to establish clear understandings of musical process, as indeed there is in seeking better understandings of medicine and health, but we should be comfortable with approaching this topic from a range of angles rather than seeking one great solution.

Concluding remarks

This opinion piece is not intended to represent a survey or even an overview picture of current music therapies and the music/medicine relationship. Instead, I hope that it can act as a catalyst towards rethinking some of the broader and richer potentialities of music within a healthier future, where music itself is potentially therapeutic. The only certainty regarding the future therapeutic role of the arts, and indeed of medicine as a whole, for humankind is that it will take on new shapes and possibilities. The rise of the brain sciences and the emergence of wholly novel ways of delivering diagnosis and care will necessitate a radical redesign of our approaches across the next generations. Knowledge about the implications of our genetic make-up and demands both for prophylactic interventions and for improved chronic illness management will likely overtake the current focus upon trauma and acute medicine.

Some of this change will occur because shifts take place within the very nature of human need itself, such as shifts in age-related disease and the rise in obesity. In the decades ahead, we can confidently assume an increased population of older people, perhaps with longer periods of disability or disease, not least as a result of reducing the impact of previously fatal diseases. Quality of life and well-being, together with enhancement of palliative and end-of-life care will become a focus for the medicine of the future, extending medicine's current interest in cure to care and the meaning of illness. In such a setting, the gentler, more empathetic qualities of the physician will need to be brought more actively into play. All of these trends will necessitate a far greater degree of self-knowledge and visible caring from health professionals, rather than an excessive focus upon competencies. The beauty of music as an intervention to alleviate suffering and enhance quality of life lies in the way that it taps into impulses and responses that are intrinsic and ancient in their provenance. These fundamental shifts undoubtedly require us to reconsider the role and delivery of music therapy, and indeed to re-evaluate the wider role of music in health and well-being.

Acknowledgments

I wish to give my thanks to Professor Pinching, who has been a tireless and immensely generous adviser to me in writing this piece. I would also like to thank Alan Bleakley whose contribution to my work is much appreciated.

Notes

1 Music *as* therapy and music therapy are not synonymous – see the distinction between 'arts for health' and 'arts therapies' in Alan Bleakley's introductory chapter within this volume.
2 See particularly the National Institute for Health and Clinical Excellence [NICE] guidelines on schizophrenia, 2009.
3 Staricoff's work was disseminated through a range of mediums – including regular reports and publications. It is also widely discussed in publications by the Arts Council England and therefore this discussion does not refer to any specific piece of literature. For a specific example of Staricoff's work see Fiona Hamilton's chapter within this volume.

14 The impact of cochlear implants on musical experience

Case study

Zack Moir and Katie Overy

Since the first attempts to stimulate the auditory system with an implanted electrode in the 1950s, there have been rapid and significant improvements in the design of cochlear implant (CI) technology. Developments in CI sound processing strategies have led to crucial improvements in the ways in which people with hearing losses and profound deafness are able to perceive speech and, in turn, communicate aurally. The success of this medical and technological revolution has resulted in a current acceptance that cochlear implantation is an 'effective and safe treatment for deafness' (McDermott 2004: 49).

These substantial improvements in CI technology and subsequent speech perception abilities mean that most CI users now tend to score very highly on tests of word/sentence recognition, perform well in open-set speech perception tests and are often even able to communicate via the telephone. However, many CI users remain dissatisfied with their perception of non-speech sounds. For example, it is common for CI users to voice complaints relating to their post-implantation perception of music. In a survey of 63 CI users, Richard S. Tyler *et al.* (2000) found that 83 per cent of participants reported a post-implantation decline in their musical enjoyment, with 51 per cent experiencing music as 'unpleasant', 'difficult to follow' or even 'painful'.

This chapter will consider the ways in which the advent and development of CI technology have impacted upon the musical experience of CI users. Two case studies will be discussed, both involving research projects that aimed to improve the musical experiences of CI users, and both reflecting ways in which current developments in music/audio processing and music technology can be utilized to counter some of the significant and varied problems associated with implant-mediated music perception.

In focusing on music and CI technology, we aim to provide an example of the interrelationship between medicine, health and music, in which medical technology can have both a positive and a negative impact. We consider the term 'health' to refer not simply to the absence of disease or infirmity, but to a state of complete physical, mental and social *well-being*, as described by the World Health Organization (WHO) and by other researchers in the area of *Music, Health and Wellbeing* (MacDonald *et al.* 2012). This conception of health is equally dependent on both how well and how ill we feel, taking a holistic view of individuals to include their physical, psychological and social health. As discussed by Raymond MacDonald *et al.* (2012), this broad definition of 'health' allows and encourages practitioners and academics from outside the field of medicine (in this case, the arts) to become legitimately involved in areas that may commonly be considered as exclusively medical. Two such examples of areas in which arts and health are linked are: (a) arts activities for hospital patients, and (b) art therapies which are often used within psychotherapeutic frameworks – both of which are intended to improve the health and well-being of the participants.

This chapter will not deal generally with the use of music in hospitals or in therapeutic contexts, but instead will explore the interrelationship between medicine, health and music via the presentation of research case studies into the musical experience of CI users. The CI population is particularly interesting in the context of this edited volume since a specific medical matter (deafness) means that medical technology (CIs) is used in everyday life, with a significant impact on musical experience. Firstly, a brief outline of the historical context in which this technology developed will be given, with an explanation of the differences that exist between the normal and the implanted auditory systems. Secondly, two case studies will be presented outlining recent research projects in this area. The first study involved the design of a software program to give CI users the opportunity to manipulate the sound of recorded music according to their individual listening preferences, and the second study involved the composition, performance and recording of an original piece of music to suit the 'average' perceptual abilities of CI users.

Historical and technological context

The electrical stimulation of the human auditory system has its origins in the early nineteenth century, when Alessandro Volta used a battery to demonstrate that electric stimulation could directly evoke auditory, visual, olfactory and touch sensations (see Zeng *et al.* 2008). However, it was not until the period between the late nineteenth century and the outbreak of the Second World War that a range of physiologists, psychologists and physicists conducted research into the nature and mechanisms of sound and hearing. For example, in 1930, Ernest G. Wever and Charles Bray discovered the 'cochlear microphonic potential', an alternating current voltage, which 'mirrors' the waveform of the acoustic stimulus stemming from the outer hair cells of the organ of corti (the organ found in the inner ear which contains the auditory sensory cells). This finding had major theoretical implications (Davis 1935) since it encouraged future research to focus on the cochlea rather than the auditory nerve. In the mid-1930s,

A. M. Andreev and colleagues presented the first direct evidence of electric stimulation of the human auditory nerve by reporting that it caused a hearing sensation in a deaf patient (Andreev *et al.* 1935).

Military developments during the Second World War led to significant improvements in many areas of technology, including electrical engineering, sonar, radar and medicine, and particularly surgical procedures and the further development of antibiotics. Importantly, much of the research conducted during this period was concerned with the miniaturization of technologies, in an attempt to render them more portable and concealable. Meanwhile, the widespread hearing damage inflicted on servicemen and women due to blasts associated with combat situations led to an increase in research associated with hearing restoration. Stephen A. Fausti *et al.* have reported that '[t]he alarming incidence of hearing loss among WWII veterans contributed largely to the creation of audiology as a novel healthcare profession' (Fausti *et al.* 2005: 48). The Cold War period fostered a culture of international scientific competition that also saw the funding of science and technological research increase dramatically (Calhoun 2002). Zeng *et al.* (2008) cite advances in the space industry during the Cold War era as having provided crucial technology such as integrated circuits, hermetical sealing and titanium encapsulation, which aided the development of CIs.

In the period directly after 1945, a number of researchers reported successful hearing using electric stimulation in totally deafened patients (for example Djourno and Eyries 1957; Djourno *et al.* 1957), which inspired intensive attempts to restore hearing to deaf people in the 1960s and 1970s (Doyle *et al.* 1964; House and Urban 1973). In the commercial arena, the House-3M single-electrode implant became, in 1984, the first device approved by the US Food and Drug Administration (FDA). Since then, CIs have continued to develop from single-electrode devices, used mostly as an aid for lip-reading and sound awareness, to a multi-electrode device that can allow an average user to talk on the telephone in quiet surroundings.

Cochlear implants and music perception

While CI-mediated speech perception is now of a very high standard, aspects of music perception can be extremely problematic for CI users. Our perception of the pitch and timbre of a sound depends on the specific location of the vibrations produced by each component frequency on the basilar membrane, within the inner ear (Helmholtz 1863). That is, the perceived pitch of a musical tone is determined by the specific places at which the basilar membrane vibrates: different regions of the basilar membrane vibrate at different sinusoidal frequencies and the auditory nerves that transmit information from these regions subsequently encode frequency 'tonotopically' (see Campbell and Greated 1987: 39–62).

In normal hearers, sound waves cause the eardrum to oscillate, which induces a series of vibrations in the ossicular chain and the cochlear fluid, eventually leading to a wave of pressure along the basilar membrane. The motion induced in the basilar membrane is detected by between 15,000 to 20,000 auditory nerve receptors, each with its own hair cell distributed along the length of the basilar membrane. In CI users, natural components of the auditory system, such as the eardrum and the ossicular chain, are bypassed and their functions are replaced by an electronic implant system. An electrical current is sent to implanted electrodes, generating an electrical field and thus stimulating auditory nerve fibres in an attempt to replicate the tonotopic stimulation of the hairs on the basilar membrane (see Wilson 2006: 23).

Thus, a major difference between the normal and the implanted auditory systems, especially with regard to music, is the accuracy of the localized stimulation of the basilar membrane. This dictates the perceived pitch of a sound (for example, high or low, C or C sharp) and also impacts upon timbre perception. A CI system's electrode array contains a maximum of only 24 electrodes (depending on the model) with the result that the localized stimulation of the auditory nerves is much less accurate than in a normal auditory system. In addition, electrical fields produced by the CI system are comparatively broad and cannot be focused as specifically as in the unimplanted auditory system, generally exciting a large population of nerve fibres instead of individual, or small groups of, fibres (Drennan and Rubinstein 2006). A metaphorical comparison would be playing middle C on a piano with one finger versus trying to play the same note while wearing a boxing glove.

Consequently, the perception of pitch in CI users is based on a degraded spatial representation that, even with the potential for up to 24 separate channels of stimulation, has sometimes been shown to yield as few as between three to nine discrete functional channels (Friesen *et al.* 2001). Additionally, the physical condition of the auditory systems of CI candidates, such as any original damage causing the deafness – compounded by the invasive/destructive nature of implant surgery – means that damage to the cochlea and surrounding areas can be an extra impediment to the accurate stimulation of the basilar membrane. Thus, CI systems face several potential problems in the accurate processing of musical sounds and these may vary widely in the CI population.

Such perceptual difficulties (with music) have been investigated experimentally, for example Gfeller and Lansing (1991) and Looi *et al.* (2004) have shown that CI users score significantly lower than normal hearers on pitch discrimination and melody recognition tasks. Timbre perception presents even more difficulties, making the discrimination and identification of musical instruments both challenging and confusing (Gfeller and Lansing 1991; Leal *et al.* 2003). For example, it has been noted that when participants with normal hearing (NH) misidentify an instrument they usually mistake it for another instrument of the same instrumental family, whereas CI users often misidentify instruments in a way that does not bear any relation to the instrumental family of the stimulus, such as confusing the sound of a flute with a piano (Gfeller *et al.* 1998, 2002b). Gfeller *et al.* (2002b) have also noted that the timbre perception of CI users is generally less accurate in the higher registers of musical instruments, compared with lower registers.

It is important to note here that CI users can often perceive rhythm about as well as normal-hearers (McDermott 2004), with rhythmic patterns being perceived much more accurately than melodic patterns (Gfeller and Lansing 1991, 1992). Rhythmic information can thus be especially helpful in the recognition of familiar music for CI users (Gfeller *et al.* 2002a; Kong *et al.* 2004). However, in general, CI users have diminished music perception abilities that can have a significant impact on their everyday music listening. In a recent questionnaire survey of 69 CI users, implantation was found to impact upon on the frequency with which participants *chose* to listen to music, with a substantial decrease in the frequency of post-implant elective music listening and, most notably, a considerable portion of participants (30 per cent) reporting that they chose not to listen to *any* music since receiving their implant (Moir 2011).

It is thus clear that, although CI technology is undoubtedly beneficial as a medical technology that is designed to improve aural communication, it can also be regarded as simultaneously detrimental to the experience of music, and indeed other arts in which music is involved (such as film, television, dance and theatre), and to social occasions in which music is involved (such as weddings, pub gatherings, parties and religious ceremonies). The following case studies outline research that was conducted in order to address some of the factors that relate to the relationship between CIs and the ways in which CI users perceive and experience music.

Case study 1: Audio mixing for individual preferences

As described above, the development of new medical technology in the form of CIs can have a negative impact on the musical experience of CI users. This case study provides an example of how parallel technological developments in sound recording/processing can be harnessed to create a system that has the potential to improve musical experience for CI users. The perception of the sound of specific musical instruments can be problematic for CI users, and in the survey mentioned above (Moir 2011) some individuals suggested that their music listening experiences might be improved if individual instruments in a piece of music could be either removed altogether, or made less prominent. Thus, our aim was to design a software program with a multi-channel mixer that could give users the opportunity to manipulate the sound of a piece of music according to their own listening preferences. Specifically, there were three main design aims: (1) the system would allow the manipulation of individual channels of audio and allow filtering on each channel; (2) the system would store the data acquired during the user's session for subsequent analysis; and (3) the system would be user-friendly and be seen as an enhancement to the musical experience of CI users.

A software program was subsequently designed to be capable of playing six channels of audio, with the user able to manipulate both the equalization (EQ) and the volume of each individual channel. The term 'equalization' refers to the way in which a combination of filters is used to boost or attenuate certain areas of the frequency spectrum of an individual sound signal, while 'volume' refers to the post-filter level of that signal. The term 'mix' then refers to the way in which the various elements of multichannel music are manipulated and combined in order to produce a composite signal: the final, combined sound of the whole musical piece.

Stereophonic recording was pioneered in the 1930 (Roads 1996: 373). Since then, most recordings in the commercial arena have been mastered in two channels. The process of multi-channel, or 'multi-track' recording has now become almost universal, but music is still generally distributed commercially as a stereophonic (stereo) recording – i.e. two-channels (left and right) – which give the impression of sound coming from more than one direction, as in natural hearing. Normally, the various volume levels, stereo positions and EQ of the original signals are fixed, defined by producers and engineers before the recording is committed to its final medium, and listeners have no control over the mix. Some home audio equipment does have EQ controls, which allow for certain frequency ranges such as bass or treble to be manipulated, but this is a 'global EQ', which is applied to the entire stereo mix, and is not the same as 'mixing EQ', which can be applied to each individual channel, for example, each instrument.[1]

The specialist multi-channel mixer system designed for this study was created using MAX/MSP (made by Cycling '74), a visual programming language for music and multimedia, which is used widely by software designers, performers and composers. MAX/MSP was chosen because it allows for the creation of clear and user-friendly graphical user interfaces and because it has the potential to allow for both the manipulation of multi-channel audio and the collection of experimental data simultaneously. Figure 14.1 shows a schematic diagram of the application's signal-path.

As illustrated, each channel of audio (the sound of an individual musical instrument) passes through a user-controlled filter bank, with three filters labelled as 'low', 'mid' and 'high'. These labels were chosen because they are used for EQ controls on most conventional domestic hi-fi systems, and are thus reasonably familiar. Three horizontal sliders on each of the channels control the EQ, where a movement of the control to the left will cut the energy in the associated frequency band, and if moved to the right, the same frequencies will be boosted.[2] The filtered signal then arrives at a gain fader that can boost or attenuate the entire (post-filter) volume of a

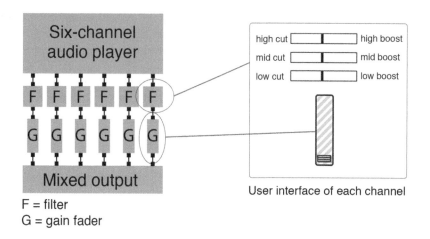

F = filter
G = gain fader

Figure 14.1 Schematic diagram of the mixer signal-path, and an example of the user interface for one channel

channel. When the audio leaves the gain fader, it is fed to the final output along with the rest of the channels; the output is, therefore, the user-created 'mix'.

A study was designed in which eight CI users and eight normal hearers used this software to create their own, preferred mix of four original pieces of music. Each piece of music was one minute long and had six channels of audio, using instruments commonly found in popular music such as bass, drums, guitar and voice. After all pieces of music had been mixed according to individual preference, participants were then presented with a comparison between two versions of one of the pieces (randomly selected) of music. They listened to their own mix and a professional mix of the same piece, (although they were not informed of this), and were asked to indicate which version they preferred. Finally, all users were asked to complete a short questionnaire relating to their experiences of using the mixer.

The individual mixes created by all participants were analyzed using long-term average spectrum (LTAS) analysis, which shows the overall frequency spectrum for each final mix. This analysis also allowed for a comparison of group averages between the CI-user and the NH group.[3] Figure 14.2 shows the LTAS for the average mixes of each group for one piece of music. As can be seen, the CI-user group's average shows less energy across the majority of the examined spectrum, only becoming similar at the very highest frequencies. The differences between the final mixes of the two groups indicate differences in listening preferences, with CI users tending to exclude certain instruments, or to make them very quiet in the final mix, compared with the NH group.

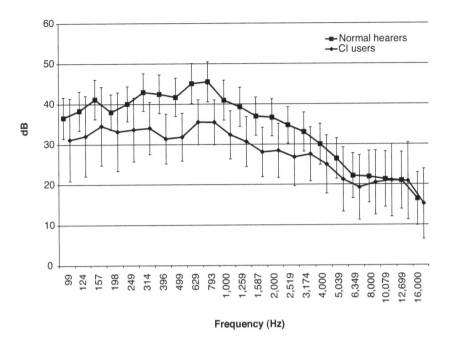

Figure 14.2 Group average long-term average spectrum of the 'personal mixes' of Piece A for normal hearers and cochlear implant users

In order to gain more detailed information regarding the treatment of specific instruments and the consequent effect on the musical character of the different mixes, LTAS analyses were conducted for each piece of music and also for each individual channel of audio. By considering the LTAS of each of these channels for Piece A, we can gain an illustration of the musical character of the group mixes. Piece A included six individual channels for drums, bass guitar, strummed guitar, lead guitar, piano and a vocalist. The average LTAS for the drums channel was much higher in volume for the CI group than for the NH group, giving the CI group's mixes a strong rhythmic character, which is consistent with reports that rhythm and drums can be heard well by CI users. The average LTAS for the bass guitar was very similar for both the CI and NH groups, which suggests that the bass guitar was well perceived by all and is consistent with evidence for the preference of low-pitched musical sounds among CI users. The average LTAS for the strummed guitar, lead guitar and piano, were considerably lower in volume across the spectrum for the CI group compared with the NH group – these instruments had been either excluded or reduced in volume. This corresponds with reports mentioned earlier that instruments producing higher pitches can be problematic for CI users, and also with reports that these instrument can have a masking effect, obscuring instruments that are easier to perceive (Moir 2011).

The vocal channel also highlighted a difference between groups, in that the CI-user group's average LTAS was much higher in energy across the whole spectrum than that of the NH group. This prominence of the voice in the mix of CI users no doubt reflects the fact that the CI is primarily designed to process speech. It also reflects a natural inclination to consider the vocal element as the focus of a song: vocals provide the lyrics of a song and often the main melody. CI users often report that musical instruments can 'drown out' or 'obscure' the vocals in music.

From a musical perspective then, this example illustrates that the character of the average CI-user's mix across all four pieces was a strong presence of bass and drums and a very prominent vocal. This outcome complements research suggesting that CI users can perceive rhythm and low-pitched musical sounds well, and confirmed that the multi-channel mixer system showed the potential to be used in a way that would be both appropriate and beneficial for CI users.

As mentioned above, after mixing each of the four pieces of music, participants were asked to listen to two versions of one of the pieces again and to select the version that they preferred. Participants were unaware that the two versions were (a) the mix that the user created during the study, and (b) a professional mix of the same piece. The outcome of these choices showed that the majority of NH users (six out of eight) preferred the sound of the professional mix, while the majority of CI users (seven out of eight) preferred the sound of their own mix. Again, this signals that the way in which most CI users encounter music, especially commercially available music, is not particularly suitable for their implant-mediated perception and that the opportunity to focus on, or make more prominent, certain aspects of the music could be beneficial.

User feedback about the software program indicated that all 16 participants: (a) found the mixer easy to use and were able to use the controls adequately; (b) found the mixer a useful tool for improving music listening; and (c) would welcome the opportunity to use the mixer when listening to music in the future. CI-user participants provided comments such as: 'bad sounds could be made quieter or even gone, if I decide'; 'it gave me more control over my listening and enjoying the different instruments'; and '[I] would like to have one for home!'. This project thus showed that although CI users may have highly individual preferences and needs that relate specifically to their implantation, as well as individual musical preferences and tastes, these can be met with a general approach: an opportunity to create unique and individualized mixes of multi-channel music. While CI technology can have a negative effect on the musical experience of CI users, music/audio technology, coupled with an understanding of the problems faced by CI users in their perception of music, can be used to provide a creative solution to some of these problems. Despite individual differences, the results of this study supported current evidence, both anecdotal and experimental, that CI users tend to prefer music with a strong rhythmic character and with lower pitched musical sounds.

The implications of this research are significant, since this technology has the potential to be developed to allow users to create individualized mixes of live performances, if individual channels of audio were made available to them.[4] While commercial music is generally released in stereo, a more advanced version of the software described here could be used to generate 'personal filter presets', with which CI users could shape an acoustic spectrum based on their own preferences. Such developments would be reasonably simple to achieve technologically.

Case study 2: Composing music for cochlear implant users

The second case study considers ways in which music can be composed for CI users, based on our understanding of the strengths and weaknesses of the implant system. As noted above, various factors relating to the perception of music – such as difficulties with pitch perception or timbre identification – can have a considerable impact on the musical experience of CI users. Such an impact, coupled with the personal relationships that individuals can have with music, and the importance that is often placed on music socially and culturally, can manifest itself in different ways with regard to engagement in musical experiences after CI implantation. For example, some individuals are extremely disheartened by their experiences of implant-mediated music, rate it poorly and wish to reject it entirely, whereas other individuals continue to, or even begin to, embrace musical experiences. By reviewing experimental research findings relating to the perception of music along with individuals' descriptions of their experiences of 'real world' music, it was possible to generate several ideas and criteria to inform a musical composition for CI users.

The composition described in this case study was commissioned by the hearing implant company MED-EL UK and was premiered to CI users and NH audience members in the Scottish Storytelling Centre in September 2009. A recording of the premier of the piece is available on CD/DVD (Moir 2010). The work was written as a quasi 'musical', involving a collection of songs with a strong central character and plot (the story of Deacon Brodie).[5] It was considered that a clear narrative thread running through the music would allow for several short pieces to be contextualized within a larger, meaningful framework. The music was written for a small ensemble of male vocalist, acoustic guitar, bass guitar, drums/percussion, cello and tenor saxophone. These instruments were were frequently reported as acceptable to listen to in the above-mentioned survey of 69 CI users, and also in discussions with CI users (see Moir 2011). The work was performed as a live concert, providing an opportunity for CI users to engage with the positive, social aspects of a live musical event.

The choices to include a strong narrative element in the composition and to perform the piece with a live audience raise some interesting aesthetic issues relating to the nature of musical experience. That is, individuals do not necessarily choose to listen to music primarily in order to have a pleasant acoustic experience in which accurate perception of the constituent signals is the primary objective – a variety of other aesthetic, emotional, social and cultural factors are usually involved. These factors can be argued to relate, in general terms, to: (a) perception of the sound and of the musicians, (b) personal response to the music, influenced by both prior experience and the current situation, and (c) awareness of the function of the music and the 'musicking' (Small 1998) person within a social, interpersonal and environmental context.

Music is present in many aspects of our social lives and concerts are a good example of an event where people meet specifically to listen to, and indeed to scrutinise, music. Music is also important in the forming of social identity during teenage years (DeNora 2000), and indeed is normally not just a passive, auditory stimulus, but an engaging multisensory, social *activity* (Overy and Molnar-Szakacs 2009: 489). It was thus considered important to offer CI users a social, cultural experience, in addition to the musical composition itself. As such, while the compositional approach to the music aimed to maximize the potential for accurate perception, this was just one aim of the composer and not an assumption that positive musical experiences are derived only from accurate auditory perception. A social occasion, good staging, lighting, good performances, visual images and subtitles were also considered central to the event.

In order to succinctly outline the way in which the music was composed for the target audience we will discuss two specific aspects of the musical composition: the treatment of rhythm and melody. The perception of these elements and their associated problems are, arguably, the most important in terms of the impact of CI technology on music perception and thus the most relevant in the current context.

The terms 'rhythm' and 'rhythmic' are often used in discussions about CI users and their successful music perception, both in anecdotal and scientific contexts. It should thus be noted that the term 'rhythm' is not used here to refer to the acoustic signals produced by drums and percussion instruments (i.e. the 'rhythm section'), but rather the rhythmic, durational, timing elements of music, regardless of instrument or context. It was decided that when composing to suit the general listening needs of CI users, rhythmic aspects of the composition should focus on the presentation of clear temporal patterns and structures that could be used to emphasize key elements of the music, promoting overall comprehensibility. For example, if a listener is generally confused or disorientated by music due to a CI – something that is frequently reported – then prominent rhythmic structures have the potential to provide valuable and aesthetically interesting musical information to attend to. This additional musical information can have the benefit of facilitating the overall comprehension and appreciation of the piece. Figure 14.3 shows an example of how layers of rhythmic organization were used to create rhythmic structures in a creative and interesting way that would allow CI users to attend to various aspects of the music depending on their individual perceptual abilities. The drums provide the rhythmic foundation for this section, with the cello emphasizing the rhythm while also implying harmony. The rhythmic foundation is built upon by the bass, which plays a contrasting rhythm, allowing it to stand out rhythmically against the foundation created by the drums and cello. The saxophone's relatively long sustained notes serve as a contrast to the overall rhythmic structure in an attempt to provide these notes with sufficient space, to be easily distinguished and thus to provide a sense of melody. Thus, the drums play an important role in this rhythmic environment, but the rhythmic content also comes from the way in which the other instruments interact with each other and combine to form structures of rhythmic information.

As discussed above, the perception of melody presents more difficulties for CI users than rhythm, and was thus dealt with in three important ways throughout the composition: the inclusion of traditional or culturally familiar melodies; repetition of melodic content; and the presentation of melodic content in a way that was distinctive from the rest of the concurrent material.

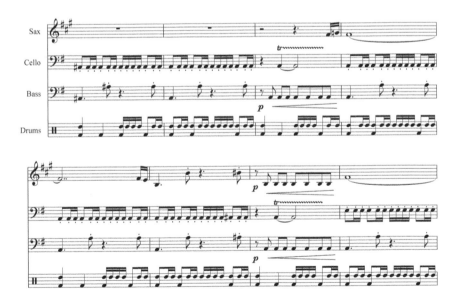

Figure 14.3 Extract of the score from 'Deacon' showing layers of rhythmic organization across the cello, bass, drums and tenor saxophone

The inclusion of melodies that are either traditional or culturally familiar was a feature of the musical style throughout the composition. The importance of this largely 'traditional' music was that it was familiar to many people, thus immediately making it more recognizable, and also placing it within a cultural framework. This approach was adopted due to numerous reports from CI users, who have reported that it is easier to perceive and recognize music known prior to implantation (Moir 2011). Melodic repetition is another simple and effective way in which to approach melody for the purposes of composition for CI users. Individuals with CIs report that in order to be able to appreciate a piece of music, they need to listen to it a number of times, each time becoming more comfortable with different musical elements (Moir 2011). With this in mind, and since familiarity can of course be gained through repetition, melodic content was often presented in the composition in a way that made use of repetition in an interesting and supportive way, such as appearing on different instruments, or with small variations.

Combining these two ideas of melodic familiarity and repetition, short excerpts of traditional Scottish music were used as the melodic basis for the music, and in some cases the original lyrics were also sung, to increase the potential of melodic recognition. In other cases original lyrics pertaining to the storyline of the musical were used. This approach provided a clear cultural framework and an explicit reference to the original sources of the melodies, something that may be particularly useful for those who find melodic and/or spectral components of music especially difficult to listen to.

The third way in which the use of melody was treated in this composition relates to attempts to foreground salient melodic information. That is, it is important to set melodic information carefully within the compositional setting in order to foreground salient aspects. The use of contrasting dynamics and timbres is a useful strategy that was used in almost all aspects of the piece. Important melodic elements were highlighted by making sure that they were either played at a louder volume, in a different pitch range from the rest of the material, or on an individual instrument to avoid any masking (see Figure 14.5). By presenting melodic information simply and prominently while still adhering to the idea that rhythmic and low-pitched musical sounds were most successfully perceived by CI users, it was anticipated that melodic components of the music would be well perceived and enjoyed.

CI technology has been developed to benefit the speech perception of its users, but the relative unsuitability of CI systems to process musical sounds has an effect on the musical experience of CI users. By researching the effect that this example of medical technology has had on music perception, it was possible to develop a musical composition that aims to circumvent known problems in the perception of music by highlighting those aspects of music that are known to be most successfully perceived by CI users. While the previous case study shows how new music technology

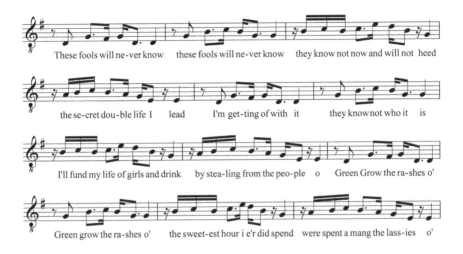

Figure 14.4 Extract of the vocal line from 'Deacon', showing the repetition of the traditional melody 'Green Grow the Rashes, O' (with melodic repetition occurring every four bars)

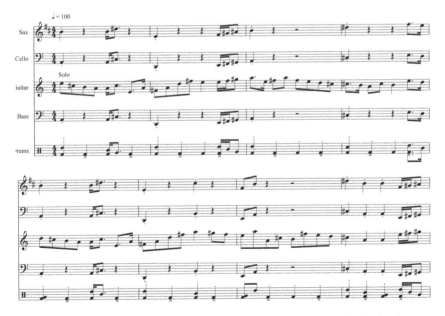

Figure 14.5 Melodic presentation to avoid masking and support rhythmic phrases

can be used to improve musical experiences; this case study shows how music can be composed specifically for CI users, based on research into the music-perception abilities and musical experiences of CI users.

Responses from audience members were generally positive and many people reported pleasure regarding both the musical social experience and the sound of the actual music itself. One participant noted:

> This is my first musical night since my cochlear implant and it is such a pleasure and a joy to be re-introduced to live music again. To be able to follow the beat and hear the change in turn and the various instruments was an absolute pleasure. Thank you so much for giving it back to me.

Participants also mentioned that they would like to have future opportunities to listen to/watch this 'musical', including a participant who stated that s/he 'will appreciate the DVD and look forward to watching it again'; and another who expressed a wish for the CD in order to be able to put it on his/her iPod. Another participant noted that this was his/her 'first venture listening to music since implant' and that s/he looked forward to listening to more.

Conclusions

The case studies presented in this chapter dealt with the way in which developments in (CI) medical technology can have an impact on musical experience, and illustrate how such difficulties have inspired measures that aim to improve musical experience. Implantation has had a profound impact on the way in which many CI users engage with and understand music and its place in their lives. For some, the implant-mediated musical experience is so poor that it has led them to reject music listening in general. For others, the ability to hear sound in any form is a delight and also helps individuals to feel more involved in social situations, religious ceremonies and family life (Moir 2011). In this sense, the effect that this example of medical technology (CIs) has on the musical experiences of its users relates not only to the accuracy with which specific elements of music are perceived, but also to the fact that it provides the opportunity to engage with music and derive musical experiences, something which has far wider implications for the well-being of CI users in a social and cultural context.

The impact of this medical technology on the musical experience of CI users is profound yet not uniform. As such, potential solutions to the problems associated with poor musical experiences need to be creative, and have the potential for individualization where possible. The music perception of CI users has become an important research topic and one that has serious implications for musical experience, well-being and health. Improvements in music listening are clearly desired by patients and, as such, are becoming an important current focus for CI design, manufacture and marketing – something that will hopefully soon have a positive effect on the musical experiences of CI users.

Acknowledgements

The authors would like to acknowledge the support of the Institute for Music in Human and Social Development, The University of Edinburgh, Professor Nigel Osborne, Dr Martin Parker, Dr Michael Edwards, Professor Simon Frith, Professor Peter Nelson, Professor Murray Campbell, Geoff Plant, MED-EL UK Ltd and the Scottish International Education Trust. We would also like to thank all the participants of the studies for their time and valuable input.

Notes

1   Rather, global EQ is designed to shape the spectrum of the stereo mix in a way that will compensate for the frequency response of the system's speakers or resonances of a particular room, for instance.
2   Each filter has the potential to cut or boost by 12 dB.
3   All LTAS analyses were conducted using a filter bank consisting of 23 1/3-octave filters (99Hz–16kHz) in Speech Filing System (University College London, 2008).
4   This could be achieved using Bluetooth or infrared technology depending on the nature of the transmitter/receiver.
5   Deacon William Brodie (1741–1788) is an infamous historical figure from Edinburgh who was a cabinet-maker and city official by day, but who maintained a secret life as a burglar and thief, by night. He is said to be the influence for Robert Louis Stevenson's *The Strange Case of Dr Jekyll and Mr Hyde*.

References

Andreev, A. M., Gersuni, G. V. and Volokhov, A. A. (1935) 'On the Electrical Excitability of the Human Ear: On the Effect of Alternating Currents on the Affected Auditory Apparatus', *Journal of Physiology USSR*, 18: 250–65.

Calhoun, C. (2002) 'Cold War', *Dictionary of the Social Sciences*, Oxford: Oxford University Press.

Campbell, M. and Greated, C. (1987) *The Musician's Guide to Acoustics*, Oxford: Oxford University Press.

Davis, H. (1935) 'The Electrical Phenomena of the Cochlea and the Auditory Nerve', *Journal of the Acoustical Society of America*, 6: 205.

DeNora, T. (2000) *Music in Everyday Life*, Cambridge: Cambridge University Press.

Djourno, A. and Eyries, C. (1957) 'Auditory Prosthesis by Means of a Distant Electrical Stimulation of the Sensory Nerve with the Use of an Indwelt Coiling', *La Presse Médicale*, 65: 1417.

Djourno, A., Eyries, C. and Vallancien, P. (1957) 'Preliminary Attempts of Electrical Excitation of the Auditory Nerve in Man, by Permanently Inserted Micro-Apparatus', *Bulletin de l'Academie Nationale de Medecine*, 141: 481–3.

Doyle, J. H., Doyal, J. B. and Turnbull, F. M. (1964) 'Electrical Stimulation of the Eighth Cranial Nerve', *Archives of Otolaryngology*, 80: 388–91.

Drennan, W. and Rubinstein, J. (2006) 'Sound Processors in Cochlear Implants', in S. Waltzmann and J. Roland (eds) *Cochlear Implant*, 2nd edn, New York: Thieme.

Fausti, S. A., Wilmington, D.A., Helt, P. V., Helt, W. J. and Konrad-Martin, D. (2005) 'Hearing Health and Care: The Need for Improved Hearing Loss Prevention and Hearing Conservation Practices', *Journal of Rehabilitation Research and Development*, 42: 45–62.

Friesen, L. M., Shannon, R. V., Baskent, D. and Wang, X. (2001) 'Speech Recognition in Noise as a Function of the Number of Spectral Channels: Comparison of Acoustic Hearing and Cochlear Implants in Noise as a Function of the Number of Spectral Channels: Comparison of Acoustic Hearing and Cochlear Implants', *Journal of the Acoustical Society of America*, 110: 1150–63.

Gfeller, K. E. and Lansing, C. R. (1991) 'Melodic, Rhythmic, and Timbral Perception of Adult Cochlear Implant Users', *Journal of Speech, Language and Hearing Research*, 34: 916–20.

Gfeller, K. E. and Lansing, C. R. (1992) 'Musical Perception of Cochlear Implant Users as Measured by the Primary Measure of Music Audiation: An Item Analysis', *Journal of Music Therapy*, 29: 18–39.

Gfeller, K. E., Knutson, J. F., Woodworth, G., Witt, S. and DeBus, B. (1998) 'Timbral Recognition and Appraisal by Adult Cochlear Implant Users and Normal Hearing Adults', *Journal of the American Academy of Audiology*, 9: 1–19.

Gfeller, K. E., Turner, C., Mehr, M., Woodworth, G., Fearn, R., Knutson, J. F., Witt, S. and Stordahl, J. (2002a) 'Recognition of Familiar Melodies by Adult Cochlear Implant Recipients and Normal Hearing Adults', *Cochlear Implants International*, 3: 29–35.

Gfeller, K. E., Witt, S., Adamek, M., Mehr, M., Rodgers, J., Stordahl, J. and Ringgenberg, S. (2002b) 'Effects of Training on Timbre Recognition and Appraisal by Postlingually Deafened Cochlear Implant Recipients', *Journal of the American Academy of Audiology*, 13: 132–45.

Helmholtz, H. (1863) *On The Sensation of Tone*, Brunswick: Vieweg-Verlag.

House, W. F. and Urban, J. (1973) 'Long Term Results of Electrode Implantation and Electronic Stimulation Of The Cochlea In Man', *The Annals of Otology, Rhinology, and Laryngology*, 82: 504–17.

Kong, Y. Y., Cruz, R., Jones, J. A. and Zeng, F. G. (2004) 'Music Perception with Temporal Cues in Acoustic and Electric Hearing', *Ear and Hearing*, 25: 173–85.

Leal, M. C., Shin, Y. J., Laborde, M. L., Calmels, M. N., Verges, S., Lugardon, S., Andrieu, S., Deguine, O. and Fraysse, B. (2003) 'Music Perception in Adult Cochlear Implant Recipients', *Acta Oto-Laryngologica*, 123: 826–35.

Looi, V., McDermott, H. J., McKay, C. and Hickson, L. (2004) 'Pitch Discrimination and Melody Recognition by Cochlear Implant Users', *International Congress Series*, 1273: 197–200.

MacDonald, R., Kreutz, G. and Mitchell, L. (2012) 'What is Music Health and Wellbeing and Why it is Important?', in R. Macdonald, G. Kreutz and L. Mitchell (eds) *Music Health and Wellbeing*, Oxford: Oxford University Press.

McDermott, H. J. (2004) 'Music Perception with Cochlear Implants: A Review', *Trends in Amplification*, 8: 49–82.

Moir, Z. (2010) *Deacon*, (CD/DVD), MED-EL UK LTD, Barnsley.

Moir, Z. (2011) 'Towards the Improvement of the Musical Experiences of Cochlear Implant Users'. Unpublished PhD thesis, University of Edinburgh.

Overy, K. and Molnar-Szakacs, I. (2009) 'Being Together in Time: Musical Experience and the Mirror Neuron System', *Music Perception*, 26: 489–504.

Roads, C. (1996) *The Computer Music Tutorial*, Boston: MIT Press.

Small, C. (1998) *Musicking: The Meanings of Performing and Listening*, Middletown, CT: Wesleyan University Press.

Tyler, R. S., Gfeller, K. E. and Mehr, M. A. (2000) 'A Preliminary Investigation Comparing One and Eight Channels at Fast and Slow Rates on Music Appraisal in Adults with Cochlear Implants', *Cochlear Implants International*, 1: 82–7.

Wilson, B. (2006) 'Speech Processing Strategies', in H. R. E. Cooper and L. C. Craddock (eds) *Cochlear Implants: A Practical Guide*, London: Whurr Publishers.

Zeng, F. G., Rebscher, S., Harrison, W. V., Sun, X. and Feng, H. (2008) 'Cochlear Implants: System Design, Integration and Evaluation', *IEEE Reviews in Biomedical Engineering*, 1: 115–42.

15 The development of clinical music therapy in adult mental health practice

Music, health and therapy

Case study

Helen Odell-Miller

Music therapy is interdisciplinary. It bridges art, science and many areas within the two including neurology, psychology, musicology, psychoanalysis, humanities and medicine. In this chapter I outline some current practices, research and changing trends in the professional practice of music therapy in Britain since 1945, and international influences upon these changes. I consider examples of how professional organizations, changing trends in clinical practice and research have contributed to the current position of music therapy as an important treatment in the twenty-first century. I then turn to examine clinical material, with a focus upon adult mental health populations for people without obvious organic brain damage. I write from the perspective of a clinician, researcher, trainer and developer of the profession.

The practice of music therapy

While most professional developments in music therapy have occurred after the Second World War, it is important to note the roots and early emergence of this phenomenon. Music therapists such as Helen Tyler (2000), Rachel Darnley-Smith (Darnley-Smith and Patey 2003) and Alison Barrington (2005, 2008) have comprehensively discussed aspects of the early history and development of the profession. Music was described in the thirteenth century as a central healing agent in connection to the liturgy of St Cecelia, who is now known as the patron saint of music. St Cecelia had been known for singing from the heart and for her passion about music as an access to emotions, an important concept in music therapy. Thomas Connolly (1955) describes the work of the Harford Group who, in 1891, formed the Guild of St Cecelia where musicians performed to sufferers of many types of medical and mental conditions, in order to alleviate symptoms. Darnley-Smith (2013) also draws attention to early twentieth-century publications such as the influential *Cambridgeshire Report on the Teaching of Music* (1933). Compiled by a panel of distinguished composers, teachers, musicians and academics, its findings advocate three important ideas that can demonstrate a link with the post-war music therapy practice that was to come. It suggests that music is good for people on an everyday basis: that it brings communities together on many levels and as 'the greatest of all spiritual forces' meets many needs (CCME 1933: 11).

After the Second World War, music therapy was defined as a form of help towards lifting mood and encouraging motivation and physical activity for war veterans in the USA and in the UK (Bunt 1994). Musicians and music educationalists discovered how performance of music made connections and sometimes appeared to even have healing potential – initially with war veterans and prisoners and for children with special needs, and later for wider populations. In the UK this work developed primarily from musical roots, for example, through the work of cellist Juliette Alvin and composer Paul Nordoff, who worked in partnership with music educator Clive Robbins. Through their work and other developments, outlined below, music therapy emerged into a registered profession.

In the immediate post-war period, UK and USA definitions of music therapy focused upon the use of music as an agent of change for educational and behavioural or remedial purposes. Such behavioural approaches remained prevalent in the USA into the late-twentieth century. In 1989 Ken Bruscia, an American pioneer of music therapy, noted that '[m]usic therapy is a process. It is a sequence of events that takes place over time, for both the client and therapist, and in both musical and non-musical areas' (Bruscia 1989: 48). This definition hinted at the relationship between patient and therapist by suggesting change in both parties, but without explicitly using psychoanalytic concepts. His sequential emphasis suggested a pattern of cause and effect, which reflected the then prevalent behavioural approaches found within treatments in the USA.

Such behavioural models did not retain their dominance in late-twentieth-century Britain, where approaches to music therapy were instead increasingly drawn from psychodynamic and psychoanalytic psychotherapies, while active music making remained central. Recent UK definitions of music therapy draw upon psychoanalytic terminology in emphasizing that music therapy provides 'a safe setting where difficult or repressed feelings may be expressed and contained. By offering support and acceptance the therapist can help the client to work towards emotional release and self-acceptance' (Odell-Miller and Sandford 2009: 2). This definition of music therapy incorporates concepts from psychoanalytic tradition and shows how its practice might concentrate on internal process and mental functioning. The use of countertransference is central to this theoretical model, including musical countertransference (Odell-Miller 2001), in enabling the music therapist to understand further the inner world of the patient.

These growing links between music therapy and psychoanalysis can be related, in part, to the devolution of psychiatric services from asylums into the community in the late 1960s. A therapeutic community movement and emphasis upon psychotherapeutic treatments for severely ill people, partly as a result of new psychotropic drug treatments and the encounter group culture from the USA, led to mainstream provision of psychotherapy within forensic and psychiatric settings, burgeoning during the 1970s and 1980s. In the UK the arts therapies developed discrete services with models such as at Fulbourn Hospital (Odell-Miller 1995; Darnley-Smith 2013). The profession became highly influenced by developments in psychotherapy, borrowing many of its concepts (Odell-Miller 2001; John 1992), while retaining music making as a central focus. Clinical supervision became central to practice, with concepts from social work (Hawkins and Sohet 1989) and general psychotherapeutic practice becoming influential. Subsequently the profession developed its own sophisticated models of supervision (Forinash 2001; Odell-Miller and Richards 2009), and in 2005 music therapy and other arts therapies were categorized in the 'major modalities' section in the *Oxford Textbook of Psychotherapy* (Schaverien and Odell-Miller 2005).

Within this psychoanalytical framework, music therapy has not only been used in an individual therapist-patient model. Music therapy in mental health services has increasingly focused upon group work, particularly through influences from the therapeutic community movement (Clark 1996; Odell-Miller 2002). 'Therapy' itself has also been broadly defined as including community change or enrichment of life (Priestley 1975; Ansdell 2002; Ansdell 1999), as helping to improve specific conditions such as communication difficulties (Alvin 1975; Nordoff and Robbins 1977) and more broadly as aiding the ability to cope with illness or stress (Wigram and De Backer 1999). Music is a social activity and when used in groups, members in music therapy can learn more about how to understand others and relate to them – both within therapy and outside in their lives (Davies and Richards 2002). Such music therapy does not resist or seek to replace medical intervention.

Although the acute medical community in the UK has not embraced music therapy in the same way as in the USA, medication works alongside music therapy and other psychological treatments in good practice. Mary Priestley (1975) advocated its use in a psychiatric in-patient setting at the outset of music therapy treatment in UK psychiatry, while more recently there has been an emphasis on Community Music Therapy approach as described by Mercédès Pavlicevic and Gary Ansdell (2004). A music therapy approach to the Tea Dance (Odell-Miller 1997) had also been established in the literature as part of music therapy tradition for some decades, which fits into the recent categorization of Community Music Therapy as described by Pavlicevic and Ansdell (2004).

Up to this point I have identified some differences between the origins and development of music therapy in the UK with that of other countries, which have also served to shape the profession and its practice in a unique way. In 2000 the Association of Professional Music Therapists (APMT) emphasized the role of musical improvisation and a flexible approach to therapy as means to bring about change for a patient. This improvisation model can include using composed and pre-composed music, as the music is adapted to suit the people undertaking therapy in the moment. Thus the intention and process rather than the end product is emphasized within music therapy, as in many forms of arts-based intervention discussed within this volume. The APMT stated that '[m]usic therapy provides a framework in which a mutual relationship is set up between client and therapist. The growing relationship enables changes to occur, both in the condition of the patient and in the form that the therapy takes' (APMT 2000: 1).

This approach is strikingly different from the USA and Australia, where receptive techniques are prevalent. Grocke and Wigram (2007) in their book *Receptive Techniques in Music Therapy* show the efficacy of receptive approaches, but their absence in UK music therapy is probably owing to a strategy and desire by early UK pioneers to use the highly musically skilled approaches that other health professionals might not be able or trained to execute. This development suggests why there has been criticism within clinical services of territorial and exclusivity arising from the professionalizing of music therapy, details of which are discussed by Barrington (2005, 2008) and Darnley-Smith (2013). However, music therapists have often worked together with artists and arts therapists, leading national initiatives and becoming involved in debates about artists and arts therapists such as within the first Standing Committee for Artists and Arts Therapists (1990), and later The Nuffield Trust initiative clarifying the roles and boundaries of different groups involved in the arts (Coats 2004).

The profession of music therapy

Music therapy is now a legally registered profession. This would not have been possible without establishing music therapy as a formal profession, demanding documentation of competencies, curricula for basic training and continuous professional development (CPD). I argue that these structures, if applied humanely and thoughtfully, provide a safe necessary boundary that helps members of the public to access music therapy, raising its profile positively. While there could appear to be direct conflict between therapy and medicine, staying close to medicine in terms of valuing the work as 'paramedical', and later 'allied to medicine', was seen as crucial by leaders of the profession. In order to achieve the 1982 Whitley Council career structure agreement for music therapists and art therapists within the National Health Service (NHS), the then main employer of music therapists, it was necessary to gain signatures from medical practitioners and to provide an evidence base that music therapy is a profession. The professional developments outlined here were facilitated through the development of professional bodies, formalization of training and pressure on government for registration – I will consider these briefly here in turn.

In the UK, the Society for Remedial Music Therapy (later the British Society for Music Therapy) was founded in 1958 by the music therapist Juliette Alvin and the Association of Professional Music Therapists in Great Britain (APMT (Great Britain)), was formed in 1976. The latter aimed to protect and fulfil the professional needs of training and qualified music therapists in the UK. These two organizations have always worked closely together and amalgamated in 2011 to form one new organization, the British Association for Music Therapy. However, such organisations were only a first step in the process of professional recognition – which also required more formalized training and a registration process.

The first training courses in music therapy were at the Guildhall School of Music and Drama (1968) and Nordoff and Robbins established short courses at the same time. The Nordoff Robbins short courses culminated in a centre and full-time course led by Sybil Beresford-Peirce and later Pauline Etkin from 1974 onwards. Such training has developed further over the last 40 years. The first MA in music therapy was established in 1994 at Anglia Polytechnic University (now Anglia Ruskin University), Cambridge. This began the development to establishing full-time MAs (two years) as the registration point for music therapists in the UK, along with Art Therapy and Dramatherapy. Higher-level research at PhD and Professorial level has also become possible in the last two decades. As of 2013 there are seven UK training courses all approved by the Health Care Professions Council (HCPC) and a well-established reputation in universities such as City University and Roehampton University in London, University of Western England in Bristol and Anglia Ruskin University in Cambridge. The process of approval by the HCPC has served to establish some uniformity within training programmes, for example, with competencies for musical standards of proficiency and core curriculum requirements. Music therapy's professionalization in the UK thus responded to specific local requirements, although taking a similar form to professionalization elsewhere in terms of a process of formalization, centralization and increasing uniformity in training.

Music therapy was first established as a profession supplementary to medicine through the Council for Professions Supplementary to Medicine (CPSM), recorded in Hansard parliamentary debates (HL Deb. 1997). From 2000, when a strategic launch of the Allied Health Professions (AHPs) took place, examples from music therapy research, career progression and clinical work were included in major documentation (DOH 2000a and 2000b). The Health Professions Council[1] later registered music therapy (from 2003), which succeeded the CPSM. While some concerns were expressed about the possible loss of freedom within the music therapeutic relationship as a result of registration, pioneers such as Diane Waller from the British Association of Art Therapists, Tony Wigram on behalf of the Association of Music Therapists, others and myself joined forces in order to negotiate with the government. We believed that establishing arts therapies as professions in their own right, and as legally registered, would provide a richer more stable and widely accessible service for the public. Through the Whitley Council agreement and later Agenda for Change (2003) – the pay system for ensuring a fairer, clearer system for all in the NHS — we also fought for the best appropriate pay and conditions for music therapists and other arts therapists. Music therapy was now firmly established as a mainstream therapy.

I do not wish to present an unproblematic teleological narrative of professionalization here. Indeed, early pioneers such as Juliette Alvin and Sybil Beresford-Peirce found it extremely difficult to see the need for professionalism, and much heated debate and argument was had within the then APMT in Great Britain in consequence. Some were concerned that the improved conditions would be too expensive and that arts therapists would be priced out of the market, a prophecy that to some extent has been realized during the economic downturn in recent years leading up to 2013. There are also counter-arguments to the benefits of state regulation and professionalism. Barrington (2005) writes from a sociological point of view and questions whether the patient's or client's view is lost while the professional aspects of music therapy are developed. She concludes that neither the patient's or client's view is lost through professional developments, but describes critiques of Procter (2004) and Ansdell (2002), the latter in a discussion about the emergence of Community Music Therapy.

Ansdell suggests that there is a danger of reducing the therapeutic and musical freedom of music therapists and imposing restraints upon them through professionalization, rather than the intended effect of protecting the client. Barrington, however, convincingly argues that professional organization and image can have a positive aspect and provide a framework within which music therapists can provide better access to treatments for patients. As one of the prime innovators of professionalization of the music therapy profession I hold an even firmer view, which is that without this professional status there would be fewer established posts and fewer people receiving music therapy in the UK.

Clinical considerations in recent thinking and practice

There is no longer any question about whether music therapy is a profession, as posed in the 1980s. However, there are now questions about the type of profession that music therapy has and should become. In her important research into the development of the music therapy profession, Alison Barrington (2005) discusses in detail how the profession moved from a small group of individual practitioners across the UK, to a professionally accredited cohesive group. It is striking that during the last half century music therapy has moved from being defined as 'remedial' practice, which sounds rather applied and clinical, to the current description on the British Association for Music Therapy website that UK arts therapists are 'reflective practitioners' who are trained in psychological development and treatment delivery. Music therapy involves the therapist and patient making music, or listening together, or one listening to the other, with an emphasis upon what can be learned, changed or alleviated by the process. Sometimes known as music psychotherapy (John 1992), it draws upon behavioural, psychoanalytic, musicological–neurological, sociological and pedagogical frameworks.

The professional practice of music therapy in the UK has always demanded that music therapists were highly skilled musicians, who often worked as performers alongside their professional work as clinical music therapists. In the late-twentieth century there has been widespread tension and debate about the extent to which music is therapeutic in itself and how much the context, application, process and non-musical elements drive the therapy. A selection of published literature from the turn of the millennium typifies debates between music therapists, which included discussions about: psychotherapy and psychoanalytical concepts; the use of verbal interpretation; whether musical technique might be impaired or interrupted by too much attention to medical, psychological or clinical phenomena; and the relative value of composed music and improvisation (for example, Aigen 1999; Ansdell 2002; Barrington 2005; Brown 1999; Odell-Miller 2001, 2003; Pavlicevic 1999; Streeter 1999). The rationale and process of music therapy that I present below must be situated in the context of such debates, as an interpretation based on the available evidence and my own experience rather than a given 'truth'.

I now wish to consider the clinical rationale, process and purpose of music therapy. It is perhaps obvious to think about why musical relationship might be helpful to a child who cannot speak, when the non-verbal qualities of musical and playful dialogue found in mother–infant interaction are the basis for encouraging development and attachment. The value of music therapy for people suffering from Alzheimer's disease may also be self-evident, in terms of connecting to an innate musicality rather than depending on cognitive function. It is perhaps less clear why music therapy is a valuable treatment for those grappling with mental illness such as schizophrenia, personality disorder or depression, in which people are often highly verbally articulate and intellectually advanced in their thinking. The answer lies in the value of music therapy for emotional engagement. Therapists can play music with patients, or listen to and experience music created by patients, to better understand their emotions and how they interact with the world. These experiences and the emotions associated with them can then be made more meaningful through subsequent discussions. Such therapy does not necessarily work in a consistent way, and this chapter later demonstrates that there may be differences in the way people need to use music depending upon their diagnoses. Self-reflection may also be unsettling for some patients, but the ultimate goal of each different process remains therapeutic. Ultimately, group members engage with music and emotions to learn how to take better care of themselves and develop concern for each other.

A case study throws up questions about the boundaries between the music for health approach and the professional practice of music therapy. In one case from my practice, a patient moved through group musical improvisation to using composed songs as a means to develop her self-confidence. The early group improvisation helped her to understand her inner world, which led to her becoming discharged from a psychatric unit, and able to live independently in the community with her three young children. She used bongo drums often to help herself think about her mood and affect, and also to connect with others in a way which, she said, relaxed her as she did not have to always talk. The patient had joined a community choir during her time as an outpatient on the unit, and sometimes she talked longingly about wanting to improve her skills as a singer. At the end of the group therapy, she asked to start singing lessons and I put her in touch with an excellent and sensitive singing teacher. In two follow-up appointments after the ending of group therapy, she brought songs to show me her progress and I accompanied her on the piano, reflecting her movement and journey into her much higher sense of worth and esteem, and towards expanding her performances to solo work within her choir. The music became what I would term an 'improvised performance', which was informed by her relationship with me as therapist and two years of individual work informed by psychoanalytical principles. The patient subsequently ceased therapy and is managing well in the community, attending the choir regularly but also drawing upon internalized processes of therapy that she developed in the group setting and through work with a music therapist.

I noted above that this case study raises some questions about the boundaries between music therapy and 'arts for health'. The approach taken with this patient could be situated within a 'music for health' framework, as the singing is a means for recovery. However, as the patient worked in collaboration with a music therapist, this case could alternatively be defined as activity-based music therapy (Odell-Miller 2007), resource-orientated music therapy (Rolvsjord 2010) or Community Music Therapy (Ansdell 2002; Pavlicevic and Ansdell 2004; Stige *et al.* 2010). This type of discourse and distinction of subtle and highly developed music therapy approaches is common in the twenty-first century, but was almost non-existent in the early post-war period in which there was virtually no clinical or theoretical research and only a few books and journal publications worldwide. While such distinctions and definitions are an important part of the professionalization process, they may also be at times restrictive and unhelpful – as indicated by the case cited above. While other contributors to this collection have noted the importance of bringing the 'arts therapies' into critical dialogue with the 'medical humanities', there is also value in acknowledging the boundaries and overlaps between different arts therapies and arts therapy frameworks.

The influence of research

At the time of writing, in relation to mental health diagnoses, there are Cochrane reviews that gather scientific evidence for the efficacy of music therapy for schizophrenia, dementia and depression. Some might be sceptical of this quantitative approach to a discipline that is related to human health and well-being, as discussed by Paul Robertson in his overview chapter for this section. However, the knowledge base provided by these reviews has also strengthened the academic and clinical profile of music therapists. Partly in response to reviews funded by the National Institute for Health Service Research (NIHR), music therapy is now included in the Clinical and Academic Careers Framework for Nurses and Midwives. In my view, such reviews do not distract or detract from the quality of the private musical and psychotherapeutic relationships with music therapists. Instead they provide a way of valuing and validating the work to the external world, while maintaining ethical discipline and protecting both patients and the public.

The process of reviewing links between mental health care and music therapy resulted in the recommendation of music therapy for people with schizophrenia and schizophrenic-type illnesses within the National Institute of Clinical Excellence (NICE) guidelines in 2009. The guideline states that:

> Arts therapies should be provided by a Health Professions Council (HPC) registered arts therapist, with previous experience of working with people with schizophrenia. The intervention should be provided in groups unless difficulties with acceptability and access and engagement indicate otherwise. Arts therapies should combine psychotherapeutic techniques with activity aimed at promoting creative expression, which is often unstructured and led by the service user.
>
> (NCCMH 2009: 257)

Within these guidelines, music therapy is described as improving symptoms of schizophrenia such as a lack of motivation, problems with socialization and difficulty making healthy relationships with others. These findings were the result of the systematic Cochrane review on schizophrenia, which included studies from Europe and China (Gold *et al.* 2005; Talwar *et al.* 2006). The nature of this review shows processes of international collaboration and transfer of knowledge between countries, which has been made much quicker and easier through new technology. The increased acceptance of music therapy within the medical profession is further indicated by the engagement of music therapists on official NICE guideline panels that determine which treatments are funded in the NHS.

Published literature on schizophrenia and music therapy is particularly prolific, but noteworthy evidence-based reviews of music therapy can also be found in relation to other aspects of mental health. Much of this literature is published across Europe and America but reaches an international audience. For example, a study of music therapy and depression was recently undertaken in Finland and published in the *British Journal of Psychiatry* (Erkkilä *et al.* 2011). The study indicated that music therapy was effective in combination with standard care, as people with depression showed a reduction in anxiety and improved general function. Another piece of new research by Catherine Carr *et al.* (2012) concludes that group music therapy appears feasible and effective for patients suffering from post-traumatic stress disorder who have not sufficiently responded to cognitive behavioural therapy.

These developments indicate that much research has linked music therapy to improvements in mental health conditions, so that 'evidence-based healthcare' should not be viewed as a threat. They also indicate that close research has differentiated between mental health conditions and their specific links to music therapy. The following research focuses upon this latter phenomenon. The case study is used to illustrate some changing trends in music therapy practice. It highlights the importance of recognizing the heterogeneity of mental health conditions and thus the variable nature of patients' responses to, and experiences of, music therapy.

Case study: Research into diagnosis and music therapy in mental health

The following case study is drawn from a doctoral research study (Odell-Miller 2007). The study was based on a survey of 23 music therapists from five established clinical music therapy services in Europe relating to the treatment of mental health, who were surveyed using purposive sampling. Many of these music therapists were – and continue to be – leaders of the field in their own countries. They had experience spanning 30 years at the time of the survey and backgrounds in at least 12 music therapy training courses across the world, drawn from the USA, Australia, Asia and countries across Europe. Therefore, while the sample is small, the results can be considered seriously and general patterns and trends in music therapy practice can be identified. The music therapists were asked whether they used the music therapy techniques and theoretical approaches commonly described in the literature (Table 15.1) and their reasons for (not) doing so. These questions were posed in relation to the use of music therapy for five diagnostic categories: schizophrenia, bipolar disorder, depression, anxiety and personality disorder.

The first finding of the doctoral study, which was complete in 2007 but for which the research surveys began in 2004, was that music therapists did not focus upon research outcomes as a driving reason for their clinical practice. The study revealed a disparity between the level of detail that different centres provided in their responses to questions, particularly their

Table 15.1 Music-therapy techniques and theoretical approaches

Techniques	*Approaches*
Singing composed songs	Supportive psychotherapy
Free improvisation with minimal talking	Psychoanalytically informed
Free improvisation and talking/interpretation	Client centred
Free improvisation with structures such as turn taking or play rules	Behavioural
Theme-based improvisation	Developmental
Activity based	Analytical music therapy
Song writing	Creative music therapy
Musical role play	Activity based
Receptive music using live music	Guided imagery in music
Receptive music using recorded music	
Imagery in music	
Music for relaxation as part of a relaxation programme	

reasons for using certain techniques or approaches with different diagnoses. Some centres provided detailed reasoning while others gave sparse and limited reasons – for example that they had received no training in a certain technique or approach so it could not be used. However, no references were made to evidence-based healthcare or to funding concerns. This outcome suggests that the profession needs to address training in order to equip music therapists to be flexible and to provide services that are needed, but that research does not necessarily directly inform clinical practice. This finding may also be indicative of changes over time and a shift towards evidence-based practice over the last decade. As noted by many of the contributors to this volume, the rise in evidence-based healthcare has led to greater levels of concern among arts therapists about the pressure to prove their worth to the NHS, funding boards and research bodies.

The second main finding of the study was that 'supportive psychotherapy' and 'psychoanalytically informed' approaches to music therapy were the most prevalent, and ranked first or second in every diagnostic category. There was agreement between centres that behavioural approaches were not a priority for any diagnostic groups, but that an approach drawing upon psychodynamic ideas, and in some cases psychoanalytic processes, was essential. These responses correspond to and support the claims made above, about the international differences between the emphasis on behavioural and psychoanalytic models of music therapy. All respondents perceived that being supportive of patients with schizophrenia, both musically and verbally, was a crucial aspect of the therapy. They were unanimous that being 'supportive' was not purely an analytic or interpretive exercise, but also an empathic one. This interpretation of support shaped the way that music was used. For example, one centre used sensorial play as a first stage of music therapy in which the therapist stayed with, mirrored and listened to the patient. The effect was supportive in maintaining the relationship while the patient was also allowed to find his or her own inner space. All results also showed that the building of a rapport with severely mentally ill patients was important.

The third important finding was that techniques of free improvisation, both with minimal talking and with talking/verbal interpretation, were ranked highest for all diagnoses. However, there were some additional differences demonstrated between psychotic disorders and non-psychotic disorders. Some centres explained the importance of the non-verbal qualities of musical improvisation and the potential for encouraging spontaneous interaction. Other centres did not justify their use of improvisation but rather took its value 'for granted'. The use of composed songs was ranked joint first with either form of free improvisation for music therapy with people suffering from schizophrenia and bipolar disorders. In such cases, therapists placed less emphasis upon using techniques requiring symbolic thinking for psychotic disorders.

The prevalence of the use of composed song reveals one of the main changes in the trend during the second half of the twentieth century and beginning of the twenty-first century. At this time, improvisation had become prevalent in Europe, especially in the UK, within a psychoanalytically informed approach to mental health and music therapy (Odell-Miller 2001 and 2003). However, the study revealed that music therapists prioritized the use of composed music for specific populations. The study thus emphasized the importance of examining music therapy in practice rather than only in theory, as music therapists took into account the specific requirements of patients with different mental health diagnoses. Barbara L. Wheeler (1987) supported this finding, showing the value of taking a more musically active approach with schizophrenic patients. Although Metzner (2003) discusses the limitations of using composed music if the patient is psychotic and might not be able to use the space to symbolize anything from the music, this seemingly referred to listening to music rather than interacting through composed songs.

The above finding was significant in showing that improvisation was not used as a 'one size fits all' approach to music therapy, as might have been expected from the published literature. The fifth finding was less surprising – that for patients with non-psychotic disorders, music therapists preferred to use techniques that require more symbolic thinking such as free improvisation with structures such as play rules, theme-based improvisation, musical role play and use of other media. These approaches were also ranked as among the best approaches to music therapy with patients suffering from anxiety, depression, eating and personality disorders. This finding confirmed an agreed awareness of the characteristics and symptoms likely to be present in some of these disorders, which was also supported in the music therapy literature. Jacqueline Robarts and Ann Sloboda (1994) discuss role play and Henk Smeijsters (1996) describes a range of more symbolic possibilities for people with eating disorders.

The roots of some of these disorders arise from early trauma and difficulty, and literature in the psychological therapies has long promoted a process of working through meaning and emotions using role play, reciprocal roles (Ryle *et al.* 1997) and 'mentalization' (Bateman and Fonagy 2004). The latter refers to the capacity to think about mental states as separate from, yet potentially causing, actions. It was referred to by three centres in the survey discussed in this chapter, which is indicative of the emerging interest in this approach to music therapy. For example, Dominik Havsteen-Franklin and Anna Maratos (Central North West London NHS Trust) have recently worked with Peter Fonagy (University College London, Professor of Psychoanalysis) to develop mentalization-based training in arts therapies.

This study indicated that music therapy is difficult to define in a precise and generic way, and continues to develop a multi-theoretical basis. Within this broad church, it would be useful to try to achieve some clarity of description between some of the many approaches. The findings of this study also highlight the potential importance of population-specific training in arts therapies. This raises a debate around specialization, particularly which aspects of music therapy would fall within 'general practice' or under more specialized approaches requiring further training prior to registration. At present such specialization is being resisted, in part because music therapy is a much smaller field than medicine. There is thus potential for future development in this area, which indicates that we are not at the end of the process of 'professionalization' outlined above.

Conclusions

It is clear that every music therapist will bring his or her own style into the therapy room and that this, in addition to training and experience, will determine the essence of the therapy. It appears that enough freedom, free thinking and creative professional practice has allowed music therapy to maintain its unique musicality and techniques of live interactive connection, while benefiting from the organization that professionalism and registration have brought. In fact the profile of music therapy is higher than it has ever been, particularly when including its influence upon other disciplines such as psychotherapy, musicology, music psychology and allied health professional clinical practice. In the twentieth and twenty-first centuries, there has been a consolidation of the clinical practice of music therapy, a rise in research and associated publications, a consolidation of training, the establishing of professional frameworks, the development of official regulation and legal registration and, finally, advances in technology in music therapy (Magee 2013).

Music therapy in adult mental health thus provides an important case study for this volume, as a form of arts and health intervention that has been clearly shaped by the context of its emergence and development. It also represents an interdisciplinary form of therapy, although this should not be unquestioningly seen as a benefit to the field. There are ongoing debates about whether music therapy has adhered too much to other disciplines and thus been in danger of diluting and detracting from the power of music as a medicine in its own right (Ansdell 2002; Barrington 2005). The debates are a sign that music therapy is established, has arrived, and is in adulthood. The profession is supported and strong enough for open debate, within and between its shifting and overlapping sub-fields relating to the adult mental health field, such as the Nordoff Robbins tradition of Creative Music Therapy (1977), Psychoanalytically Informed Music Therapy (Odell-Miller 2001), Music Psychotherapy (John 1992), and most recently, Cognitive Analytical Music Therapy (Compton-Dickinson *et al.* 2013). The influence of music therapy within the music psychology and musicology fields is demonstrated and represented within recent literature (Hallam *et al.* 2009; Malloch and Trevarthen 2009; Barnard 2012). Debates now focus on the place of music therapy in the field and the type of framework within which it should be applied, but there is little question that it can be a form of robust treatment – or, dare I say, a form of 'medicine'.

Note

1   The Health Professions Council (HPC) was set up following the under the National Health Service Reform and Health Care Professions Act 2002, to replace the Council for Professions Supplementary to Medicine, in 2003. In 2012 it became the HCPC to include Social Care.

References

Aigen, K. (1999) 'The True Nature of Music-Centred Therapy Theory', *British Journal of Music Therapy*, 13: 77–82.

Alvin, J. (1975) *Music Therapy*, London: Hutchinson.

Ansdell, G. (1999) 'Challenging Premises', *British Journal of Music Therapy*, 13: 72–6.

Ansdell, G. (2002) 'Community Music Therapy and the Winds of Change', in C. Kenny and B. Stige (eds) *Contemporary Voices in Music Therapy: Communication, Culture and Community*, Oslo: Unipub.

Association of Professional Music Therapists (APMT) (2000) 'Careers Leaflet', unpublished.

Barrington, A. (2005) 'Music Therapy: A Study in Professionalisation', unpublished thesis, University of Durham.

Barrington, A. (2008) 'Challenging the Profession', *British Journal of Music Therapy*, 22: 65–72.

Barnard, P. (2012) 'What Do We Mean by the Meanings of Music?', *Empirical Musicology Review*, 7: 1–2.

Bateman, A. and Fonagy, P. (2004) *Psychotherapy for Borderline Personality Disorders: Mentalization Based Treatment*, Oxford: Oxford University Press.

Brown, S. (1999) 'Some Thoughts on Music, Therapy, and Music Therapy', *British Journal of Music Therapy*, 13: 63–71.

Bruscia, K. (1989) *Defining Music Therapy*, Philadelphia: Spring House Books.

Bunt, L. (1994) *Music Therapy: An Art Beyond Words*, London: Routledge.

Cambridgeshire Council of Musical Education (CCME) (1933), *Music and The Community: The Cambridgeshire Report on the Teaching of Music*, Cambridge: Cambridge University Press.

Carr C., d'Ardenne P., Sloboda A., Scott C., Wang D. and Priebe S. (2012) 'Group Music Therapy for Patients with Persistent Post-Traumatic Stress Disorder – An Exploratory Randomized Controlled Trial with Mixed Methods Evaluation', *Psychology and Psychotherapy: Research and Practice*, 85: 179–202.

Clark, D. (1996) *The Story of a Mental Hospital*, London: Free Associations.

Coats, E. (ed.) (2004) *Creative Arts and Humanities in Healthcare: Swallows to other Continents*. London: The Nuffield Trust.

Compton-Dickinson, S., Odell-Miller, H. and Adlam, J. (2013) *Forensic Music Therapy*, London: Jessica Kingsley.

Connolly, T. (1995) *Mourning into Joy: Music, Raphael, and Saint Cecilia*, New Haven and London: Yale University Press.

Darnley-Smith, R. (2013) 'What is the Music of Music Therapy? An Enquiry into the Aesthetics of Clinical Improvisation', unpublished thesis, University of Durham.

Darnley-Smith, R. and Patey, H. (2003) *Music Therapy*, London: Sage Publications.

Davies, A. and Richards, E. (eds) (2002) *Music Therapy and Group Work*, London: Jessica Kingsley.

Department of Health (DOH) (2000a) *Meeting the Challenge: A Strategy for the Allied Health Professions*, London: DOH.

DOH (2000b) *Allied Health Professions-Building Careers*, London: DOH.

Erkkilä, J., Punkanen, M., Fachner, J., Ala-Ruona, E., Pöntiö, I., Tervaniemi, M., Vanhala, M. and Gold, C. (2011) 'Individual Music Therapy for Depression: Randomised Controlled Trial', *British Journal of Psychiatry*, 199:132–9.

Forinash, M. (2001) *Music Therapy Supervision*, Philadelphia: Barcelona.

Gold, C., Heldal, T. O., Dahle, T. and Wigram, T. (2005) 'Music Therapy for Schizophrenia or Schizophrenia-Like Illnesses', *Cochrane Database of Systematic Reviews*, 2: DOI: 10.1002/14651858.CD004025.pub2.

Grocke, D. and Wigram, T. (2007) *Receptive Methods in Music Therapy: Techniques and Clinical Applications for Music Therapy Clinicians, Educators, and Students*, London: Jessica Kingsley.

Hallam, S., Cross, I. and Thaut, M. (2009) *The Oxford Handbook of Music Psychology*, Oxford: Oxford University Press.

Hawkins, P. and Sohet, R. (1989) *Supervision in the Helping Professions*, Milton Keynes: Open University Press.

HL Deb. (1997) 578 col. 2026–29.

John, D. (1992) 'Towards Music Psychotherapy', *Journal of British Music Therapy*, 6: 10–13.

Magee, W. L. (2013 [in press]) *Music Technology in Therapeutic and Health Settings*, London: Jessica Kingsley Publishers.

Malloch, S. and Trevarthon, C. (2009) *Communicative Musicality*, Oxford: Oxford University Press.

Metzner, S. (2003) 'The Significance of Triadic Structures in Patients Undergoing Therapy for Psychosis in a Psychiatric Ward', in S. Hadley (ed.) *Psychodynamic Music Therapy Case Studies*, Philadelphia: Barcelona Publishers.

National Collaborating Centre for Mental Health (NCCMH) (2009) *Schizophrenia. Core Interventions in the Treatment and Management of Schizophrenia in Adults in Primary and Secondary Care*, Updated Edition, Leicester and London: The British Psychological Society and The Royal College of Psychiatrists.

Nordoff, P. and Robbins, C. (1977) *Creative Music Therapy*, New York: John Day.

Odell-Miller, H. (1995) 'Why Provide Music Therapy in the Community for Adults with Mental Health Problems?', *British Journal of Music Therapy*, 9: 4–10.

Odell-Miller, H. (1997) 'Music Therapy and the Functions of Music with Older Mentally Ill People in a Continuing Care Setting', in M. Denham (ed.) *Continuing Care for Older People*, London: Stanley Thornes Publishers Ltd.

Odell-Miller, H. (2001) 'Music Therapy and its Relationship to Psychoanalysis', in Y. Searle and I. Streng (eds) *Where Analysis Meets the Arts*, London: Karnac Books.

Odell-Miller, H. (2002) 'One Man's Journey and the Importance of Time: Music Therapy in an NHS Mental Health Day Centre', in A. Davies and E. Richards (eds) *Music Therapy and Group Work*, London: Jessica Kingsley.

Odell-Miller, H. (2003) 'Are Words Enough? Music Therapy as an Influence in Psychoanalytic Psychotherapy', in L. King and R. Randall (eds) *The Future of Psychoanalytic Psychotherapy*, London: Whurr.

Odell-Miller, H. (2007) 'The Practice of Music Therapy for Adults with Mental Health Problems: The Relationship between Diagnosis and Clinical Method', unpublished thesis, Aalborg University Denmark.

Odell-Miller, H. and Richards, E. (2009) *Supervision of Music Therapy*, London: Routledge.

Odell-Miller, H. and Sandford, S. (2009) 'Music Therapy in the United Kingdom', *Voices*. Online. Available: https://normt.uib.no/index.php/voices (accessed 5 January 2013).

Pavlicevic, M. (1999) 'Thoughts, Words and Deeds: Harmonies and Counterpoints in Music Therapy Theory', *British Journal of Music Therapy*, 13: 59–62.

Pavlicevic, M. and Ansdell, G. (2004) *Community Music Therapy*, London: Jessica Kingsley.

Priestley, M. (1975) *Music Therapy in Action*, London: Constable.

Procter, S. (2004) 'Playing Politics: Community Music Therapy and the Therapeutic Redistribution of Music Capital for Mental Health', in M. Pavlicevic and G. Ansdell (eds) *Community Music Therapy*, London: Jessica Kingsley.

Robarts, J. and Sloboda, A. (1994) 'Perspectives in Music Therapy with People Suffering from Anorexia Nervosa', *Journal of British Music Therapy*, 8: 7–14.

Rolvsjord, R. (2010) *Resource-Oriented Music Therapy in Mental Health Care*, Gilsum, NH: Barcelona Publishers.

Ryle, A., Leighton, T. and Pollock, P. (1997) *Cognitive Analytic Therapy of Borderline Personality Disorders*, Chichester: Wiley.

Schaverien, J. and Odell-Miller, H. (2005) 'The Arts Therapies', in G. Gabbard, J.

Beck and J. Holmes (eds) *Oxford Textbook of Psychotherapy*, Oxford: Oxford University Press.

Smeijsters, H. (1996) 'Music Therapy with Anorexia Nervosa: An Integrative Theoretical and Methodological Perspective', *British Journal of Music Therapy*, 10: 3–13.

Standing Committee of Arts Therapies Professions (2000), *Artists and Arts Therapists: A Brief Discussion of their Roles within Hospitals, Clinics, Special Schools and in the Community*, London: Carnegie United Kingdom Trust.

Stige, B., Ansdell, G., Elefant, C. and Pavlicevic, M. (2010) *Where Music Helps: Community Music Therapy in Action*, Aldershot: Ashgate.

Streeter, E. (1999) 'Finding a Balance between Psychological Thinking and Musical Awareness in Music Therapy Theory – A Psychoanalytic Perspective', *British Journal of Music Therapy*, 13: 5–20.

Talwar, N., Crawford, M. J., Maratos, A. (2006) 'Music Therapy for Patients with Schizophrenia: Exploratory Randomised Controlled Trial', *British Journal of Psychiatry*, 189: 405–9.

Tyler, H. (2000) 'The Music Therapy Profession in Modern Britain', in P. Horden (ed.) *Music as Medicine: The History of Music Therapy since Antiquity*, Aldershot: Ashgate.

Wheeler, B. L. (1987) 'Levels of Therapy: The Classification of Music Therapy Goals', *Music Therapy*, 6: 39–49.

Wigram, T. and De Backer J. (eds) (1999) *Clinical Applications of Music Therapy in Psychiatry*, London: Jessica Kingsley.

Appendix

A timeline of the medical humanities

Alan Bleakley and Therese Jones

1937	*USA*	At Vanderbilt University School of Medicine, E. E. Reinke calls for 'leavening technical training with a liberal education'.
1944–45	*UK*	The medical humanities 'begin' as the nascent art therapy movement. Adrian Hill publishes *Art Versus Illness* about using art to treat patients in a tuberculosis sanatorium.
1947	*USA*	George Sarton coins the term 'medical humanities' in the journal that he founded: *Isis*, the official publication of the History of Science Society.
1952–57	*USA*	Case Western Reserve medical school introduces a history of medicine innovation during an extended curriculum overhaul.
1967	*USA*	The first Department of Humanities in any medical school is established, at Pennsylvania State University's College of Medicine.
1970	*USA*	The Society for Health and Human Values (SHHV) is officially established as a membership organization.
1973	*USA*	The Institute of Medical Humanities is founded at the University of Texas, Galveston with content emphases in history, literature and religious studies.
1976	*Australia*	Anthony R. Moore, a surgeon working at the University of Melbourne, first uses the term 'medical humanities' in the medical education literature.
	Argentina	The University of La Plata medical school develops an optional medical humanities provision.
1979	*USA*	*Journal of Medical Humanities* launched.

1982	*USA*	The journal *Literature and Medicine* is launched.
1984	*USA*	Eric Cassell publishes an influential Hastings Center commissioned report *The Place of the Humanities in Medicine.*
1990	*USA*	The Center for Literature and Medicine is established at Hiram College including the *Literature and Medicine* book series.
1991	*USA*	Kathryn Montgomery Hunter publishes *Doctors' Stories*, arguing that doctors' clinical reasoning can be seen as a narrative process within the detective genre.
1993	*UK*	The Wellcome Foundation organizes a seminar on the arts in health.
		The General Medical Council publishes *Tomorrow's Doctors.*
1994	*USA*	The first medical humanities website is established at the New York School of Medicine.
1994	*New Zealand*	The first medical humanities conference is organized: 'The Science and Art of Medicine'.
1995	*UK*	The Royal Society of Medicine organizes a symposium entitled 'Art in Hospitals: Past, Present and Future'.
		I. C. McManus, based at St Mary's Hospital (Imperial College) London, writes an article in *The Lancet* highlighting the importance of incorporating the humanities into medical education.
1996	*New Zealand*	The University of Auckland, New Zealand, hosts the first Pacific Rim conference on narrative-based medicine.
1998	*USA*	The Society for Health and Human Values, Society for Bioethics Consultation and American Society for Bioethics and Humanities merge to form the American Society for Bioethics and Humanities.
1998–99	*UK*	Two landmark medical humanities conferences are organized with the aim of broadening the interests of the medical humanities beyond arts therapies: 'Windsor I' and 'Windsor II'.
1998	*UK*	The first UK medical humanities conference is organized. The conference proceedings refer to UK medical humanities initiatives as 'twenty years behind' the Galveston model (see 1973).

		The Medical Humanities Unit is established at the Royal Free and University College Medical School, London.
1999	*UK*	The Nuffield Trust helps to establish a Centre for the Arts and Humanities in Health and Medicine at the University of Durham and a new Institute of Medical Humanities.
2000	*UK*	The *British Medical Journal* publishing group launches a new journal – *Medical Humanities* – as a sister publication to the established *Journal of Medical Ethics*.
2000	*USA*	The Program in Narrative Medicine is established at Columbia University.
2002	*UK*	The inaugural meeting of the UK Association for Medical Humanities is held at the University of Birmingham.
		Peninsula Medical School (Universities of Exeter and Plymouth) is the first UK medical school to integrate the medical humanities as core curriculum.
2003	*USA*	A special edition of the journal *Academic Medicine* is devoted to the state of the art of medical humanities in medical education, dominated by USA medical schools.
2004	*Canada*	*Ars Medica,* a biannual journal, exploring 'what makes medicine an art' is launched.
2008	*UK*	The Wellcome Trust awards two large grants to set up centres for research in the medical humanities, at the University of Durham and the University of London King's College.
		In the USA, electronic medical humanities journal *Hektoen International* is founded in Chicago by the Hektoen Institute of Medicine (first edition published in 2009).
2009	*UK*	An updated version of *Tomorrow's Doctors* removes specific recommendations concerning the humanities in the undergraduate medicine curriculum, but maintains an emphasis on communication skills.
2011	*Canada*	The inaugural conference of the Canadian Health Humanities network is held in Toronto.
2014	*USA*	The first *Health Humanities Reader* is published by Rutgers University Press.

References

Cassell, E. J. (1984) *The Place of the Humanities in Medicine*, New York: The Hastings Center Publications.

Hill, A. (1945) *Art versus Illness: A Story of Art Therapy*, London: Allen & Unwin.

Hurwitz, B. and Dakin, P. (2009) 'Welcome Developments in UK Medical Humanities', *Journal of the Royal Society of Medicine*, 102: 84–5

Jones, T., Wear, D. and Friedman, L. D. (eds) (2013 [in press]) *Health Humanities Reader*, New Jersey: Rutgers University Press.

McManus, I. C. (1995) Humanity and the Medical Humanities, *The Lancet*, 346: 1143–5.

Montgomery Hunter, K. (1991) *Doctors' Stories: The Narrative Structure of Medical Knowledge*, Princeton, NJ: Princeton University Press.

Moore, A. R. (1976) 'Medical Humanities: A New Medical Adventure', *New England Journal of Medicine*, 295: 1479–80.

Reinke, E. E. (1937) 'Liberal Values in Premedical Education', *The Journal of the Association of American Medical Colleges*, 12: 151–6.

Index